Ferenc Kuhn

Ocular Traumatology

Ferenc Kuhn

Ocular Traumatology

With 190 Figures and 74 Tables

Springer

Ferenc Kuhn, MD
President, American Society of Ocular Trauma
Executive Vice President, International Society of Ocular Trauma
Associate Professor of Clinical Ophthalmology, University of Alabama at Birmingham
Professor, Department of Ophthalmology, University of Pécs, Hungary
Associate Director of Clinical Research, Helen Keller Foundation for Research and Education
1201 11th Avenue S., Suite 300
Birmingham, AL 35205
USA

Library of Congress Control Number: 2007936598

ISBN 978-3-540-33824-6 Springer Berlin Heidelberg New York

Springer is a part of Springer Science+Business Media
springer.com

Editor: Marion Philipp, Heidelberg, Germany
Desk Editor: Martina Himberger, Heidelberg, Germany
Reproduction, typesetting and production: LE-TEX Jelonek, Schmidt & Vöckler GbR, Leipzig, Germany
Cover design: Frido Steinen-Broo, EStudio, Calamar, Spain

Printed on acid-free paper 24/3180/YL 5 4 3 2 1 0

Preface

This handbook on ocular traumatology[1] follows one I jointly edited/authored with D. Pieramici (Santa Barbara, California) about 5 years ago. When asked recently whether the current book represents a second edition to Ocular Trauma: Principles and Practice[2], my answer was both no and yes.

I can answer *no* because so much has changed since the previous book was published that much in this book is new material;[3] and *no* because the current book was mostly written by myself alone to assure uniformity in substance as well as style.

Yes because Ocular Traumatology uses similar content-, structure- and formatting-related guidelines[4] that were introduced in the previous book. General management principles are prominently featured here (see Chap. 1.8), and they precede the detailed discussion of specific treatment issues. I can answer *yes* because the latter guidelines are categorized by tissue instead of (the traditional) method of dividing the eye into anterior vs

1 This book is dedicated solely to the eyeball ("*ocular* traumatology"); adnexal trauma ("*ophthalmic* traumatology") is not discussed.

2 Thieme, New York, 2002.

3 Every new idea presented here has first undergone rigorous, real-life-testing by teams of experts.

4 Such as the utilization of highlighted text ("Pearl", "Cave", "Pitfall", "Controversial") or the incorporation of all abbreviations into a single section.

posterior segments – which elective cases permit[5] but with which injuries are irreconcilable. I can answer *yes* also because the patient's perspective is included, as is the science and art of counseling, an all too often neglected field in medicine; *yes* because this book emphasizes the importance of the surgeon's self-test, which must be conducted in the planning phase of any and every intervention: Am I capable of doing an optimal job? – because if not, instant referral is usually preferable to an intervention that is limited by the capabilities of the surgeon or the facility[6]; and *yes* because this book discusses the "why"[7] as much as the "when," "what," and "how."

Analyzing the "why" is brought to the next level, as explained in Chap. 1.8. The surgeon should always plan for the intervention (strategy and tactics), and do so with the end point in sight. When closing a corneal wound, the goal is not simply the creation of a watertight seal. The anatomy of the entire globe must be restored to as close to its pre-injury condition

---

5 Even encourage: such specialization involves greater expertise in a certain field, albeit a narrower one. The ocular traumatologist, however, is best characterized by the innovative term coined by the great Italian ophthalmologist/artist Cesare Forlini from Ravenna: "POPEYE": pole to pole of the eyeball.

6 "Nil nocere" (i.e., do no harm); in other words: just as there is no such thing as being a "little pregnant," there is no such thing as a job half done. Suboptimal management is unacceptable if it is the result of a procedure for which the ophthalmologist's training or available equipment was known to be insufficient yet he decided to go ahead with it anyway. The ophthalmologist's job is not simply to make the eye's condition better than what it would be without his intervention; the job is to perform surgery/treatment that approximates the ideal, the optimal, the maximum as close as objectively possible.

7 i.e., the rationale of why something is done one way as opposed to another. I once was visited by a young ophthalmologist eager to learn vitreoretinal surgery. She kept asking "Why did you do this?" for 2 weeks, often challenging my reply. Toward the end of the study period, after receiving an exhaustive answer to a complex question, her facial expression morphed into that of a wife who thinks she has caught her husband's mischief when he comes home late one evening, but the husband provides a reasonable answer and escapes being caught. The visiting ophthalmologist said: "You have an explanation for everything!" My answer was: "No, not everything. But I feel uncomfortable doing anything without knowing why I am doing it; I am trying to identify such an explanation for everything I do. The adage that 'because that's how it always has been done' isn't sufficient."

as possible.[8] The question is not "When and how am I going to suture this corneal wound?" but "What does it take to fully rehabilitate this injured eye?"[9] The answer includes, but is not restricted to, watertight and function-oriented closure of the corneal wound[10]. If additional pathologies (hyphema, iris laceration, etc.) are present, carry a realistic risk to have formed (vitreous hemorrhage, retinal break, etc.), or can reasonably be expected to occur in the future (retinal detachment, PVR, etc.), the surgeon should carefully weigh all of these abnormalities and determine the best strategy (number, scope, and timing of the intervention) before details of the surgical tactics (number and introduction sequence of the corneal sutures, their type, etc.) are even contemplated. A surgeon who does not understand this is only a "pseudosurgeon": he may be an expert in a given tissue pathology, but he is not a true trauma specialist who treats the injured organ or, preferably, the person who sustained an injury.[11]

---

8 The surgeon can restore anatomy only; functional recovery always follows the anatomical one, and while anatomical reconstruction may be promised to the patient in many cases, the promise of functional improvement should not be given lightheartedly: whether anatomical restoration indeed brings improved function is a more complex issue with several unknowns.

9 This explains why I do not like to use the term "damage control surgery." What the ocular traumatologist really aims for is not damage control but complete functional rehabilitation of the injured eye – and person.

10 See Chap. 2.2.

11 This mismentality is so often seen in real life when a patient with a posterior segment IOFB is treated. For the "pseudosurgeon" it is the removal of the IOFB that receives priority, and addressing the coexisting pathologies is of secondary importance. The question of expected, longer-term complications, such as PVR, is not even raised at this point. Conversely, for the "real" surgeon the coexisting pathologies take priority over IOFB removal, and longer-term complications are seriously considered as the management plan (strategy) is designed.

Ocular traumatology is a difficult field for many reasons:

1. It offers a number of general guiding principles but relatively few specific, ready-to-apply instructions that are applicable in the very case that the ophthalmologist must treat next.[12]
2. It has a success rate that is nowhere comparable to that of cataract surgery – yet the effort that goes into trying is incomparably greater.
3. Treatment of the injured eye requires longer sessions spent in the early-morning hours in an OR that may be ill-equipped for such surgery.
4. The patient is very worried to lose vision – yet he can harbor an unreasonable expectation of functional recovery.
5. The physician–patient relationship is established by chance, not by choice: the trust of the patient, an absolutely integral part of an optimal physician–patient relationship,[13] must be earned. Earning this trust is not easy, and the "bedside manner" (i.e., the act of counseling) exhibited by the ophthalmologist is as important in this process as are his treatment results.

Surgery on the traumatized eye can also be uniquely difficult because of visibility issues. In most elective surgeries the visibility problem is usually related to a narrow pupil. In ocular traumatology this is often compounded by corneal edema, lens opacity, and, most importantly, a vitreous with severe hemorrhage. In eye surgery the surgeon almost never benefits from tactile or audible feedback, only visual. In a serious vitreous bleeding or infection, even this feedback is greatly challenged: distinction between vitreous and retina may be almost impossible, requiring special surgical tactics

12 Don't ever forget: It is never the dexterity of the traumatologist that determines the outcome of the case. The hands are simply servants of the brain, executors of the brain's commands: unless the brain carefully selects the best possible treatment option, concerning both strategy and tactics, even the most delicate hands are unlikely to achieve the most optimal result.

13 Which, in turn, is mandatory if the physician wants full cooperation from the patient, including the taking of medications, positioning, returning for follow-up, etc. (see Chap. 1.4).

(see Chaps. 2.9, 2.17). Another example of the need for a major paradigm shift is the management of the injured lens: whether the traditional, and otherwise optimal, method of phacoemulsification is deemed acceptable, a series of questions need to be answered.[14]

These are just a few of the difficulties an ocular traumatologist faces; the often significant financial implications, or the constant threat of becoming the target of a malpractice suit, are not even mentioned here.

The sum of these difficulties is increased stress for the ocular traumatologist. Stress is known to be harmful to the human being, but I firmly believe that this is actually a positive type of stress.[15] The lower surgical success rate is more than compensated for by those hard-earned victories, but the surgeon must learn to consciously appreciate and cherish these successes. Even in the developing countries, where there may be a shortage of equipment and material, so much more is achieved today than only a few years ago.[16] True, very few questions in ocular traumatology can be binary because there are more “it depends” than straight “yes” or “no” answers, but it is exactly this challenge that makes the field so exciting and fulfilling.[17]

In the U.S., less than one-third of medical schools require formal training in ophthalmology. Among those who receive such training, and among ophthalmology residents throughout the world, only few are willing to undertake the challenging field of trauma. For those who do, however, nothing can compete with the gratification offered by the successful management of a “hopeless” injury. I am confident that future generations of patients will not be deprived of the same “caring cure” today’s ocular trauma experts provide.

Last but not least, I gratefully acknowledge the support, encouragement, inspiration, and friendship of those without whom this book could never have been written. This is a long list, and I can name only a few of these

---

14 See Chap. 2.7.

15 Remember that laboratory animals have a shorter life span if they are kept in a completely stress-free environment.

16 See Paudyal G et al.: Ophthalmology (2005); 112:319–26.

17 It is true no more that “we know just enough to know that we don’t know enough.”

people because of space limitations.[18] In Birmingham, Robert Morris and C. Douglas Witherspoon have, for almost two decades, been my "trauma soul mates" professionally as well as the greatest of friends. In Hungary, I found vitrectomy as a specialty at the suggestion of Bálint Kovács, and was fortunate enough to work with the dedicated and talented Viktória Mester for many years. My assistant in Birmingham, LoRetta Mann, has provided not only data for the book but also moral support. I also thank Marion Philipp and Martina Himberger at Springer and Anne Strohbach at LE-TEX, who made the job of transforming this material into a book as easy as possible.

Finally, I thank my family[19] for their nonwavering support and love, and I apologize for the countless hours, days, weeks, and months that I spent "on the job," instead of being with them.

Ferenc Kuhn

18 I nevertheless want to mention Cesare Forlini, Giampaolo Gini, Bowes Hamill, and Wolfgang Schrader.

19 Mary, my wife, and my two daughters, Sophia and Judy.

Contents

Section II

Section III

Contributors

Yaniv Barkana
Department of Ophthalmology
Assaf Harofe Medical Center
Zerifin 70300
Israel
E-mail: yaniv.barkana@yahoo.com

Michael Belkin
Eye Technologies Laboratory
Goldschleger Eye Research Institute
Tel Aviv University
Sheba Medical Center
Tel Hashomer 52621
Israel
E-mail: belkin@netvision.net.il

Claude Boscher
Unité d'Ophtalmologie
Hopital Américain de Paris
63 Boulevard Victor Hugo
92 200 Neuilly sur Seine
France
E-mail: cboscher@wanadoo.fr

Gábor Kocsis
Kiscenki utca 50/c
Nagycenk, 9485
Hungary
E-mail: kocsisszommer@mail.datanet.hu

Ferenc Kuhn
University of Alabama at Birmingham
1201 11th Avenue S., Suite 300
Birmingham, AL 35205, USA
E-mail: fkuhn@mindspring.com

LoRetta Mann
University of Alabama at Birmingham
Helen Keller Foundation for Research and Education
1201 11th Avenue South, Suite 300
Birmingham, AL 35205, USA
E-mail: lorettamann@useironline.org

Viktória Mester
Sheikh Khalifa Medical City
Health Services for the Emirate of Abu Dhabi
Abu Dhabi
United Arab Emirates
E-mail: viktoriamester@hotmail.com

Robert Morris
Founder, United States Eye Injury Registry
Associate Professor of Clinical Ophthalmology, University of Alabama at Birmingham
President, Helen Keller Foundation for Research and Education
President, International Society of Ocular Trauma
1201 11th Avenue South, Suite 300
Birmingham, AL 35205, USA
E-mail: bobmorris@helenkellerfoundation.com

Dante Pieramici
California Retina Research Foundation
Santa Barbara California
Doheny Eye Institute
Los Angeles California
California Retina Consultants
Santa Barbara, California
E-mail: dpieramici@yahoo.com

Wolfgang Schrader
Department of Ophthalmology
University of Wuerzburg
Josef-Schneiderstrasse 11
97080 Würzburg
Germany
E-mail: w.schrader@augenklinik.uni-wuerzburg.de

Norbert F. Schrage
Department of Ophthalmology Cologne Merheim
Ostmerheimer Street 200
51109 Cologne
Germany
E-mail: Schrage@acto.de

C. Douglas Witherspoon
United States Eye Injury Registry
University of Alabama at Birmingham
Helen Keller Foundation for Research and Education
1201 11th Avenue South, Suite 300
Birmingham, AL 35205
USA
E-mail: cdw529@mac.com

Abbreviations

Acronym	Stands for
A	Appendix
AC	Anterior chamber
AIDS	Acquired immune deficiency syndrome
AION	Anterior ischemic optic neuropathy
ALK	Automated lamellar keratoplasty
ALT	Argon laser trabeculoplasty
APD	Afferent pupillary defect
ASTM	American Society for Testing and Materials
BB	A 0.18-in. diameter pellet (for air gun or shotgun)
BETT	Birmingham Eye Trauma Terminology
BSS	Balanced salt solution
C3F8	Perfluoropropane gas
CAI	Carbonic anhydrase inhibitor
CCD	Charge couple device
CDC	Centers for Disease Control and Prevention
CF	Count fingers
CME	Cystoid macular edema
CNS	Central nervous system
CNV	Choroidal neovascularization
CT	Computed tomography
DSAEK	Descemet's stripping automated endothelial keratoplasty
EAV	Endoscopy-assisted vitrectomy
ECCE	Extracapsular cataract extraction

ECH	Expulsive choroidal hemorrhage
EDTA	Ethylen-diamine-tetraacetic acid
EEM	External electromagnet
EIRA	Eye Injury Registry of Alabama
EMP	Epimacular proliferation (macular pucker)
EOM	Extraocular muscle
ER	Emergency room
ERG	Electroretinogram
ETDRS	Early Treatment Diabetic Retinopathy Study
EVS	Endophthalmitis Vitrectomy Study
FA	Fluorescein angiography
FB	Foreign body
FDA	Food and Drug Administration
FILMS	Fluidic internal limiting membrane separation
FLAG	Fluorescein angiography
GFLI	Gas-forced liquid infusion
GRIN endoscope	Gradient-index endoscope
HEIR	Hungarian Eye Injury Registry
HM	Hand motion
IBO	Indirect binocular ophthalmoscope/y/ic
ICCE	Intracapsular cataract extraction
ICD	International Classification of Diseases
ICG	Indocyanine green
ICIDH	International Classification of Impairments, Disabilities, and Handicaps
ICR	Intrastromal corneal ring
ICU	Intensive care unit
ILM	Internal limiting membrane
IOFB	Intraocular foreign body
IOM	Permanent intraocular magnet
IOP	Intraocular pressure
IR	Infrared
ISOT	International Society of Ocular Trauma
J	Joule

LASIK	Laser in-situ keratomileusis
LMA	Laryngeal mask airway
LP	Light perception
MMP	Matrix metalloproteinase
mph	Miles per hour
MVC	Motor vehicle crash
MVR	Microvitrectomy (e.g., blade)
MRI	Magnetic resonance imaging
NA	Not applicable
NEI	National Eye Institute (U.S.)
NETS	National Eye Trauma System
NLP	No light perception
OCT	Optical coherence tomography
OR	Operating room
PK[1]	Penetrating keratoplasty
PMMA	Polymethyl methacrylate
PRK	Photorefractive keratectomy
psi	Pounds per square inch
PTK	Phototherapeutic keratectomy
PVD	Posterior vitreous detachment
RBC	Red blood cells
RK	Radial keratotomy
RPE	Retinal pigment epithelium
RR	Relative risk
SCH	Suprachoroidal hemorrhage
SF6	Sulfur hexafluoride gas
SO	Sympathetic ophthalmia
sp.	Species
TA	Triamcinolone acetonid
TKP	Temporary keratoprosthesis
TON	Traumatic optic neuropathy
TPA	Tissue plasminogen activator
U	Unit
UBM	Ultrasound biomicroscope/y

USEIR	United States Eye Injury Registry; URL: www.useironline.org
UV	Ultraviolet
VEP	Visual evoked potential
VGEF	Vascular endothelial growth factor
VKH	Vogt–Koyanagi–Harada syndrome
WEIR	World Eye Injury Registry; URL: www.weironline.org
YAG laser	Neodymium-doped yttrium aluminium garnet (Nd:YAG) laser
WHO	World Health Organization

1 "Penetrating" here is not a BETT definition: the surgical incision is full thickness in this case.

SECTION I

1.1 Terminology of Mechanical Injuries: the Birmingham Eye Trauma Terminology (BETT)

Ferenc Kuhn, Robert Morris, Viktória Mester,
C. Douglas Witherspoon

1.1.1 If the Terminology Is Not Standardized

Akin to two people not speaking a common language (Fig. 1.1.1), ophthalmologists are unable to unambiguously communicate with each other if the terms they use to describe an eye injury are not standardized. If the terms used do not have straightforward definitions, practitioners cannot understand each other when discussing an ocular trauma case, nor can research be conducted, and its results published, without the risk of the data being misinterpreted.

There are very few publications in the literature that provide definitions for the terms used, and those that do may not enforce its own definitions [1]. Consequently, inconsistencies are often found even within the same publication. Common problems include:

- Use of different terms to describe the same injury ("double penetrating" [15], "double-perforating" [17] and "perforating" [7])
- Use of the word "blunt" without specifying whether it refers to the agent or to the resulting injury [8]
- Alternatively using, even within the same publication, two different terms (penetrating, perforating) to describe the same injury [11]
- Use of the term "penetrating" to describe any open globe injury [3]
- Use of the term "rupture" to describe any open globe injury [16]
- Lack of indicating the tissue of reference when using the term "perforating" [4]

These misnomers are summarized in Fig. 1.1.2, and in Tables 1.1.1 and 1.1.2.

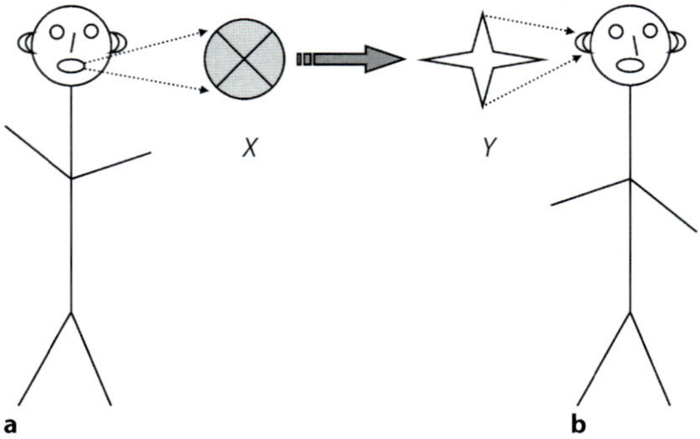

Fig. 1.1.1 Miscommunication if two people do not speak the same language. Individual "**a**" is communicating message "*X*"; however, this is understood by individual "**b**" as "*Y*." The reason for misinterpretation is the nonstandardized methods of coding and decoding the message

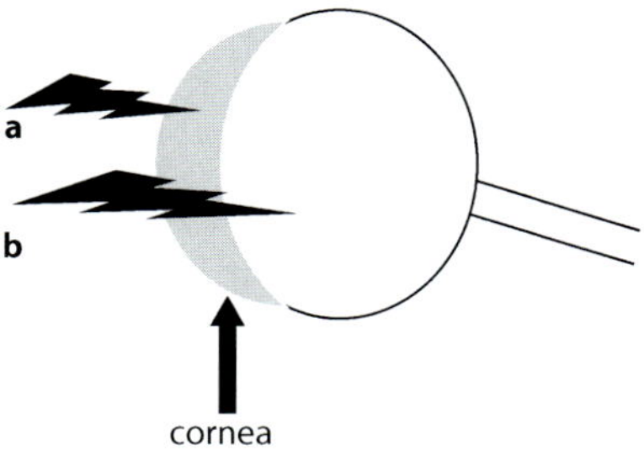

Fig. 1.1.2 The importance of indicating the tissue of reference when defining an eye injury term. Injury **a** is a *closed globe* injury but a penetrating injury of the *cornea* (i.e., not of the *globe*): the object violated the cornea but did not cause a through-and-through wound. Injury **b** is an open globe trauma; it is a *perforating* (through-and-through) injury of the *cornea* but a *penetrating* (into, not through) injury of the *globe*

1.1.2 Characteristics of an Ideal Eye Trauma Terminology System

In an ideal eye trauma terminology system, the following criteria must be satisfied:

- The tissue of reference must always be obvious.
- Each term must have a unique definition.

Table 1.1.1 A selection of confusing eye injury terms in the literature and their recommended substitutes

Term and reference	Controversy	Clinical implication	Recommendation
Blunt injury [8]	The inflicting object is blunt The consequences of the trauma are "blunt"	Open globe injury (rupture) Closed globe injury (contusion)	The word "blunt" should be replaced by one of the more appropriate terms: "contusion" or "rupture"
Blunt nonpenetrating globe injury [9]	Can an injury occur that is sharp but nonpenetrating?	Probably a closed globe injury	This term should be replaced by "contusion"
Blunt penetrating trauma [10]	How can an injury be both blunt and penetrating?	Open globe injury probably by a blunt object	This term should be replaced by "rupture"
Blunt rupture [13]	Are not all ruptures blunt?	Open globe injury by a blunt object	This term should be replaced by "rupture"
Contusion rupture [5]	How can an injury be both a contusion and a rupture?	Probably an open globe injury	This term should be replaced by "rupture"
Sharp laceration [2]	Is there a laceration that is not sharp?	An open globe injury caused by a sharp object	This term should be replaced by "penetrating" or "perforating"

- No term can be applied for more than a single injury type.
- No injury may be described by different terms.
- All injury types must be included.

1.1.3 The Birmingham Eye Trauma Terminology (BETT)

The key to this system is that all definitions refer to the entire globe, not to a specific tissue. (There is no need, therefore, to include reference to a

Table 1.1.2 Inappropriately used ocular trauma terms in the literature

Term and reference	Intended meaning by author	Likely interpretation by reader	Comment
Penetrating [3]	All types of open globe injury	Injury with an entrance wound	All penetrating injuries are open globe but not all open globe injuries are penetrating
Penetrating [6]	No distinction between penetrating and perforating trauma	Injury with an entrance wound	Penetrating and perforating injuries must be distinguished as they have different management and prognostic implications
Rupture [12]	All types of open globe injury, including IOFB injuries	Open globe injury caused by a blunt object	All ruptures are open globe but not all open globe injuries are ruptures
Perforating [4]	Injury with a single (entrance) wound [13]	Questionable	Unless the tissue of reference is also indicated, it is not possible to determine which injury type is described
	Injury with both entrance and exit wounds [14]	Questionable	

tissue in the term.) If a tissue is specified, it refers to *location* and is not a modifier of the term. In Fig. 1.1.2, injury "B" shows a penetrating trauma; if it is described as a "penetrating corneal injury", it means that the wound is corneal. (Prior to BETT, it could have meant either a *closed globe* injury (penetrating into the *cornea*) or an *open globe injury* (penetrating into the *globe*). BETT is described in detail in Table 1.1.3, and in Figs. 1.1.3 and 1.1.4. Traumatic enucleation of the eye is shown in Fig. 1.1.5.

There are cases in which the injury occurs by a complex mechanism. For instance, if the patient falls onto a glass table that has a sharp edge, the *wound* may be a laceration (penetrating injury), but the *injury* has a rupture component (major tissue loss) as well as a contusion element (maculopathy). In such cases the worst injury type (rupture, in this example) is the one that best describes the consequences and implications of the case.

Table 1.1.3 Terms and definitions in BETT

Term	Definition	Comment
Eye wall	Sclera and cornea	Though the eye wall has three layers posterior to the limbus, clinical and practical purposes dictate that violation of only the most external tissue (sclera) is to be considered
Closed globe injury	No full-thickness wound of eye wall	The cornea and the sclera are not breached through and through
Open globe injury	Full-thickness wound of the eye wall	The cornea and/or sclera is breached through and through
Contusion	No wound of the eye wall	The damage may be due to direct energy delivery/shock wave by the object (e.g., choroidal rupture), or to changes in the shape of the globe (e.g., angle recession)
Lamellar laceration	Partial-thickness wound of the eye wall	The wound in the eye wall is not "through" but "into"
Rupture	Full-thickness wound of the eye wall, caused by a large blunt object	Since the eye is filled with incompressible liquid, the impact results in instant IOP elevation. The eye wall yields at its weakest point (rarely at the impact site, rather, for instance, along an old cataract wound); the actual wound is produced by an inside-out mechanism, and tissue prolapse is almost unavoidable

Some injuries have a complex mechanism and are thus difficult to classify (e.g., an intravitreal BB pellet is technically an IOFB injury, but since this blunt object requires great force to enter the eye, the wound is created as if it were a rupture; see the text for more details). In such situations, the ophthalmologist can describe the injury as "mixed" (i.e., rupture with an IOFB) and select the more serious type (rupture), or the one that dominates the acute management (IOFB). Complete destruction of the eye and traumatic enucleation (see Fig. 1.1.5) are not included in the system

Table 1.1.3 *(continued)* Terms and definitions in BETT

Term	Definition	Comment
Laceration	Full-thickness wound of the eye wall, caused by a sharp object	The wound is at the impact site and is created by an outside-in mechanism; since IOP elevation is unavoidable, tissue prolapse is common
Penetrating injury	An entrance wound is present	If more than one wound is present, each must have been caused by a different object
IOFB	One or more foreign objects are present	Technically a penetrating injury, but grouped separately because of different clinical implications (management, prognosis)
Perforating injury	Both an entrance and an exit wound are present	The two wounds caused by the same agent

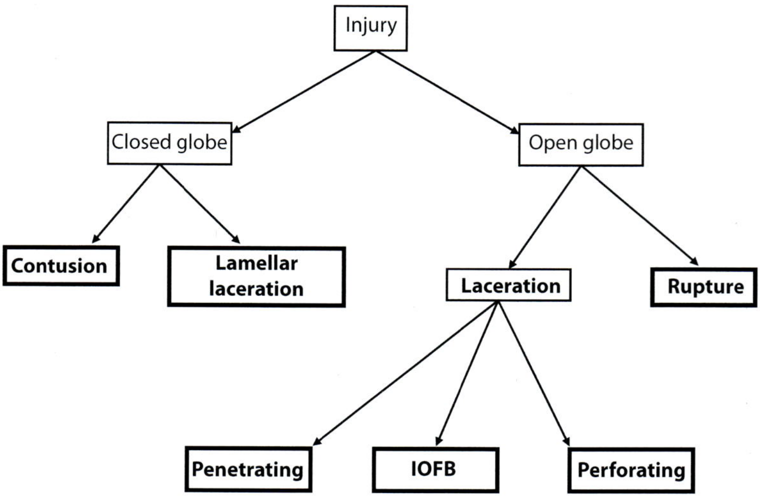

Fig. 1.1.3 BETT. The *bold boxes* indicate those diagnoses that are used as clinical entities

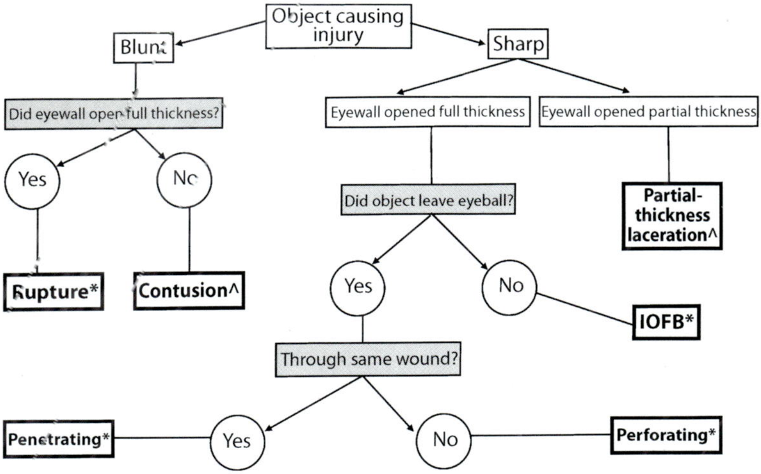

Fig. 1.1.4 Practical guide to classifying mechanical eye injuries in BETT. The *bold boxes* indicate those diagnoses that are used as clinical entities. Injuries marked with an *asterisk* are open globe, those with a *caret* are closed globe

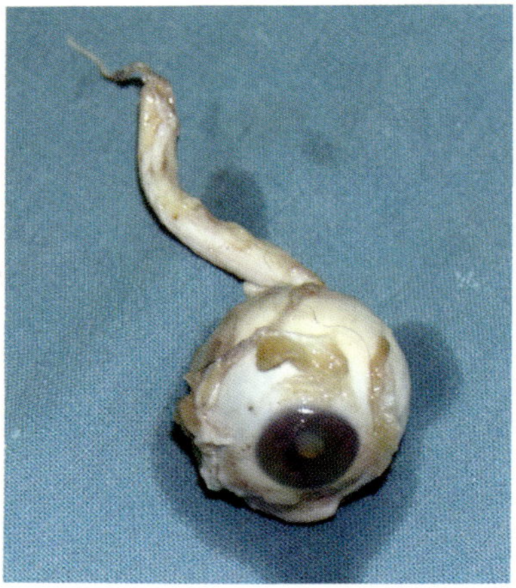

Fig. 1.1.5 Enucleation caused by an animal attack. This 45-year-old man was attacked by his dog. A traumatic enucleation occurred, but the eye itself is intact. (Courtesy of Z. Slezak, Varasdin, Croatia)

DO:

- apply BETT in your clinical practice as well as in your research

DON'T:

- elect randomly the term to describe the eye injury

Summary

Using a standardized language in ocular traumatology is mandatory to avoid ambiguity between health care professionals, regardless of the type of communication.

References

[1] Alfaro V, Liggett P (1998) Vitrectomy in the management of the injured globe. Lippincott Raven, Philadelphia
[2] de Juan E, Sternberg P, Michels R (1983) Penetrating ocular injuries: types of injuries and visual results. Ophthalmology 90: 1318–1322
[3] de Juan E, Sternberg P, Michels R, Auer C (1984) Evaluation of vitrectomy in penetrating ocular trauma. A case-control study. Arch Ophthalmol 102: 1160–1163
[4] Eagling EM (1976) Perforating injuries of the eye. Br J Ophthalmol 60: 732–736
[5] Eide N, Syrdalen P (1987) Contusion rupture of the globe. Acta Ophthalmol 182S: 169–171
[6] Hassett P, Kelleher C (1994) The epidemiology of occupational penetrating eye injuries in Ireland. Occup Med 44: 209–211
[7] Hutton WL, Fuller DG (1984) Factors influencing final visual results in severely injured eyes. Am J Ophthalmol 97: 715–722
[8] Joseph E, Zak R, Smith S, Best W, Gamelli R, Dries D (1992) Predictors of blinding or serious eye injury in blunt trauma. J Eye Trauma 33: 19–24
[9] Liggett P, Gauderman W, Moreira C, Barlow W, Green R, Ryan S (1990) Pars plana vitrectomy for acute retinal detachment in penetrating ocular injuries. Arch Ophthalmol 108: 1724–1728
[10] Meredith T, Gordon P (1987) Pars plana vitrectomy for severe penetrating injury with posterior segment involvement. Am J Ophthalmol 103: 549–554
[11] Moisseiev J, Vidne O, Treister G (1998) Vitrectomy and silicone oil injection in pediatric patients. Retina 18: 221–227

[12] Pump-Schmidt C, Behrens-Baumann W (1999) Changes in the epidemiology of ruptured globe eye injuries due to societal changes. Ophthalmologica 213: 380–386
[13] Punnonen E, Laatikainen L (1989) Prognosis of perforating eye injuries with intraocular foreign bodies. Acta Ophthalmol 66: 483–491
[14] Ramsay R, Knobloch WH (1978) Ocular perforation following retrobulbar anesthesia for retinal detachment surgery. Am J Ophthalmol 86: 61–64
[15] Ramsay RC, Cantrill HL, Knobloch WH (1985) Vitrectomy for double penetrating ocular injuries. Am J Ophthalmol 100: 586–589
[16] Rudd J, Jaeger E, Freitag S, Jeffers J (1994) Traumatically ruptured globes in children. J Pediatr Ophthalmol Strab 31: 307–311
[17] Topping T, Abrams G, Machemer R (1979) Experimental double-perforating injury of the posterior segment in rabbit eyes: the natural history of intraocular proliferation. Arch Ophthalmol 97: 735–742

1.2 Classification of Mechanical Eye Injuries

Ferenc Kuhn and Dante Pieramici

1.2.1 The Need for a Standardized System to Describe Characteristics of a Serious Eye Injury

Several variables (e.g., tissue abnormalities, functional consequences) can be used to describe the injury. A system that provides meaningful yet concise information is extremely helpful for clinicians, researchers, and patients.

1.2.2 The Development of the Classification[1] System

A group of trauma specialists[2] was gathered to develop the system based on their clinical experience, using the Delphi process[3] and Likert questions[4]. The fundament for the classification system was BETT (see Chap. 1.1).

---

1 The name "classification" reflects the fact that the system breaks down the findings into a few categories and has several options in each.

2 The initiative came from Paul Sternberg; other members of the *Ocular Trauma Classification Group* included: Thomas Aaberg, William Bridges, Antonio Capone, Jose Cardillo, Eugene deJuan, Ferenc Kuhn, Travis Meredith, William Mieler, Timothy Olsen, Patrick Rubsamen, and Timothy Stout.

3 A question is asked from the group; discussion follows and a consensus is reached. The group moves to the next question, and the procedure is repeated until all agree that the final product is the best and most useful that can be achieved.

4 The possible answer to the yes-or-no question ranges from "strongly agree" to "strongly disagree."

Table 1.2.1 Classification of open and closed globe injuries

	Injury type		Grade	Pupil		Zone	
	Open globe	Closed globe	Open and closed globe	Open and closed globe		Open globe	Closed globe
A	Rupture	Contusion	≥20/40	Positive	I	Cornea and limbus	External Bulbar conjunctiva Cornea Sclera
B	Penetrating	Lamellar laceration	20/50 to 20/100	Negative	II	Limbus to 5 mm posterior into sclera	Anterior segment Anterior chamber Iris Angle Lens Pars plicata
C	IOFB	Superficial FB	19/100 to 5/200		III	Posterior to 5 mm from the limbus	Posterior segment Ciliary bod Choroid Vitreous Retina Optic nerve
D	Perforating	Mixed	4/200 to LP				
E	Mixed		NLP				

[a]Presence (positive) or absence (negative) of APD in the injured eye

1.2.3 The Classification System for Mechanical Eye Injuries

A separate classification system is used for open and for closed globe injuries [11]. The system evaluates four variables:

- Type (based on the mechanism of injury) [3, 6, 7, 9]
- Grade (based on the initial visual acuity) [2–4, 7, 12, 13]
- Pupil (depending on the presence or absence of an afferent pupillary defect) [3, 8]
- Zone (based on the location of the wound in open globe injuries and on what the most posterior tissue that has been damaged is in closed globe injuries) [2–4, 6, 7, 12]

Table 1.2.1 shows the details of the system.

Pearl

It is possible to determine almost all elements of the system during the ophthalmologist's initial examination of the eye or during primary surgery; special testing may be necessary if an IOFB or an occult scleral wound is suspected.

DO:

- determine the classification system's elements during work-up and surgery

DON'T:

- forget to base your findings on the BETT system

Summary

The classification system provides a simple method of conveying important information about an eye injury, and it has been proven to carry prognostic information as well [1, 5].

References

[1] Bajaire B, Oudovitchenko E, Morales E (2006) Vitreoretinal surgery of the posterior segment for explosive trauma in terrorist warfare. Graefe's Arch Clin Exp Ophthalmol 244: 991–995

[2] Brinton G, Aaberg T, Reeser F, Topping T, Abrams G (1982) Surgical results in ocular trauma involving the posterior segment. Am J Ophthalmol 93: 271–278

[3] De Juan E, Sternberg P, Michels R (1983) Penetrating ocular injuries: types of injuries and visual results. Ophthalmology 90: 1318–1322

[4] Eagling EM (1976) Perforating injuries of the eye. Br J Ophthalmol 60: 732–736

[5] Ersanli D, Unal M, Aydin A, Gulecek O, Kalemoglu M (2005) Results of pars plana vitrectomy in closed-globe injuries. Ophthal Surg Lasers Imaging 36: 182–188

[6] Gilbert CM, Soong HK, Hirst LW (1987) A two-year prospective study of penetrating ocular trauma at the Wilmer Ophthalmological Institute. Ann Ophthalmol 19: 104–106

[7] Hutton WL, Fuller DG (1984) Factors influencing final visual results in severely injured eyes. Am J Ophthalmol 97: 715–722

[8] Joseph E, Zak R, Smith S, Best W, Gamelli R, Dries D (1992) Predictors of blinding or serious eye injury in blunt trauma. J Eye Trauma 33: 19–24

[9] Martin D, Meredith T, Topping T, Sternberg PJ, Kaplan H (1991) Perforating (through-and-through) injuries of the globe. Surgical results with vitrectomy. Arch Ophthalmol 109: 951–956

[10] Park S, Marcus D, Duker J, Pesavento R, Topping P, Frederick A, D'Amico D (1995) Posterior segment complications after vitrectomy for macular hole. Ophthalmology 102: 775–781

[11] Pieramici D, Sternberg JP, Aaberg ST, Bridges JWZ, Capone JA, Cardillo JA, DeJuan JE, Kuhn F, Meredith TA, Mieler W, Olsen TW, Rubsamen P, Stout T (1997) A system for classifying mechanical injuries of the eye (globe). Am J Ophthalmol 123: 820–831

[12] Sternberg P, de Juan E, Michels RG, et al. (1984) Multivariate analysis of prognostic factors in penetrating ocular injuries. Am J Ophthalmol 98: 467–472

[13] Williams DF, Mieler WF, Abrams GW et al. (1988) Results and prognostic factors in penetrating ocular injuries with retained intraocular foreign bodies. Ophthalmology 95: 911–916

1.3 Predicting the Severity of an Eye Injury: the Ocular Trauma Score (OTS)

Ferenc Kuhn, Robert Morris, Viktoria Mester,
C. Douglas Witherspoon, LoRetta Mann

1.3.1 Forecasting[1] the Final Outcome of a Serious Injury

A serious eye injury is a major psychological trauma to the patient and family. The most pressing issue for them is to learn about the long-term visual consequence as soon as possible ("Will I go blind?"). Having prognostic information is equally important for the ophthalmologist while he is making triaging decisions (see Chap. 1.8) and as he is counseling the patient (see Chap. 1.4).

1.3.2 Prognostic Information: a Literature Review

Many authors have published studies that have identified variables making the likely outcome of the injury favorable or unfavorable. Unfortunately, much of information in these studies is controversial (Table 1.3.1), and none of the reports present a digital system (i.e., measurable, numerical, objective).

1.3.3 Characteristics of an Ideal Forecasting System

The characteristics of an ideal forecasting system are as follows:

1 Nobel laureate Niels Bohr (1885–1962) once said that "Forecasting is easy... unless it's about the future."

Table 1.3.1 Contradictory prognostic information in the literature. (Modified after [4])

Variables reported both as with and without prognostic significance[a]	Boundary signaling prognostic significance	Surgical interventions reported as either with or without prognostic significance[b]
Age	Anterior vs posterior	No. of operations
Cause of injury	Sclera vs limbus	Prophylactic cryopexy
Endophthalmitis	Limbus vs cornea	Prophylactic scleral buckling
Extent of wound	Limbus vs cornea or sclera	
Facial fracture		Timing of vitrectomy[c]
Hyphema	Cornea vs sclera anterior to muscle insertion	Prophylactic antibiotics[d]
Initial visual acuity		PPV vs tap for endophthalmitis[e]
Injury type		Silicone oil vs gas[e] for PVR
IOFB	Sclera: anterior to vs posterior to muscle insertion	PPV vs external magnet for IOFB
IOFB location		IOL implantation: primary vs secondary
Laterality of eye injured		
Lens injury	Equator	
NLP initial vision	Sclera vs limbus or cornea	
Perforating injury		
Retinal detachment	Sclera, posterior vs scleral	

[a]These variables were determined to have prognostic significance in some studies but to not have any prognostic value in other studies.

[b]"Early" was defined as 3 days in one study [2] and 14 days in another [1]

[c]The type of drug used is important

[d]In posttraumatic infections tap should not be considered as an option [5] (see Chap. 2.17)

Table 1.3.1 *(continued)* Contradictory prognostic information in the literature. (Modified after [4])

Variables reported both as with and without prognostic significance[a]	Boundary signaling prognostic significance	Surgical interventions reported as either with or without prognostic significance[b]
Sex		
Tissue prolapse	Wound length: 2, 3, 4, 5, 6, 9, 10, 11, 12, 15 mm	
VEP, ERG		
Vitreous hemorrhage		
Wound location		

[e]The type of intravitreal gas used is important

- Sufficient data can be collected during the evaluation of the injured person or the initial surgery to allow the prognosis to be predicted.
- The variables used are those that would be part of the normal management process.
- The prognostic information is quantitative rather than qualitative.
- The value is simple and easy to calculate.
- The system is reproducible and reliable.

1.3.4 The Ocular Trauma Score (OTS)

A system that appears to satisfy all criteria described above has been developed using over 2,500 cases from the USEIR [3].[2] Based on one functional

2 Developed by USEIR researchers using a grant from the National Center for Injury Prevention at the CDC

Table 1.3.2 Calculating the OTS and predicting the visual outcome

Step 1: Determining the raw points	Variable	Raw point value
Initial vision	NLP	60
	LP/HM	70
	1/200–19/200	80
	20/200–20/50	90
	≥20/40	100
	Rupture	−23
	Endophthalmitis	−17
	Perforating injury	−14
	Retinal detachment	−11
	APD	−10

Step 2: Conversion of the raw points into the OTS, and identifying the likely visual outcome (%)						
Sum of raw points	OTS	NLP	LP/HM	1/200–19/200	20/200–20/50	≥20/40
0–44	1	74	15	7	3	1
45–65	2	27	26	18	15	15
66–80	3	2	11	15	31	41
81–91	4	1	2	3	22	73
92–100	5	0	1	1	5	94

If none of the five pathologies are present, the visual acuity determines the OTS (initial visual acuity)[3] and five anatomical (rupture, endophthalmitis, perforating injury, retinal detachment, APD) characteristics, the OTS value is immediately available at the conclusion of the evaluation/initial surgery with reasonably reliable prognostic implications (Table 1.3.2).

1.3.5 Use of the OTS in Clinical Practice

A small card can easily be prepared and carried in the ophthalmologist's pocket. On the front of the card is printed the system to calculate the OTS, and on the back side the visual acuity table. Early clinical experience utilizing the OTS is favorable [6, 7].

Pearl:

One of the benefits of reporting serious eye injury cases to a standardized database (see Chap. 1.7) is that on the USEIR and WEIR websites (www.useironline.org, www.weironline.org) the OTS calculation is immediately available.

DO:

- have the OTS available and use it during counseling and decision-making; it gives more accurate information than visual acuity alone

DON'T:

- imply to the patient that the OTS is specifically for him; rather, that this is statistical information, which may or may not apply in his individual case

Summary

Its is extremely useful for both patient and ophthalmologist to have reliable prognostic information about the injury

3 The most important, albeit not independent, variable

References

[1] Brinton G, Aaberg T, Reeser F, Topping T, Abrams G (1982) Surgical results in ocular trauma involving the posterior segment. Am J Ophthalmol 93: 271–278

[2] Coleman D (1982) Early vitrectomy in the management of the severely traumatized eye. Am J Ophthalmol 93: 543–551

[3] Kuhn F, Maisiak R, Mann L, Mester V, Morris R, Witherspoon C (2002) The Ocular Trauma Score (OTS). Ophthalmol Clin North Am 15: 163–166

[4] Kuhn F, Maisiak R, Mann L, Morris R, Witherspoon C (2002) The Ocular Trauma Score (OTS): Prognosticating the final vision of the seriously injured eye. In: Kuhn F, Pieramici D (eds) Ocular trauma: principles and practice. Thieme, New York, pp 14–12

[5] Mittra RA, Mieler WF (1999) Controversies in the management of open-globe injuries involving the posterior segment. Surv Ophthalmol 44: 215–225

[6] Sarrazin L, Averbukh E, Halpert M, Hemo I, Rumelt S (2004) Traumatic pediatric retinal detachment: a comparison between open and closed globe injuries. Am J Ophthalmol 137: 1042–1049

[7] Sobaci G, Akin T, Erdem U, Uysal Y, Karagul S (2006) Ocular trauma score in deadly weapon-related open globe injuries. Am J Ophthalmol 141: 760–761

1.4 Counseling the Injured Individual and the Family

Ferenc Kuhn and Robert Morris

1.4.1 Definition

If a patient with a nonemergency (elective) medical condition consults an ophthalmologist, the physician will typically spend time with the person, explaining:

- The nature of the condition
- The available management options (including observation, i.e., natural history)
- The benefits and risks/complications of each option
- The patient's expected experience with each option (e.g., pain, inconvenience)
- The possibility of multiple surgeries and protracted recovery
- The likely functional and anatomical outcome[1]
- If applicable, the need for, and availability of, rehabilitation services

Counseling is the process during which the physician provides information (Fig. 1.4.1) for the patient (family) about the medical condition and

1 For the patient, the prognosis is the most important information (see Chap. 1.3). The ophthalmologist must ensure that his message is neither too optimistic nor too pessimistic. Based on the long list of potential complications a serious injury may cause, a *mildly pessimistic* prognosis is preferable to an optimistic one.

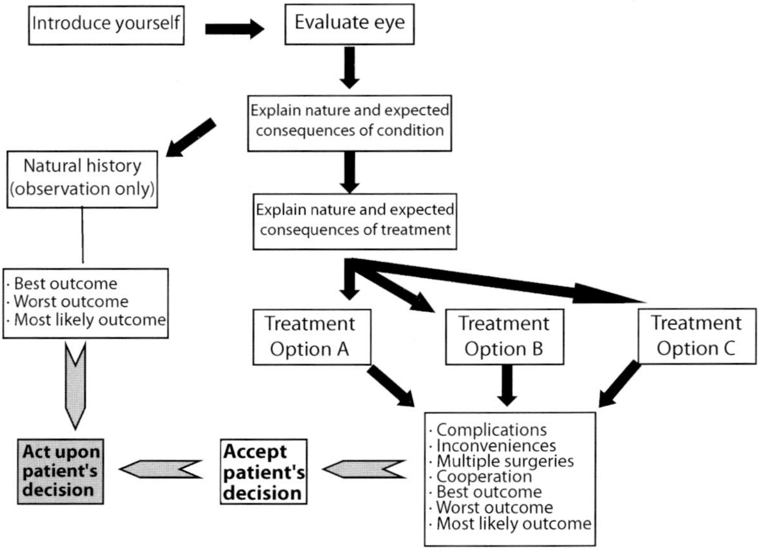

Fig. 1.4.1 Flowchart showing the elements of counseling. This is not a blueprint that would be valid for every encounter or situation; individualize the scenario described here as the situation demands it

its treatment to aid informed decision making.[2] Counseling is not a monologue but a discussion; the patient's input is not tolerated but encouraged.

Counseling should be no different regardless of whether the pathology is caused by a disease such as diabetes or an eye injury.

2 The patient *wants* to have answers to the many questions he has. If the attending ophthalmologist won't adequately answer them, the patient will look for answers from another ophthalmologist (who has only limited information about the case) or turn to a neighbor or an internet page.

1.4.2 "Whose Eye Is it?"

The answer is simple: the eye belongs to the patient, not to the physician.[3]

Pearl

The counseling ophthalmologist's role is to help the patient make the treatment decision, not to make the decision for (instead of) the patient.

- If the condition is a true emergency (i.e., a chemical injury), counseling (even detailed history-taking) is deferred so as to facilitate the intervention (see Chaps. 1.10, 3.1).
- If the patient is unconscious, a minor, or not of sound mind, and the prognosis would likely to worsen with treatment delay (so that proper consent from the family or a guardian can be obtained), the ophthalmologist should initiate treatment according to his best judgment.

1.4.3 The Goals of Counseling

Poor communication is a common source of problems such as misunderstanding, ignorance, lack of cooperation, suspicion, mistrust, and, if the outcome is perceived as suboptimal, litigation. Effective communication is crucial for several reasons.

- Gaining the patient's confidence. Chance, rather than choice, brings the injured patient to the ophthalmologist: the patient's trust is not automatic, it must be earned.

---

3 *"Every human being of adult years and sound mind has a right to determine what shall be done with his own body; and a surgeon who performs an operation without his patient's consent, commits an assault, for which he is liable in damages"* (Justice Benjamin Cardozo, Court of Appeals of New York; Schloendorff vs. The Society of the New York Hospital, 211 N.Y. 125; 105 N.E. 92 (1914).

- Establishing and maintaining a partnership. Patient and ophthalmologist must cooperate throughout the entire treatment and follow-up period. The process can last several years, and loss of cooperation reduces the chance of success.
- Making the patient understand and endorse the objective of treatment. Restoring the eye's anatomy to as close to normal as possible is all a physician can attempt.

Cave

A physician should not promise functional recovery but make the patient understand that restoring the anatomy is *conditio sine qua non* to improve vision.

1.4.4 The Elements of Proper Counseling

Proper counseling is as much an art as it is a science. Counseling is difficult to teach: its learning curve is long and steep, and practicing it requires considerable experience and patience. Counseling demands:

- Expert knowledge of ophthalmology in general and of ocular traumatology in particular
- Empathy (understanding,[4] compassion, distance-keeping sympathy)
- Ability to listen

4 Understanding, among others, that the eye's anatomy, the significance and consequences of the injury, and the implications of the treatment are new and mysterious to the patient, although they all are common and obvious to you, the ophthalmologist. Most patients, for instance, would not know that no pain is expected during slit-lamp examination, that tearing is natural after taking a photograph with bright flash, or that a small puncture of eye wall with a wire can cause disastrous complications and immediate intervention is needed even if the visual acuity remained unaffected after the injury.

- Ability to observe, perceive, and appropriately react to the patient's communication and metacommunication, tailoring the message to the patient's unique situation, needs, and education and intelligence level
- Ability to effectively communicate through words and gestures (Table 1.4.1)
- Time and patience

Table 1.4.1 Selected elements of metacommunication

What	How
Intonation	Should be congruent with content
Body language (kinesis)	Facial expression
	Attentive, not "empty"
	Serious but not "dramatic"
	Encouraging
	Head position (turn toward patient, not away)
	Phatic signaling[1]
	Hand gestures (modest but present)
Eyes	Look into patients' (not into distance)
Distance	Close enough without breaching privacy[2]
Physical contact	Holding/touching hand/arm/shoulder, done appropriately, conveys understanding, support[3]

As a general rule, there should be no contradiction

[1] Empathically nodding: feedback signaling that the ophthalmologist remains connected to the patient.

[2] Societal issues must also be taken into consideration: in certain societies a much larger physical distance ("personal space") is required than in others.

[3] Societal issues must also be taken into consideration: certain religions discourage physical touch while other religions are neutral. Unwritten nonreligious rules also exist in this regard.

Pearl

The "target" in the counseling process is never the eye: it is the patient, who must at the end have a reasonably good understanding of the eye's condition so that he can make an informed decision regarding treatment.

The initial counseling step is evaluation (see Chap. 1.9) of the patient and the eye to allow the ophthalmologist to have a decent understanding of the globe's condition. The actual counseling consists of:

- Providing information about the eye's condition
- Explaining to the patient and, preferably, to the family, the treatment options and the benefits and risks of each option (Fig. 1.4.2)[5]
- Answering the questions of the patient
- Arriving at a mutually acceptable decision regarding the choice of treatment

The ophthalmologist's presentation must be in a language and format that the patient can understand. This is especially difficult because the patient is under tremendous anxiety: worried about the long-term impact of the eye injury on his vision, on his own quality of life as well as on that of his family, on his future income, etc.

The ophthalmologist should not be "coaching" and should not force on the patient his own, preselected, preferred option[6] (Fig. 1.4.3). The possibility of sympathetic ophthalmia must always be discussed (see Chap. 1.8).

Once the patient makes his choice, actual treatment follows. Counseling, however, does not end there: it should be *continuous* up to the last follow-up visit. Ideally, counseling is done in the presence of a witness (e.g., nurse) and a family member. A written record should always be taken, and taken simultaneously.

5 This should include details such as postoperative posturing.

6 Reasonable alternatives are almost always available.

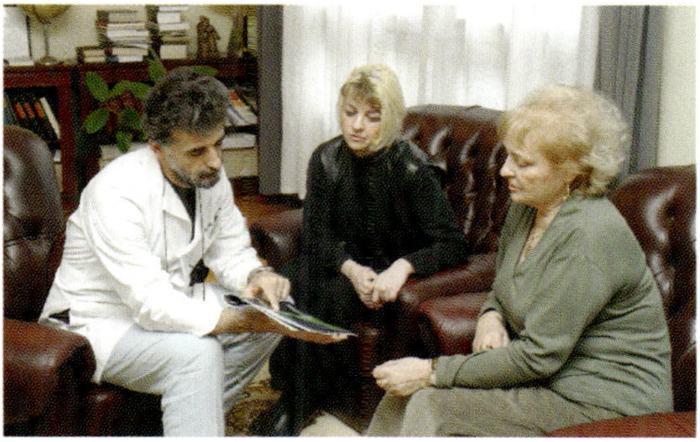

Fig. 1.4.2 Counseling in real life. The patient (*right*) and her daughter listen to the ophthalmologist as he uses illustrations to explain the therapeutic options available for the patient's injured right eye.

1.4.5 The Benefits of Proper Counseling

The benefits of proper counseling are as follows:

- It is much easier for the ophthalmologist to earn the trust of the patient if he is appreciated as a physician who is not only knowledgeable but one who cares.
- A patient who is treated as a *partner* in, rather than simply a *target* of, the treatment process is more likely to adhere to physician instructions and return for follow-ups.
- A patient who was honestly told the risks of injury and treatment, and the difficulties associated with the option he himself chose, is less likely to "be surprised" if the outcome is suboptimal and is thus less likely to initiate legal action against the ophthalmologist (see Chap. 1.8).

- Patient presents with a 6-h-old injury
- Hit with a fist
- Visual acuity: NLP
- Findings: scleral rupture; subconjunctival blood; total vitreous hemorrhage; no IOFB; retinal detachment; subretinal blood accumulation
- Patient conscious, alert, denies alcohol or drug consumption

"Coaching" ← Counseling options → **"Noncoaching"**

"Coaching"

- You have an injury from which there is virtually no chance for recovery.
- Surgery may be attempted, and should you want me to, I will try it, but I am not sure that even stitching the eye together is possible.
- Another problem is that such injuries have been found to cause a very severe inflammation, which can involve your good eye and cause blindness in the good eye.
- The only certain method to prevent this is by removal of your injured eye as soon as possible, but no later than within 2 weeks.
- Again, remember that this eye probably won't function anyway.

Patient's likely choice: enucleation

"Noncoaching"

- You have a very serious injury.
- I can perform reconstructive surgery (or refer you to a colleague for it). Based on the best available data, this surgery has an estimated 50% chance to improve your vision, and even an unsuccessful surgery reduces the otherwise real risk that your eye will start shrinking in the future.
- You also have to know that unless your injured eye is removed now, there is a possibility of your good eye later developing a potentially blinding inflammation.
- The chance of this complication is no more than 1/1,500.
- With early recognition – and I will describe to you the symptoms – and proper treatment, however, your good eye has a better than 50% chance of maintaining reading vision.

Patient's likely choice: reconstruction

Fig. 1.4.3 The "coaching" and "noncoaching" versions of counseling. For further details see Chap. 1.8. Only a condensed version of each counseling option is provided here as an illustration

1.4.6 Giving Up the Fight for the Eye

The surgical interventions may cause too much pain and inconvenience[7], the medications may cause secondary complications (cushingoid face after systemic corticosteroid therapy), the therapy may be very costly, and the visual gain may appear to be minimal. The surgeon should encourage the patient to not give up the fight while there is reasonable hope to improve, however small that improvement may be.[8] Conversely, he must understand and accept if the patient eventually cannot bear it anymore and wants to discontinue treatment.

Cave

According to Murphy's law, any future disaster will strike the healthy fellow eye. Every effort should be made to save as much vision in the injured eye as possible, even if this eye will be no more than a "spare tire".[9] This reconstruction is time-dependent: when the fellow eye loses vision years later, it will be too late to improve on the injured eye's condition.

7 Inconvenience is much more than suffering from the actual injury, raising crucial quality of life questions. For instance, hospitalization, however brief, can prevent someone from being able to feed his animals, whether they are pets or means of livelihood. Even if this may appear as a mundane issue to the ophthalmologist who is fighting for vision, this is not mundane but crucially important to the patient.

8 Those who have 20/20 vision in both eyes may have difficulty understanding why an improvement from hand motion to 5/200 means a huge difference to the patient.

9 As have many other ocular traumatologists, the authors treated several patients in whom that minimal vision, saved in the severely injured eye years earlier through persistent reconstruction efforts against poor odds, became *the* vision when the fellow eye became blind.

DO:

- make a concerted effort to truly understand what it means to suffer a sight-threatening eye injury
- learn basic psychology to be able to "decode" the patient's metacommunication and apply this knowledge when communicating with the patient
- encourage the patient to take every reasonable measure to improve the eye's condition and not give up while there is still hope
- treat the injured patient, not a traumatized eye or a damaged tissue

DON'T:

- hurry the communication; this is not time wasted, even if occasionally more time is spent on explanation than on treatment
- let your pessimism show even if you consider the situation rather discouraging; even seemingly insignificant signs, such as a drooped mouth, can lead to major anxiety, and convey to the patient that he has no hope since his physician has none
- underestimate the power of empathy and effective communication: the patient will be grateful when he sees the effort you have put into trying to improve the injured eye's condition
- force a preconceived treatment option on the patient by "coaching," but instead examine all available treatment options, even if this includes referral of the patient to another specialist

Summary

Counseling is as important a part of treatment as surgery. Making the patient a partner in the management process is beneficial to everyone involved. Learning how counseling can be conducted effectively is not easy, but the "return on the investment" far outweighs the difficulties.

1.5 From the Other Side: the Patient's* Viewpoint

Gábor Kocsis

*This chapter was written by a patient who sustained a very serious eye injury. It is an "eye opener" even for an experienced ocular traumatologist to be confronted with the description of the entire management process as seen from the other side.

I am 41 years old, 180 cm tall, and I weigh 100 kg[1]. I love sports and the outdoors, and work out with my friends every week, even playing some mild contact sports occasionally.

This is what we had on our mind on that day, 3 May 2005. We had just finished our warm-up and I leaned forward to adjust my clothing as my friend, who was standing next to me, raised his hand. His finger somehow hit my left eye, I felt sudden pain and my vision was gone. My lid immediately became swollen and I could not open my eye.

My friends, visibly scared, quickly took me to the county hospital. Here the chief of ophthalmology told me that I needed surgery instantly to save my eyeball. I did not even have time to truly realize what was happening to me as I was taken for emergency surgery, which lasted several hours. When I woke up I had no idea about my eye's condition, but I was somehow hopeful that all was well and one day I would be able to see again.

The next day, my ophthalmologist told me that the operation was successful but that I needed further surgery or surgeries. These surgeries would require special equipment, which this hospital could not offer. He promised to find for me an ophthalmologist who specialized in ocular trauma and who would hopefully be able to help me.

This promise did give me some encouragement initially, but with time I was getting more and more desperate. I had absolutely no vision in my eye, and although I had no pain, it slowly started to sink in that I was going to

1 6 feet, 220 lbs

lose my eye. It was getting increasingly difficult to sleep at night, I just kept on rolling in bed, thinking about what the future was going to bring.

I understood that my ophthalmologist did everything he could to keep my eyeball alive, but the pressure in the eye was falling and the vision was not coming back. I had been a healthy young man, with so many plans for my life – and this was all gone forever in a split of a second. I became a patient, a sick man, who was at the mercy of the disease and the physicians. It was impossible for me to comprehend and accept this.

After a few weeks, I was finally given some good news. My hometown ophthalmologist was able to reach a specialist who split his work between two countries and was thus not always available. The specialist agreed to immediately see me. As I said thank you and good-bye to my physician, he encouraged me not to lose hope and to believe in miracles and miracle doctors. To this day, I remember his words.

I was taken to a hospital in another city. The specialist examined my eye and told me that he was going to be honest and straightforward with me. The eye's condition was very severe and required immediate surgery, he said, and he could not promise anything except that he would do everything he could to help. His words were truly shocking to me; up until then, I had not truly realized how serious the situation was. All I could think about was how my life was going to change. "What will happen to me?" I kept thinking. How can I keep on living under such conditions? Will I be able to continue my work? Will I be able to earn enough money to support my family? Can I play with my children? Can I ever go back to playing sports again?

I was hundreds of kilometers from family and friends, with the phone as the only way of communicating with them. It was my wife who had kept the hope alive so that I did not give up but rather continue fighting for my eye. I needed all her encouragement, because what followed was a series of tests and operations, and a lot of inconvenience.

During the next year I underwent no less than five surgeries; the injured eye's overall condition has improved, but I am increasingly overwhelmed by what's happening to me. My blood pressure is now high and I have to take medication. It is difficult to wake up in the morning to face the real world. I have become mentally imbalanced, and I have to take tranquillizers so that I can sleep at night. I was able to keep my job, but between periods of work I spend a lot of time at home, recuperating. I was hopeful that going back to work would help keep my mind occupied with work-related issues. Thanks to my co-workers, this indeed helps a little, but my anxiety has only subsided, never disappeared. It is difficult for me to accept what has happened to me. I often fight myself over it, even though I know I have to accept it. I, who had spent so much time with my family building our home, gardening, cooking, now cannot find my place in society. Nothing can keep my mind occupied enough. I am impatient with those who are close to me. I gave up sports and the outdoors, which has further reduced my spirits. I am afraid that any physical strain will make my condition worse, even though I was informed that this is not the case. Now all I want is to live a simple, uneventful life.

I am a religious person, and I often turn to God to guide me, to give my sight back, and to allow me to live in peace with myself. I know that the healing process takes a long time, and I appreciate the honesty coming from my eye trauma specialist. I know that I still may have several surgeries ahead of me, and I know that the outcome is uncertain. I may have some vision left when this is all over, or I may lose not only my vision but also my eyeball. I am grateful for the treatment I have been given, but I wish that my country had not a single – but several – specialists available at any time to intervene without delay if somebody were to have an injury like mine.

It was difficult for me to put my thoughts on paper, as this forced my mind to again focus on what has happened to me. But I do hope that those who read my story will benefit from it.[2]

2 The patient suffered a posterior scleral rupture with extensive tissue extrusion, total vitreous hemorrhage, and retinal incarceration; his initial vision was NLP. The eye's comprehensive reconstruction was delayed because the only surgeon who agreed to attempt secondary reconstruction was unavailable for almost 3 weeks. When the eye finally underwent vitrectomy and chorioretinectomy, PVR was already present. Several reoperations were performed, the eye is prephthysical, and the recurring PVR-retinal detachment keeps pushing the silicone oil against the cornea, causing zonular opacity. Visual acuity improved to CF, and additional surgeries are planned as needed.

1.6 Myths and Truths in Ocular Traumatology*

Ferenc Kuhn and Dante Pieramici

*In this chapter, we provide a brief list of selected dogmas and their rebuttals. All physicians employ a few dogmas in their daily practice because this is what they were taught and may not have had the opportunity to challenge them. Patients also have beliefs that originate in the media, or come from the parents or the next-door neighbor.

The interest of this book's author in ocular traumatology was established on his very first day of residency. A young man with a fresh IOFB presented to the emergency service. The object entered the eye through the sclera and, causing neither lens damage nor vitreous hemorrhage, came to rest on the retinal surface. The visual acuity remained 20/20.

By tradition, decisions in such "challenging cases" were always made by the department chairman. He determined that in this case the IOFB required so urgent a removal that surgery could not be delayed for general anesthesia to become available. All ophthalmologists at the department were present in the OR, and collectively held their breath, as the chairman manipulated the EEM giant "head" – a sphere larger than the patient's head (Fig. 1.6.1). Its conical tip was moved closer to the eye until contact, then the chairman stepped on the pedal, activating the electromagnetic field. When the IOFB presented at the wound a few seconds later, ophthalmologists in the OR sighed with relief – it was only the patient who screamed "I lost my vision!".

This author assumed that a vitreous hemorrhage had occurred, which in those previtrectomy days[1] was often fatal. Indeed, this eye became blind, yet no ophthalmologist raised doubts regarding the validity of the chosen treatment method.

1 At the time, vitrectomy was rarely used in trauma surgery anywhere, and it was unavailable in the particular country.

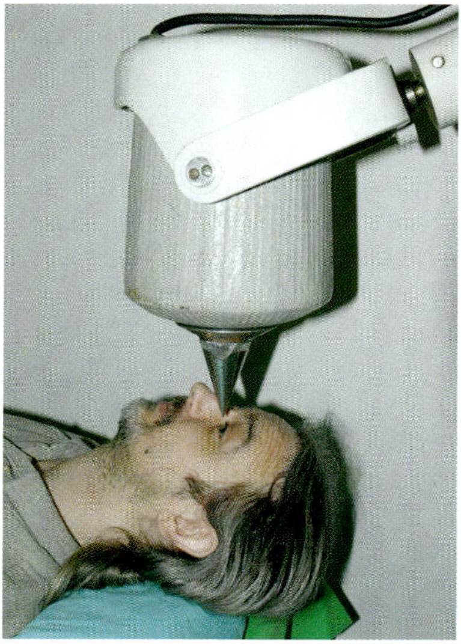

Fig. 1.6.1 The external (electro-) magnet (EEM) in use. The EEM weighs more than a ton; its working end, a cylinder with a conical attachment, is much larger than the patient's head. The magnet's working end, which contains the magnetic pole, must be lowered so that the tip of the cone actually touches the eye. It is easy to understand that the conscious patient's anxiety reaches new highs when the device is brought down onto the eye. (Photograph courtesy of G.Takács, Pécs, Hungary)

After a similar case a few weeks later, the author gathered all his courage and asked the chairman, in the privacy of his office: "Why are we pleased when the patient is not?" The short reply "*How dare you challenge what we have been doing for a hundred years!*" was one of the *myth*s of the day: an IOFB must be removed from the eye, regardless of the risk of severe (often irreparable) iatrogenic complications. The dogma went like this: Even if IOFB removal poses a higher risk of vision loss than no intervention, the patient cannot leave an ophthalmology department with a retained object in his eye.[2]

2 True, it is extremely rare that a fresh IOFB is not removed today – but this is an entirely different proposition in the era of vitreous surgery (see Chap. 2.13).

Pearl

Never accept dogmas. Always try to find a rational answer to the "Why?" question.

Such myths have been driving medicine for many centuries. Most of them have been eliminated/denied/corrected over the years, but some still linger, often blindsiding treatment decisions. Many of these myths come from inertia: "You should do this or avoid that because that's how it has always been done." Such myths are especially prevalent in trauma management: no prospective, randomized, double-masked trials are available to give us scientifically solid guidance. Nevertheless, these myths should be confronted with *truths*, which should be based on utilizing the best available scientific knowledge. Such knowledge comes from a careful analysis of published case reports or series, personal experience, and common sense. Challenging these myths[3] must be encouraged: always answering the "Why?" question[4] is the most important source of improving on current routine.

Table 1.6.1 provides a summary of myths (and truths) from the patients' side. These myths are generally addressed during counseling. For the surgeon, it is important not only to base his own decisions on reason, rather than emotion, but to also help the patient make the same transition.

Myths, as seen above, are not unique to patients; Table 1.6.2 shows those that originate from health care providers.

3 You can often call them axioms or dogmas.

4 e.g., Why medications and not surgery? Why surgery 10 days later and not now? Why phacoemulsification and not lensectomy? Why monomanual and not bimanual surgery? Why segmentation and not delamination?

Table 1.6.1 Myths and truths concerning the patient

Myth	Truth
The patient's satisfaction after an injury is determined by the outcome	The patient's expectation differs from that of the surgeon; the patient tends to compare the outcome with what vision in that eye used to be, while the surgeon bases it on personal experience and literature data.[1] It is during counseling that the surgeon should try to inform the patient about the prognosis. After proper counseling, the following equation should characterize the patient's anticipation: expectation = hope – reality
Loss of vision in one eye means that the fellow eye is "overused," strained	The workload of one eye is independent of that of the fellow eye. No restriction should be placed on the use of the remaining eye, but greater attention should be paid to protecting it from injury
There is no logic in trying to salvage an eye if the chance of visual improvement is small (e.g., from LP to HM)	While the decision whether to seek reconstruction or give up on the eye is the patient's, the ophthalmologist should encourage reconstruction (see Chap. 1.4), even if the chance of improvement is small. Should vision be lost in the fellow eye in the future, it may be too late to reconsider surgery in the injured eye
Physical activity should be severely restricted if one eye suffered serious visual loss due to injury or disease	Retinal detachment will not be caused by strain (e.g., jogging, lifting weights). Valsalva maneuver, however, may theoretically cause decreased oxygen supply to the eye or lead to necrotic peripheral retinal holes that can lead to retinal detachment in the presence of vitreoretinal traction or to macular detachment in eyes with optic pit. Valsalva maneuvers should be discouraged[2] as should sports with direct or indirect contact (e.g., boxing, judo, parachuting)

[1] In other words, the patient takes a personal approach, the ophthalmologist a statistical approach.

[2] The authors ask their patients to keep on breathing while exercising (akin to some tennis players who audibly exhale with each shot).

Table 1.6.1 *(continued)* Myths and truths concerning the patient

Myth	Truth
If an air bag deploys during an MVC, the risk of severe eye injury increases, justifying deactivation	Even if air bags occasionally cause serious ocular trauma,[3] the risk of eye injury is 2.5 times higher if there is no air bag deployment during an MVC (see Chap. 1.7)

Table 1.6.2 Myths and truths concerning the ophthalmologist

Myth	Truth
Ocular trauma experts understand each other even if they do not use the BETT system	Experience is no substitute for using standardized, unambiguous terms to describe an injury. "Blunt trauma", for instance, remains a meaningless, uninterpretable term if it is unclear whether a rupture or a contusion has occurred
The preoperative evaluation should strive for identifying every tissue pathology so that the surgeon is able to fully prepare for all contingencies	Not only is it impossible to preoperatively confirm the presence/absence of each tissue pathology, it is often dangerous: tissue prolapse or even ECH can result. The evaluation is best restricted to the establishment of those factors that are crucial in planning surgery,[4] and leave the additional details to be determined during the operation
Counseling is less important if the tissue damage is caused by injury since the choice of treatment is fairly straightforward	Even if those rare cases when only a single treatment option is applicable, observation is always an alternative; it is the patient's right to determine what should happen to the eye[5]
Should only minimal visual gain be expected, there is no justification for investing effort, time, and resources into reconstruction, especially if multiple surgical sessions are likely necessary	Only the patient can make such a decision, after proper (i.e., unbiased) counseling; if the anatomical normalcy is not restored, the eye is much more likely to go into phthisis and be eventually removed, which is a major psychological trauma to the patient

[3] The patient who sustained eye injury from the air bag could have died without air bag deployment.

[4] e.g., presence of an IOFB or retinal detachment. See Chap. 1.8 for further details.

[5] See Chapter 1.4 for further details.

Table 1.6.2 *(continued)* Myths and truths concerning the ophthalmologist

Myth	Truth
Because of the threat of sympathetic ophthalmia, it is advisable to remove an eye if it has no hope for functional improvement (e.g., NLP vision at presentation) as well as eyes whose injury "looks really bad"	Sympathetic ophthalmia is rare enough not to make it a decisive factor in the triaging process; the patient should be properly counseled and allowed to make the ultimate decision.[6] An eye whose vision is NLP vision but the injury is recent may significantly improve with proper treatment (see Chap. 1.8), and an eye's appearance should never justify enucleation
There is no effective weapon in our armamentarium against phthisis	Phthisis cannot be reversed but can be halted if timely scar removal or cyclodialysis treatment is performed; if the ciliary body is destroyed, implantation of a permanent keratoprosthesis or complete pressure-filling of the eye with silicone oil may help (see Chap. 1.8)
Even if inexperienced, the surgeon should attempt surgical reconstruction of an injured eye: if a problem that is beyond his capabilities is encountered, he can simply stop surgery and refer the patient at that point	Unless the surgeon is convinced that he is prepared to deal with all major pathologies that may have occurred, it is usually advisable to refer the patient for comprehensive reconstruction elsewhere instead of attempting half solutions or making the eye's condition worse
Follow the advice of your teachers; their longer experience make them right	Your teachers probably indeed have much more experience, but this does not automatically mean that they are right in every case; challenging their recommendations and waging a healthy debate can only improve the treatment plan

[6] The editor has yet to see a single patient who chose enucleation of a freshly injured eye if eye preservation is also offered as an option – even if the eye is never expected to regain any function (see Chap. 1.4).

Table 1.6.2 *(continued)* Myths and truths concerning the ophthalmologist

Myth	Truth
Patients with certain conditions (such as a traumatic macular hole or EMP) should not be operated on unless visual acuity drops to a predetermined certain level (e.g., 20/40)	There is no justification for the ophthalmologist to have a paternalistic attitude and determine for the patient what his visual needs are; instead of a predetermined cut-off visual value (which, incidentally, has no scientific basis anyway), the indication is up to the patient, based on proper counseling
Use of an "antidote" is recommended when irrigating for a chemical injury: i.e., use an acid if the agent was an alkali	Dilution of the agent is the goal; this is much more effective and less risky than balancing two agents against each other;[7] certain fluids, however, are more effective than water (see Chap. 3.1)
Even if surgery is urgent, it should be delayed until general anesthesia becomes available	If an emergency presents,[8] other forms of anesthesia, even if they involve some compromise regarding the operation, may be preferred to deferral (see Chap. 1.8)
Lacerations involving the upper canalicular system need not be repaired since the upper canaliculus has an insignificant role in tear transport	In some people the upper canalicular system is more important in tear transport than the lower one; since this cannot be determined before/during reconstruction, both lid's canaliculus must be repaired
Patching a corneal erosion results in faster healing	Although patching may be preferred by the patient, it can extend the healing process by causing corneal temperature elevation
Bilateral patching of the patient with a monocular open globe injury reduces ocular motility and thus the risk of further injury	In a cooperative patient, unilateral shielding is sufficient to prevent further tissue extrusion and ECH; uncooperative patients should be restrained or sedated; bilateral patching can be counterproductive by increasing anxiety even though this can indeed facilitate retinal reattachment

[7] Remember, both agents are harmful if applied alone.

[8] e.g., an ECH can be prevented by wound closure under topical/peribulbar anesthesia.

Table 1.6.2 *(continued)* Myths and truths concerning the ophthalmologist

Myth	Truth
A breached lens capsule is synonymous with cataract formation	Even if an intralenticular FB is present or the lens has been traversed, the lens opacity may remain localized and stationary;[9] in addition, primary lens removal has side effects and potential risks, which should be carefully weighed before lens removal is performed (see Chap. 2.7)
If the vitreous hemorrhage is organized and the presence of retinal detachment cannot be ruled out, the surgeon should proceed in a "horizontal", layer-peeling fashion to avoid iatrogenic retinal injury	The risk of extensive retinal injury is much greater with "horizontal" sweeping; "vertical digging" on the nasal side may indeed create a small retinectomy, but once the retina is identified, progression is easier, and the risk of additional retinal damage is much smaller (see Chap. 2.12)
Blind cryopexy over a Zone III injury helps prevent retinal detachment	Blind cryopexy implies that the surgeon is unable to visualize the pathology and thus control probe placement[10] or freezing time. This in turn means that the intervention is not only ineffective but outright dangerous since the increased inflammation involves a higher PVR risk
To prevent retinal detachment, all posterior retinal breaks should be treated with laser	If the vitreous has been completely removed from the edges of the break and in its vicinity,[11] the RPE is healthy, and there is no posterior staphyloma, detachment from a posterior retinal break is extremely unlikely. Conversely, anterior breaks require (laser) treatment as it is impossible to completely remove the vitreous at the base

[9] The younger the patient, though, the more likely that cataract will not only develop but do so rapidly.

[10] Thecryopexy spots should be placed over healthy retina (i.e., *not* over the break itself) and completely surround the break (see Chap. 2.9).

[11] Complete prior vitreous removal is mandatory if an intentional break is created, e.g., for the removal of subretinal pathology.

Table 1.6.2 *(continued)* Myths and truths concerning the ophthalmologist

Myth	Truth
The advent of vitrectomy did not improve the prognosis of eyes with serious trauma	An eye has a much higher chance of recovering vision today than in the previtrectomy era – provided that the posterior retina and the optic nerve had not been destroyed at the time of injury
If the vitreous hemorrhage is caused by contusion, it is safe to observe the patient and consider vitrectomy after 3 months	The "3 months" is an unscientific, artificial waiting period; retinal detachment can occur early; therefore, either surgery should be considered sooner than 3 months if the hemorrhage does not rapidly resolve. Following the case with serial ultrasonography to detect vitreous organization may not be feasible. Vitrectomy achieves early visual rehabilitation and allows prevention of secondary complications (see Chap. 2.9)
Rupture has a better prognosis than contusion since the risk of subfoveal choroidal rupture is smaller	It is true that subfoveal choroidal rupture is much less common in ruptures than in contusions, but a ruptured eye still has a much higher risk of losing vision than a contused eye
Orbital FBs should be removed to prevent secondary complications	Removal of deep FBs involves significant risk; unless they do cause secondary complications (i.e., infection, compression of the optic nerve), they should be left in situ
Orbital floor fractures invariably require surgical repair and this should be done as soon as possible	Many orbital floor fractures do not result in significant enophthalmos or diplopia and thus do not require surgical repair; early repair of an orbital fracture in the presence of associated intraocular injury (i.e., a posterior scleral wound) may result in additional iatrogenic trauma and should be deferred

1.7 Clinical Epidemiology, Prevention, and Rehabilitation

Ferenc Kuhn

1.7.1 Introduction

No matter how effective the treatment of an eye injury proves to be, prevention is always preferred. Effective prevention, in turn, must be based on data collected and analyzed in a scientifically rigorous manner. Ideally, such data are population-based, instead of representing a survey of patients presenting to a single institution over a limited period of time (snapshot).[1] An overview of different study characteristics is given in Table 1.7.1.

Any data collection system has to answer at least the most elementary questions in epidemiology: who; when; where; and how. It is immensely useful if clinical data are included so that the short- and long-term significance of the injury are also known.

Pitfall

Designing a good survey questionnaire is not an easy task. Asking for too little information reduces usefulness; asking for too much results in a low response rate with low scientific credibility.

Rehabilitation of the eye trauma victim is similar to the process employed for those losing sight from other etiologies in many respects, but in others

1 This does not imply that snapshots do not yield useful information; their value, however, is more circumscribed than that of an ongoing surveillance system whose catch area and duration are greater.

Table 1.7.1 Analysis of recent epidemiological studies

Country	Study design and duration, subjects	Most important findings	Reference
India	Retrospective; population-based; three rural-areas-based; epidemiological + clinical; all injury types included; 5-year survey	Workplace injuries were the most common; vegetable matter the most frequent cause	[37]
Australia	Retrospective; population-based; single-institution-based; epidemiological + clinical; all injury types included; 8-year survey	Overall injury incidence and alcohol use significant cause among Aboriginals; initial visual acuity correlates with final vision	[71]
USA	Retrospective; national database reviewed; only gun-related injuries analyzed; epidemiological; 10-year survey	The rate of gun-related eye injuries declined in the observed period; most occur at home and are unintentional; blacks are at the highest risk for ocular trauma from firearms	[51]
USA	Retrospective; single-institution-based; open-globe trauma studied; epidemiological; 3-year survey	Men are typically injured from projectiles (penetrating trauma), women from falls (rupture)	[36]

Selected publications that provide an international perspective from the last decade

Table 1.7.1 *(continued)* Analysis of recent epidemiological studies

Country	Study design and duration, subjects	Most important findings	Reference
India	Prospective; single-institution-based; single etiology studied; epidemiological + clinical; 1-year survey	The bottle rocket is the most devastating firework; poor initial visual acuity, open globe trauma, APD, and endophthalmitis are poor prognostic factors	[70]
India	Prospective; rural-population-based; epidemiological; history-based	4.5% of persons with monocular and 0.4% of bilateral trauma prevalence in lifetime; higher than for glaucoma, AMD, or diabetic retinopathy	[59]
Cote d'Ivoire	Prospective; single-institution-based; pediatric population studied; epidemiological + clinical; 16-month survey	Most injuries occur during unsupervised play; 55% final monocular blindness rate	[54]
Poland	Retrospective; single-institution-based; all injury types included; epidemiological + clinical; 9-year survey	The injury incidence rate did not decline during the study period; 40% of eyes lose useful vision	[46]

Selected publications that provide an international perspective from the last decade

Table 1.7.1 *(continued)* Analysis of recent epidemiological studies

Country	Study design and duration, subjects	Most important findings	Reference
Germany	Retrospective; data from two institutions compared; open globe trauma studied; epidemiological; 18-year survey	The risk of open globe trauma (i.e., rupture) in older people has been increasing; the overall rate has remained steady	[66]
Croatia	Retrospective; single-institution-based; adult population studied; epidemiological + clinical; 5-year survey	The home is the place of injury in 41%; 18% final monocular blindness rate	[30]
Nepal	Prospective; single-institution-based; all injury types included; epidemiological + clinical; 6-year survey	Delay of care is a major cause of poor outcome	[34]
Colombia	Retrospective; single-institution-based; pediatric population studied; epidemiological + clinical; 5-year survey	Only 8% of closed but 55% of open globe injuries caused severe visual impairment	[67]
France	Retrospective; single institution-based; all injury types included; epidemiological; 11-year survey	Ophthalmological emergencies should not be treated at general ERs but at ophthalmic emergency centers	[23]

Selected publications that provide an international perspective from the last decade

Table 1.7.1 *(continued)* Analysis of recent epidemiological studies

Country	Study design and duration, subjects	Most important findings	Reference
Singapore	Prospective; single institution-based; all injury types included; epidemiological; 3-month survey	Low rate of protective goggle use at the workplace	[75]
Singapore	Retrospective; nationwide; only severe trauma studied; epidemiological; 6-year survey	The rate of trauma occurrence did not decline during the study period but the rate of hospitalization did; the incidence peaks in young adults and in those over 70 years	[78]
Hungary, USA	Prospective; nationwide; only severe trauma studied; epidemiological + clinical; 15-year survey (ongoing data collection)	The spectrum of trauma varies considerably in the two countries; comparison helps highlight certain unique characteristics	[38]

Selected publications which provide an international perspective from the last decade

it is different: the person is often young; therefore vocational issues play an increased role.

1.7.2 Clinical Epidemiology

Several studies have been published on the incidence and prevalence of ocular trauma. The data vary greatly, based on study design as well as geographical and societal factors. Table 1.7.2 shows the findings from selected reports.

Table 1.7.2 Incidence and prevalence rates of eye injuries; a literature review

Finding	Country and study design	Reference
Incidence rate for eye injury: 65 for males, 38 for females	Nepal, districtwide	[34]
Incidence rate for persons hospitalized with eye injury: 8.1	Scotland; nationwide	[17]
Incidence rate for persons hospitalized with eye injury: 12.6	Singapore; nationwide	[78]
Incidence rate for persons hospitalized with eye injury: 13.2	USA; nationwide	[35]
Incidence rate for persons hospitalized with eye injury: 15.2	Sweden; countywide	[6]
Incidence rate for persons hospitalized with eye injury: 23.9	Croatia, countywide	[30]
Cumulative lifetime prevalence: 860	Nepal; nationwide	[7]
Cumulative lifetime prevalence: 14,400	USA; citywide	[32]
Incidence of "penetrating" eye injuries: 3.6	Australia; hospital-based	[21]
Incidence rate of eye injuries requiring hospitalization: 15.2	Australia; hospital-based	[21]
Incidence rate of open globe injuries: 3	Germany; hospital-based	[66]
Incidence rate of "perforating" eye injuries: 3.3	Sweden; hospital-based	[10]
Incidence rate of monocular blindness caused by injuries: 4.1	Croatia, countywide	[30]

Incidence rates are per 100,000 population and per year unless otherwise indicated

Table 1.7.2 *(continued)* Incidence and prevalence rates of eye injuries; a literature review

Finding	Country and study design	Reference
Of all monocular blindness cases, 40% caused by trauma	US; population-based	[15]
Incidence rate of hospitalized cases of eye injuries: 13.2	U.S.; hospital-based	[73]
Prevalence of trauma-related bilateral blindness: 200	Nepal; interview-based	[7]
Incidence rate of eye injuries requiring medical treatment: 975	U.S; interview-based	[24]
Incidence rate of acute, hospital-treated eye injuries: 423	US; ER and hospital records	[31]
One-year cumulative incidence of blinding outcome from serious ocular trauma: 0.41	Scotland; hospital-based	[17]
Incidence rate of eye injuries among professional boxers: 17.1 per 100 matches	USA, statewide	[5]
Annual incidence rate of ER-treated eye injuries: 315	USA, nationwide	[52]
Annual incidence of ocular trauma per 100,000 employees: 537	USA, statewide	[26]

Incidence rates are per 100,000 population and per year unless otherwise indicated

1.7.2.1 The USEIR

The USEIR is the world's largest database of serious eye injuries system (http://www.useironline.org/). Headquartered in Birmingham, Alabama, it collects initial and follow-up, epidemiological, and clinical information on all types of serious injury (defined as *trauma resulting in permanent and significant structural or functional change to the eye or adnexa*). The USEIR encourages participation of individual ophthalmologists as well as institutions. Its customized software allows entering data over the Internet; the data are not incorporated into the database before undergoing multiple layers of quality checks. The data are secure: only those who entered them can access them, and no individual patient can be identified in the database. An identical database (http://www.weironline.org/) is available, free, for ophthalmologists working in any other country in the world.

While it is true that "eye injury can happen to anyone at any time," certain risk factors exist. Selected risk factors and injury occurrence characteristics are discussed below.

1.7.2.2 Age

- The majority of those injured are young adults, with an average age around 30 years [38, 48, 65, 73].
- Those sustaining a serious eye injury over the age of 60 years (see Chap. 2.16) have different etiologies (rate of fall: 23% if over 60 years, 2% if under 60 years, $p<0.001$), injury types (rate of rupture: 31% if over 60 years, 11% if under 60 years, $p<.001$), and thus prognosis (poor final vision statistically significantly more common).[2]

1.7.2.3 Gender

- The typical male:female ratio is 4:1 [11, 18, 22, 23, 25, 30, 34, 36, 38, 43, 50, 53, 56, 60].
- In the USEIR, 79% of injured persons are males (male:female ratio: 3.8:1). Figure 1.7.1 shows a detailed breakdown of age and gender in the USEIR.

1.7.2.4 Socioeconomic Status

- The lower on the societal "ladder" a person is, the higher his risk of suffering an eye injury is [24, 43].

2 The report on this study from the USEIR and supported by a grant from the EyeSight Foundation in Birmingham, Alabama, is in press.

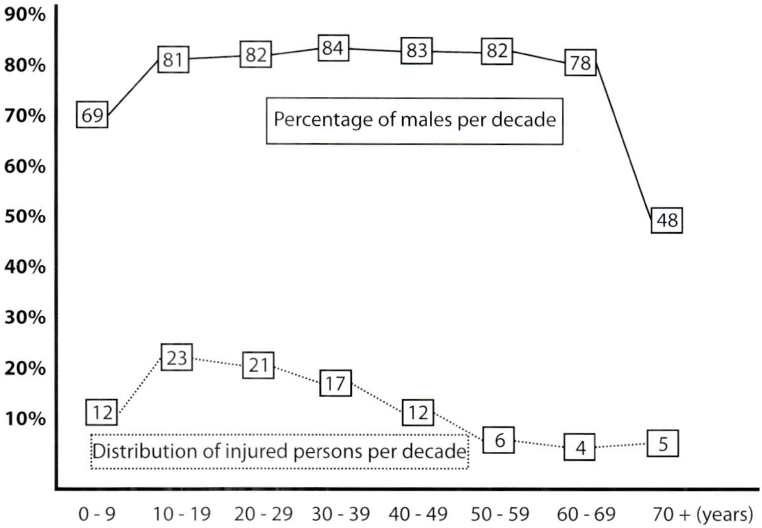

Fig. 1.7.1 Analysis of age and gender in the USEIR, based on 15,296 cases. In most age categories, a strong male preponderance is found. The lower figure in the first decade of life and the reversed figure among those over 70 years is probably due to behaviors that are less prominently different early and late in life; in the latter category it is also important to note that women live approximately 7 years longer than men.[1] The most-at-risk period is between 10 and 40 years: 61% of all injuries occur in these three decades

[1] http://www.cdc.gov/nchs/data/series/sr_02/sr02_129.pdf

- The breaking of rules/laws (e.g., traffic violations, alcohol, or drug use) or unsettled social status (e.g., unemployment) also signifies an elevated risk [24, 58].

1.7.2.5 Race

- Among those aged 25–65 years in the U.S., blacks and Hispanics have a 40–60% higher risk than whites [73].

- Race is an especially important risk factor in becoming a victim of assault: in the U.S., blacks have a risk twice as high as whites [73] and a more than twice as high risk of having visual impairment from injury [32].
- Even an activity such as driving has its racial component: per mile traveled, 13- to 19-year-old black and Hispanic male teenagers have a nearly twice as high risk of dying in an MVC than white teenagers of the same age [2].
- Race and socioeconomics have a combined effect.

1.7.2.6 Place

- The significant shift from the workplace to the home, identified first by USEIR researchers [38] in the context of a large, multicenter study, has been confirmed in several subsequent studies [30, 34, 52, 66]. In some rural areas in developing countries the workplace remains the most important site [37]. Figure 1.7.2 shows a detailed breakdown of the place of injury in the USEIR.
- The proportion of workplace injuries is relatively low (19% in the USEIR database),[3] and it shows a continuing downward trend: it was 28% prior to 1989 [77] and 12% in 2005. This reduction is due to the fewer number of workers in industry [12], the availability of proper eye-protective devices [74], and the employee-enforced laws requiring to actually wear them (see below).[4]
- The increase in the rate of injuries occurring at home is dramatic. Two societal facts appear to contribute to this development: the rising number of elderly people (in the U.S. in 2003, the average 75-year-old person

3 Nevertheless, among all nonfatal occupational injuries, ocular trauma results in the highest percentage of days missed from works on the first and second days after the injury (45 and 23%, respectively; U.S. Department of Labor, 27 March 2003, Washington).

4 In addition, the importance of public education should not be neglected. This author operated on a car mechanic who presented with an IOFB he sustained as he was working on a car in his garage. When asked whether he wore eye protection, the mechanic explained that he does wear it at the his workplace – where it is mandatory – but not when he is doing the very same work at home.

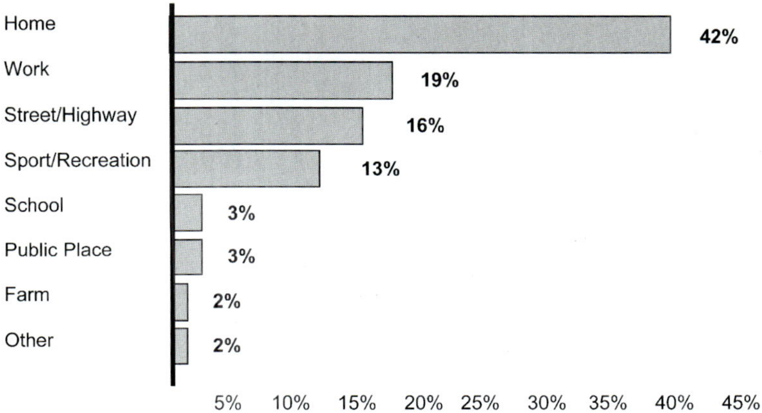

Fig. 1.7.2 The place of injury in the USEIR, based on 13,645 cases (See the text for further details.)

could still expect to live another 11.8 years[5]) and the rising popularity of the do-it-yourself movement: the use of power tools, for instance, is a well-known risk factor for eye injury.

- Street and highway as the site of injury increased from 15% in 1995 to 19% in 2005 in the USEIR. The reason is not an increase in MVCs but, sadly, violence.

1.7.2.7 Source

- What the most common object causing a serious eye injury is largely depends on the location of the study; for instance, in one report from India hypodermic needles were found to the most significant culprit [27]. The significance of the study site is also shown by the very different national scenes (U.S., Hungary, Mexico) when comparing injuries caused by pressurized bottles [39] or by the proportion of injuries inflicted by champagne bottle corks (Fig. 1.7.3).

5 http://www.cdc.gov/nchs/data/hus/hus05.pdf#027

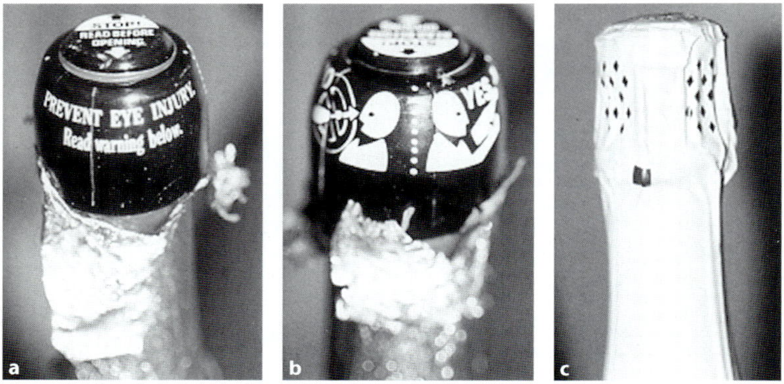

Fig. 1.7.3 Typical champagne bottles in the U.S. and Hungary. In the USEIR, 0.06% of all serious eye injuries are caused by champagne bottle corks; in the HEIR, 2.2% ($p<0.00001$). Since Hungarians do not consume significantly more champagne than Americans, the explanation is most likely found in the presence of warning labels on the bottles in the U.S. (**a,b**) and their omission on the bottles sold in Hungary (**c**). These findings highlight the efficacy of a well-designed preventive measure

- Figure 1.7.4 shows a detailed breakdown of the source of injury in the USEIR, which includes data from rural as well as urban areas.
- Various *blunt objects* remain the most frequent cause (33%). Their significance would be even higher if not for the “fall” category (5%): this injury typically happens to elderly people getting injured at home, and the culprit is usually a blunt object such as a door knob or the edge of a piece of furniture.
- Among *sharp objects*, nails represented 21%. This is explained by the widespread use of wood as construction material in the U.S. (forestry, carpentry).
- Among those who are injured as a result of a *fall*, the likelihood of a prescription glass contributing to the injury was significantly higher in the those over 65 years of age [69].

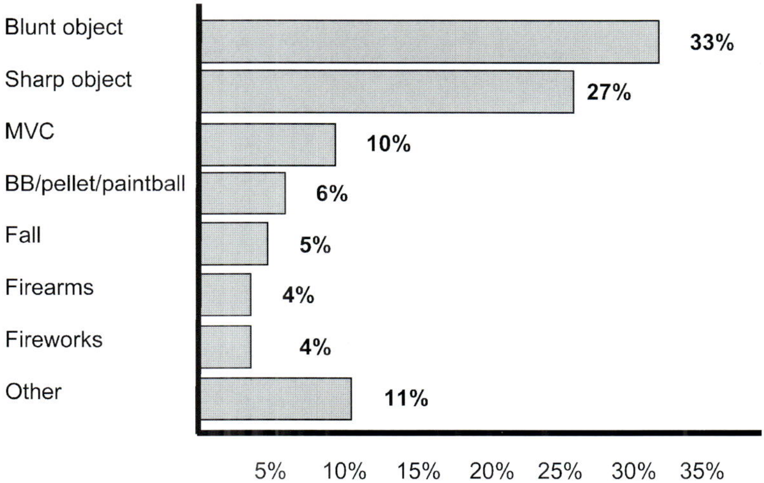

Fig. 1.7.4 The source of injury in the USEIR, based on 15,031 cases (See the text for details.)

- Although the individual's own risk is impossible to estimate,[6] it is interesting to review which types of sports cause the most number of injuries (Fig. 1.7.5). *Paintball* is an emerging menace in the non-powder-gun category [61, 72].

1.7.2.8 Intent

- Assault was the cause in 19% of injuries in the USEIR (Fig. 1.7.6); 1% was self-inflicted.

6 No data are available about the number of players or the duration of participation.

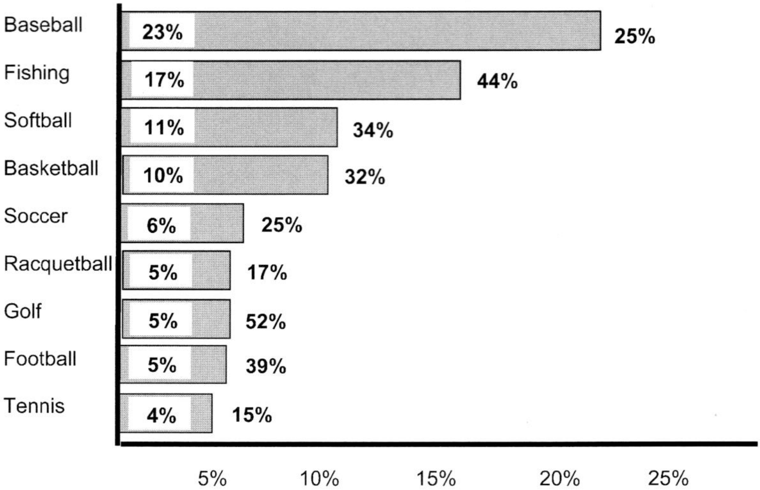

Fig. 1.7.5 Sport-related ocular trauma in the USEIR, based on 1,075 cases. The *bars* and the *numbers on the left within the bars* show the proportion of each sport among all sports injuries. The *numbers to the right of the bars* show the percentage of eyes with a final visual acuity of worse than 20/40 in each sport

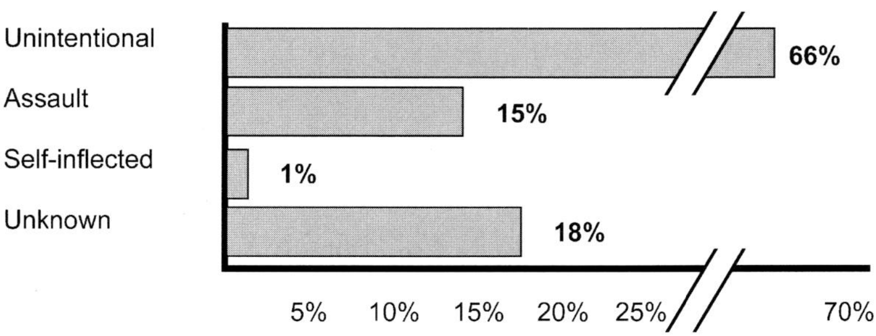

Fig. 1.7.6 The intent of injury in the USEIR, based on 12,559 cases

- Firearms were responsible for 71% of all self-inflicted ocular trauma. Surprisingly, the enucleation rate was more than three times higher (25 vs 7%) in this group than among those who were assaulted.

1.7.3 Prevention

Pearl

It is human nature to presume that although "eye injuries happen, they happen to somebody else." To be effective, it is this mindset that prevention must change.

All ophthalmologists have a responsibility to contribute to the fight for preventing eye injuries by identifying risk factors in general and risky behaviors in particular. The contribution can range from warning a single individual of the dangers in a given situation (Fig. 1.7.7) to initiating legislation against a more general threat. Using common sense in daily life is also crucial; everyone should realize, for instance, how dangerous a bungee cord is (Fig. 1.7.8).

Several published reports have identified areas amenable for the introduction of preventive measures and showed the benefits of such measures.

1.7.3.1 MVC-related Deaths and Injuries

- Although the number of drivers increased sixfold between 1925 and 1997 in the U.S., the annual death rate has declined from 18 to 1.7 per 100 million vehicle miles traveled (a 90% decrease) in the same period.[7] Several factors (e.g., better road design, improved driver education, energy-absorbing vehicle systems, the use of laminated, not heat-toughened, windshields [45]) contributed to the improvement, but it was primarily the introduction of seat belts and air bags that must be credited.

7 http://www.cdc.gov/mmwr/preview/mmwrhtml/mm4818a1.htm

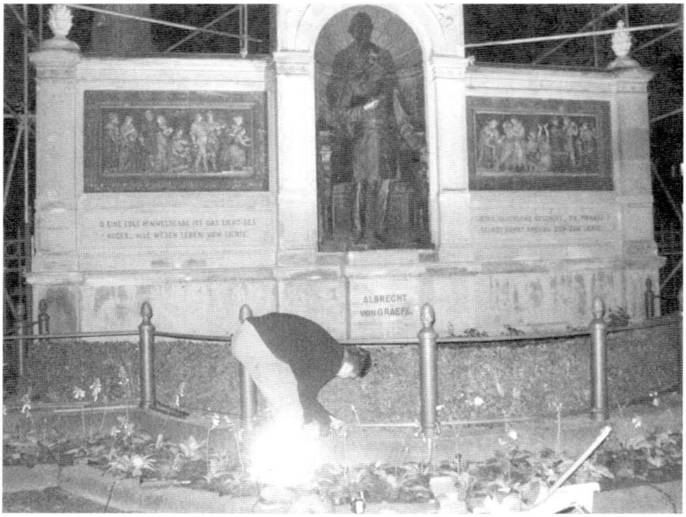

Fig. 1.7.7 Risky activity: a scene from everyday life. The author took this picture in Berlin, Germany, during a large ophthalmology conference in 2005. The worker was repairing a metallic fence: hammering, chiseling, welding, and using power tools to cut and strip. He did not wear eye protection. The sad irony of the scene is that it occurred at the memorial of Albrecht von Graefe

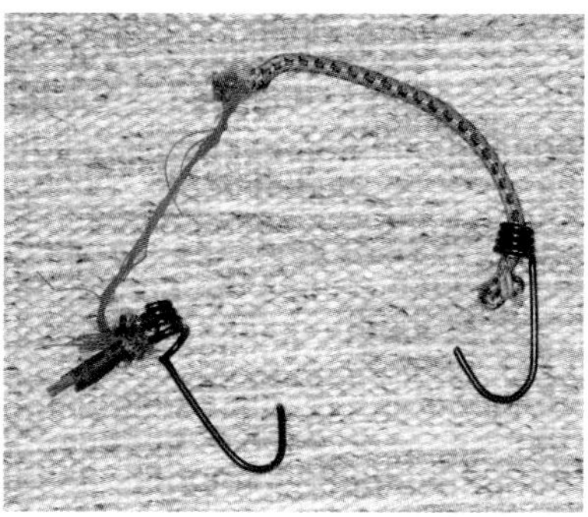

Fig. 1.7.8 A worn bungee cord. Bungee cords are very useful around the house to fasten/clamp/anchor/secure/tie/fix various objects. They can cause very severe injury, including loss of the eye, if they become loose on the opposite end from the user. The risk is compounded by the fact that the cords can also disintegrate with time; this specimen is from the author's own collection

Table 1.7.3 Rate of facial fracture among 3,731 patients injured during a motor vehicle crash. (From [68])

No restraint	Seat belt only	Air bag only	Seat belt and air bag
380 of 2295 (17%)	97 of 1147 (8%)	9 of 84 (11%)	11 of 205 (5%)
Risk reduction	53%	36%	71%

- Seat belt laws reduced the number of eye injuries by 47–65% [8, 13][8] and facial fractures by 9 percentage points [68] in the U.S., where 82% of drivers buckle up.[9] The effect of legislation is shown by the fact that the rate is significantly higher in states with primary, rather than secondary, law.[10]
- Air bags reduce the risk of sustaining an eye injury during a crash by 2.5 times [40].
- Although air bags may themselves be a source of ocular trauma, this risk is minimal, especially when compared with the risk of death in the crash [41, 63].
- Air bags are supposed to *supplement*, not substitute, seat belt use (Table 1.7.3).
- The increase in the number of air bags per vehicle and the decrease of air bag deployment force are expected to further reduce the injury risk.
- In the USEIR, the rate of MVC-related serious eye injuries decreased from 12% in 1995 to 8% in 2005.

8 Seat belts saved an estimated 12,000 lives in the U.S. in 2001; two-thirds of those killed did not wear them (http://www.nhtsa.dot.gov/people/injury/airbags/buasbteens03).

9 http://www.cdc.gov/mmwr/preview/mmwrhtml/mm4818a1.htm

10 A *primary* seat belt law allows police to stop a vehicle when an unbelted driver/passenger is seen; a *secondary* seat belt law means that another infraction must also have occurred.

1.7.3.2 Sports-related Ocular Trauma[11]

- Ice hockey is a prototype success story. Among Canadian youth players, 283 eye injuries were seen in the 1974–1975 season; after face visors were mandated, the number of eye injuries dropped by 68%, and not a single eye was injured if the player wore full-face protection [62].
- Baseball is a major source (Fig. 1.7.5) in the U.S. In one study, a 28% reduction was achieved with a protective device [16].
- Racquetball and squash. The proportion of these games among all sport-related injury cases was reduced from 73% in 1982 to 38% in 1987 as proper protective devices[12] were introduced [19].
- Paintball, an increasingly popular sport, represents a very significant risk of causing permanent visual loss.[13] Proper eye protection is very efficient in preventing it–if the device is actually worn [44].
- Golf is not a common cause of eye injury, but if either the club or, more often, the ball does cause injury, it is very serious, resulting in a 40% enucleation rate [9, 28, 55, 76].

1.7.3.3 War-related Trauma

Although the rate of eye injuries among all war-related trauma has steadily increased since the mid-19th century (1.76% in the Crimean War [1854–1856], 6.8% in the Lebanon War [1982], 16% in Iraq [2004]) [3, 47], not a single eye injury occurred among Israeli Defense Forces soldiers wearing proper goggles (Fig. 1.7.9).

11 In 2000, over 42,000 persons were injured in the U.S. during sports; 72% of these persons were younger 25 years (Sports and recreational injuries, U.S. Consumer Product Safety Commission, 2000). In general, females had a twice as high risk as males to sustain a sports injury.

12 e.g., CRS 300 in Canada

13 Its rate among all injuries in the USEIR was 0.5% in 2000, increasing to 1.8% in 2005.

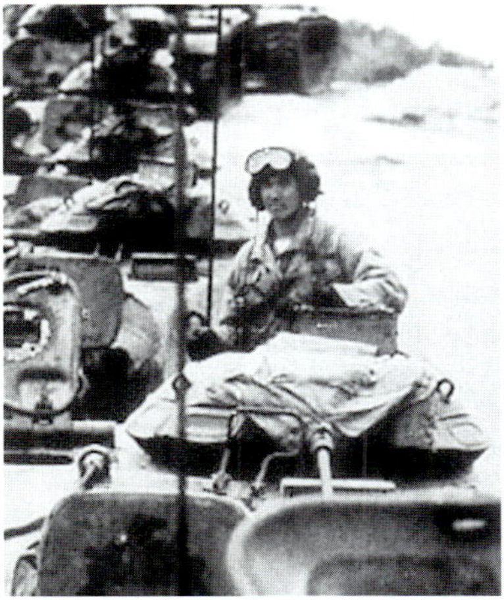

Fig. 1.7.9 Eye protection is effective only if it is actually worn. This photo shows a soldier from the Israeli Defense Forces, who was issued a proper goggle to protect him from eye injury; he obviously is not reducing his risk of ocular trauma (Courtesy of M. Belkin, Tel Aviv, Israel)

1.7.3.4 Fireworks-related Ocular Trauma

In the USEIR database, 4% of cases are caused by fireworks, and 80% of these result from bottle rockets [42]. States that prohibit private fireworks[14] have a 50-fold reduction in the rate of injuries as compared to states without such regulation [4]. Fireworks can result in very severe injury (see Fig. 2.12.1).

1.7.3.5 Hammering

In the USEIR database, 4% of all serious trauma are sustained while hammering; in the HEIR, 9% [38]. This statistically significant difference is most probably due to increased public awareness in the U.S., emphasizing the danger of this activity and the benefits of protective devices [29].

14 Public displays are still allowed.

1.7.3.6 Protective Eyewear

The ideal device[15] is:

- Tailored to a specific purpose (i.e., different designs are necessary for soccer and for racquetball)
- Resistant against major impact (made of 3- or even 4-mm polycarbonate) as well as against scratching
- Held by a proper frame that does not break or let go
- Offering frontal as well as side protection without interfering with the field of view
- Designed to prevent fogging
- Readily available (e.g., prominently displayed at the checkout counter in home-improvement stores)
- Affordable

Controversial

The answer as to whether a *regular prescription glass* contributes to the injury risk since it can shatter [33] or offers at least some protection [49], is not straightforward. The finding that only 27,152 people were estimated to be treated at the ER in the U.S. due to such injury in a 2-year period[16], and that only 3.8% of these persons had to be admitted [69], appears to support the protective theory.

1.7.4 Rehabilitation

If complete restoration of the injured eye's visual functions cannot be achieved, rehabilitation becomes necessary so that the person can utilize his remaining vision to the fullest extent possible. If vision cannot be im-

15 The SG-1 (Wiley X Eyewar, Livermore, Calif.), a versatile, multifunctional, antiballistic eyewear issued for personnel in the U.S. military, satisfies most criteria listed here.

16 An estimated 96 million people in the U.S. wear prescription glasses.

proved, the person needs rehabilitation (e.g., vocational training, psychological support; see below).

Pearl

Therapy and some form of rehabilitation ideally occur simultaneously; use of the OTS allows the ophthalmologist to make a reasonable prediction regarding the long-term visual prognosis of the injured eye(s), and initiate rehabilitation early. This rehabilitation ranges from the ophthalmologist encouraging positive patient attitude to "building" and utilizing a new fovea [20].

Impairment of vision is typically measured in distance visual acuity (Table 1.7.4), even if reading ability better reflects the impairment's impact on quality of life [64]. While acuity remains the most readily measured function and is the basis for classification (Table 1.7.5), other tests measure reading speed [57] or assess function related to vision (AFREV) by incorporating visual field loss as well as the ability to perform everyday tasks [1]. While society has an official "translation" for calculating what degree of vision loss corresponds to what degree of impairment to the whole person (Table 1.7.6), this certainly varies with individual needs.

If an eye injury is vision-threatening, the person faces several short- and long-term challenges:

- Significant initial anxiety
- Psychological adaptation to a new, unfavorable reality[17]
- Loss of, or major changes in, career opportunities
- The potential of severe financial loss[18]
- The need to accept an altered lifestyle

---

17 With a chronic problem such as glaucoma or age-related macular degeneration, the person has a much longer period of time to prepare himself for life with visual impairment; this is significantly less difficult than facing the implications of an *acute* ("out of the blue") visual loss.

18 Cost of treatment itself and/or the loss of a well-paying job.

Table 1.7.4 Visual acuity and the corresponding central vision loss in percentage

Visual acuity				Loss of central vision
Decimal	Metric 6	Metric 4	USA	(%)
1.33	6/5	4/3	20/15	0
1.0	6/6	4/4	20/20	0
0.8	6/7.5	4/5	20/25	5
0.6	6/10	4/6	20/30	10
0.5	6/12	4/8	20/40	15
0.4	6/20	4/10	20/50	25
0.3	6/22	4/12	20/60	35
0.28	6/24	4/14	20/70	40
0.25	6/24	4/16	20/80	45
0.2	6/30	4/20	20/100	50
0.15	6/38	4/25	20/125	60
0.13	6/50	4/30	20/150	70
0.1	6/60	4/40	20/200	80
0.07	6/90	4/60	20/300	85
0.05	6/120	4/80	20/400	90
0.02	6/240	4/160	20/800	95

Table 1.7.5 Classification of visual performance, distal and near; aids of vision enhancement and substitution

Vision	Visual acuity level	Person's visual performance	Reading distance	Aids
Normal	20/12–20/25	Full	≥33 cm (binocular)	None/prescription glasses

Vision substitution means that tactile (e.g., Braille) or audible (e.g., computer-generated, audiotape) input replaces it.

Table 1.7.5 *(continued)* Classification of visual performance, distal and near; aids of vision enhancement and substitution

Vision	Visual acuity level	Person's visual performance	Reading distance	Aids
Near normal	20/30–20/60	Almost full	33–20 cm (binocular)	Stronger prescription glass, low-powder magnifier (≤5 D)
Moderately low	20/70–20/160	Very good, but educational assistance often needed	16–10 cm (binocular)	Strong (half) prescription glass (with prisms for binocularity); strong magnifier (>8 D); videomagnifier
Severely low	20/200–20/400	Reasonable good with visual aids	8–5 cm (monocular)	High-power reading lens (12–20 D); high-power magnifier (>16 D); videomagnifier
Profoundly low	20/500–20/1000	Poor and laborious	4–2 cm (monocular)	Very high-power reading lens (24–48 D); very high-power magnifier (>28 D); videomagnifier; vision substitution

Table 1.7.5 *(continued)* Classification of visual performance, distal and near; aids of vision enhancement and substitution

Vision	Visual acuity level	Person's visual performance	Reading distance	Aids
Near blindness	20/1250–20/2500	Very poor, serves as an adjunct to nonvisual input/skills	–	Videomagnifier; vision substitution
Blindness[1]	NLP	–	–	Videomagnifier; vision substitution

Vision substitution means that tactile (e.g., Braille) or audible (e.g., computer-generated, audiotape) input replaces it (*continued*)

Table 1.7.6 Loss of vision and its implication to the impairment of the whole person

Impairment of visual system (%)	Impairment of whole person (%)
25 (loss of vision in one eye)	24
50	47
75	71
100 (loss of vision in both eyes)	85

[1] In the true sense of the word, "blindness" means NLP, although terms such as "legal blindness" – applied for legal, rather than medical, purposes – are still used in everyday practice.

- An increased risk of further injury [14][19]

19 The risk of sustaining another injury (e.g., falling down the stairs) is greater if the person's vision is poor, especially if this occurred only recently; a vicious circle can also ensue since the eye can be reinjured during a fall.

- An impaired quality of life[20]
- Occasionally permanent physical disfigurement

To minimize the effects of these challenges, rehabilitation must aim at both maximizing the eye's remaining potential (low vision specialist[21]) and additional experts [20] such as psychologists, vocational advisers, occupational therapists, nurses, educators, mobility therapists, social workers. The ophthalmologist should be the initiator for the entire process and remain available for advice and leadership.[22] A file on such patients should be kept so that if a new therapeutic option becomes available, the patient can be contacted.[23]

---

20 e.g., a diabetic patient may become unable to accurately draw and inject insulin without somebody's help

21 e.g., to develop and utilize to the maximum the function of a new macula; to use movement, rather than binocular parallax for stereopsis

22 Throughout the entire treatment/rehabilitation process, the ophthalmologist must emphasize the positives, not the negatives, to the patient. Focusing on what can be achieved, rather than on what was lost, improves patient attitude, cooperation, and outcome.

23 The author is forever indebted to Donald C. Fletcher, MD, San Francisco, Calif., for his invaluable contributions. Tables 1.7.5 and 1.7.6 are based on his previous works.

DO:

- collect information on your eye injury cases, utilizing the standardized system (www.useironline.org, www.weironline.org)
- think of prevention, whether this concerns an individual case or a major societal risk factor
- consider initiating proper rehabilitation as soon as it becomes clear that vision cannot be restored in the injured eye

DON'T:

- think that collection of epidemiological and clinical information on all your patients with serious eye injury is a waste of time: this is the basis for prevention and the improvement on current treatment approaches
- downplay the possibility of visual rehabilitation if an injured patient has poor vision; with proper techniques, the eye's functional capability can be increased substantially

Summary

Collecting epidemiological data on the occurrence of eye injuries allows identification of trends and societal risk factors. This information can then serve as the basis for designing and implementing preventive measures. Continuing data collection is necessary for the evaluation of the efficacy of the preventive measure. If the eye's functional capability remains seriously depressed despite all reasonable treatment efforts, the eye and person must be rehabilitated to utilize to the maximum the eye's remaining capabilities and help the person cope with the situation.

References

[1] Altangerel U, Spaeth G, Steinmann W (2006) Assessment of function related to vision (AFREV). Ophthal Epidemiol 13: 67–80

[2] Baker S, Braver E, Chen L, Pantula J, Massie D (1998) Motor vehicle occupant deaths among Hispanic and Black children and teenagers. Arch Pediatr Adoles Med 152: 1209–1212

[3] Belkin M, Treister G, Dotan S (1984) Eye injuries and ocular protection in the Lebanon War, 1982. Isr J Med Sci 20: 333–338

[4] Berger L, Kalishman S, Rivara F (1985) Injuries from fireworks. Pediatrics 75: 877–882

[5] Bledsoe G, Li G, Levy F (2005) Injury risk in professional boxing. South Med J 98: 994–998

[6] Blomdahl S, Norell S (1984) Perforating eye injury in the Stockholm population: an epidemiological study. Acta Ophthalmol 62: 378–390

[7] Brillant GE (1988) The epidemiology of blindness in Nepal. Report of the 1981 Nepal Blindness Survey. The SEVA Foundation, San Rafael

[8] Briner A (1976) Penetrating eye injuries associated with motor vehicle accidents. Med J Aust 1: 912–914

[9] Burnstine MA, Elner VM (1996) Golf-related ocular injuries. Am J Ophthalmol 121: 437–438

[10] Byhr E (1994) Perforating eye injuries in a western part of Sweden. Acta Ophthalmol 72: 91–97

[11] Casson R, Walker J, Newland H (2002) Four-year review of open eye injuries at the Royal Adelaide Hospital. Clin Exp Ophthalmol

[12] Catalano R, Maus M (2004) Economic antecedents of temporal variation in the incidence of ocular trauma. Ophthalmol Epidemiol 11: 279–289

[13] Cole MD, Clearkin L, Dabbs T, Smerdon D (1987) The seat belt law and after. Br J Ophthalmol 71: 436–440

[14] Coleman A, Stone K, Ewing S, Nevitt M, Cummings S, Cauley J, Ensrud K, Harris E, Hochberg M, Mangione C (2004) Higher risk of multiple falls among elderly women who lose visual acuity. Ophthalmology 111: 857–862

[15] Dana M, Tielsch J, Enger C, et al. (1990) Visual impairment in a rural Appalachian community. J Am Med Assoc 264: 2400–2405

[16] Danis R, Hu K, Nell M (2000) Acceptability of baseball face guards and reduction of oculofacial injury in receptive youth league players. Inj Prev 6: 232–234

[17] Desai P, MacEwen C, Baines P, Minassian D (1966) Incidence of cases of ocular trauma admitted to hospital and incidence of blinding outcome. Br J Ophthalmol 80: 592–596

[18] Desai P, MacEwen C, Baines P, Minassian D (1996) Epidemiology and implications of ocular trauma admitted to hospital in Scotland. J Epidemiol Community Health 50: 436–441

[19] Easterbrook M (1988) Ocular injuries in racquet sports. Int Ophthalmol Clin 28: 232–237

[20] Fletcher D, Colenbrader A (2002) Rehabilitation of patients with ocular trauma. In: Kuhn F, Pieramici D (eds) Ocular trauma: principles and practice. Thieme, New York, pp 27–32

[21] Fong L (1995) Eye injuries in Victoria, Australia. Med J Austral 162: 64–68
[22] Framme C, Roider J (1999) Epidemiology of open globe injuries. Klin Monatsbl Augenheilk 215: 287–293
[23] Girard B, Bourcier F, Agdabede I, Laroche L (2002) Activity and epidemiology in an ophthalmological emergency center. J Fr Opthalmol 701–711
[24] Glynn R, Seddon J, Berlin B (1988) The incidence of eye injuries in New England adults. Arch Ophthalmol 106: 785–789
[25] Gothwal V, Adolph S, Jalali S, Naduvilath T (1999) Demography and prognostic factors of ocular injuries in South India. Austral N Z J Ophthalmol 27: 318–325
[26] Islam S, Nambiar A, Doyle EV, AM , Biswas R, Ducatman A (2000) Epidemiology of work-related burn injuries: experience of a state-managed workers' compensation system. J Trauma 49: 1045–1051
[27] Jalali S, Das T, Majji A (1999) Hypodermic needles: a new source of penetrating ocular trauma in Indian children. Retina 19: 213–217
[28] Jayasundera T, Vote B, Joondeph B (2003) Golf-related ocular injuries. Clin Experiment Ophthalmol 31: 110–113
[29] John G, Witherspoon C, Morris R, White M, Feist R (1988) Field evaluation of polycarbonate versus conventional safety glasses. Southern Med J 81: 1534–1536
[30] Karaman K, Gverovic-Antunica A, Rogosic V, Lakos-Krzelj V, Rozga A, Radocaj-Perko S (2004) Epidemiology of adult eye injuries in Split-Dalmatian county. Croatian Med J 45: 304–309
[31] Karlson T, Klein B (1986) The incidence of acute hospital-treated eye injuries. Arch Ophthalmol 104: 1473–1476
[32] Katz J, Tielsch J (1993) Lifetime prevalence of ocular injuries from the Baltimore Eye Survey. Arch Ophthalmol 111: 1564–1568
[33] Keeney A, Fintelmann E, Renaldo D (1972) Clinical mechanisms in non-industrial trauma. Am J Ophthalmol 74: 662
[34] Khatry S, Lewis A, Schein O, Thapa M, Pradhan E, Katz J (2004) The epidemiology of ocular trauma in rural Nepal. Br J Ophthalmol 88: 456–460
[35] Klopfer J, Tielsch J, Vitale S, et al. (1992) Ocular trauma in the United states, eye injuries resulting in hospitalization, 1984 through 1987. Arch Ophthalmol 110: 838–842
[36] Koo L, Kapadia M, Singh R, Sheridan R, Hatton M (2005) Gender differences in etiology and outcome of open globe injuries. J Trauma 59: 175–178
[37] Krishnaiah S, Nirmalan PK, Shamanna BR, Srinivas M, Rao GN, Thomas R (2006) Ocular trauma in a rural population of southern India: the Andhra Pradesh Eye Disease Study. Ophthalmology 113: 1159–1164
[38] Kuhn F, Mester V, Berta A, Morris R (1998) Epidemiology of serious ocular trauma: The United States Eye Injury Registry (USEIR) and the Hungarian Eye Injury Registry (HEIR). Ophthalmologe 95: 332–343

[39] Kuhn F, Mester V, Morris R, Dalma J (2004) Serious eye injuries caused by bottles containing carbonated drinks. Br J Ophthalmol 88: 69–67

[40] Kuhn F, Morris R, Witherspoon C (1995) Eye injury and the air bag. Curr Opin Ophthalmol 6: 38–44

[41] Kuhn F, Morris R, Witherspoon C, Byrne J, Brown S (1993) Air bag: Friend or foe? Arch Ophthalmol 111: 1333–1334

[42] Kuhn F, Morris R, Witherspoon CD, Mann L, V M, Modis L, Berta A (2000) Serious fireworks-related eye injuries. Ophthalmic Epidemiol 7: 139-148

[43] Liggett P, Pince K, Barlow W, Ragen M, Ryan S (1990) Ocular trauma in an urban population. Ophthalmology 97: 581–584

[44] Listman D (2004) Paintball injuries in children: more than meets the eye. Pediatrics 11: 5–8

[45] MacEwan C, Naines P, Deasi P (1999) Eye injuries in children: the current picture. Br J Ophthalmol 83: 933–936

[46] Mackiewicz J, Machowicz-Matejko E, Salaga-Pylak M, Piecyk-Sidor M, Zagorski Z (2004) Penetrating eye trauma epidemiology in own material. Klin Oczna 106 (Suppl): 448–449

[47] Mader T, Aragones J, Chandler A, Hazlehurst J, Heier J, Kingham J, Stein E (1993) Ocular and ocular adnexal injuries treated by United States military ophthalmologists during Operations Desert Shield and Desert Storm. Ophthalmology

[48] Maltzman B, Pruzon H, Mund M (1976) A survey of ocular trauma. Surv Ophthalmol 21: 285–290

[49] May D, Kuhn F, Morris R, Witherspoon C, Danis R, Matthews P, Mann L (2000) The epidemiology of serious eye injuries from the United States Eye Injury Registry. Graefe's Arch Clin Exp Ophthalmol 238: 153–157

[50] McCarty C, Fu C, Taylor H (1999) Epidemiology of ocular trauma in Australia. Ophthalmology 106: 1847–1852

[51] McGwin GJ, Hall T, Xie A, Owsley C (2006) Gun-related eye injury in the United States, 1993–2002. Ophthal Epidemiol 13: 15–21

[52] McGwin GJ, Owsley C (2005) Incidence of emergency department-treated eye injury in the United States. Arch Ophthalmol 123: 662–666

[53] Mela E, Dvorak G, Mantzouranis G, Giakoumis A, Blatsios G, Andrikopoulos G, Gartaganis S (2005) Ocular trauma in a Greek population: review of 899 cases resulting in hospitalization. Ophthal Epidemiol 12: 185–190

[54] Mensah A, Fany A, Adjorlolo C, Toure M-L, GM K, Mihluedo K, Diallo A, Coulibaly F, Berete R (2004) Epidemiology of eye injuries in Abidjanian children. Sante 14: 239–243

[55] Mieler WF, Nanda SK, Wolf MD, Harman J (1995) Golf-related ocular injuries. Arch Ophthalmol 113: 1410–1413

[56] Mönestam E, Björnstig U (1991) Eye injuries in northern Sweden. Acta Ophthalmol 69: 1–5

[57] Morris R, Scharper P, Fletcher D, Witherspoon C, Kuhn F, Harrill M (2006) Removal of epimacular proliferation (EMP) in eyes. Retina 26: 589

[58] Negrel A, Thylefors B (1998) The global impact of eye injuries. Ophthalmic Epidemiol 5: 143–169

[59] Nirmalan P, Katz J, Tielsch J, Robin A, Thulasiraj R, Krishnadas R, Ramakrishnan R (2004) Comprehensive eye survey. Ocular trauma in a rural south Indian population: the Aravind Comprehensive Eye Survey. Ophthalmology 111: 1778–1781

[60] Oner A, Kekec Z, Krakucuk S, Ikizceli I, Sozuer EM (2006) Ocular trauma in Turkey: a 2-year prospective study. Adv Ther 23: 274–283

[61] Parker J, Simon H (2004) Eye injuries due to paintball sports: a case series. Pediatr Emerg Care 20: 602–603

[62] Pashby T, Pashby R, Chisholm L, Crawford J (1975) Eye injuries in Canadian hockey. Can Med Assoc J 113: 663

[63] Pieramici D, Kuhn F (2003) Frontal air bags and eye injury patterns in automobile crashes. Arch Ophthalmol 121: 1807–1808

[64] Richter-Muenksch S, Stur M, Stiffer E, Radner W (2005) Differences in reading performance of patients with Drusen maculopathy and subretinal fibrosis after CNV. Graefe's Arch Exp Cin Ophthalmol 244: 154–162

[65] Schein O, Hibberd P, Shingleton B (1988) The spectrum and burden of ocular injury. Ophthalmology 95: 300–395

[66] Schrader W (2004) Epidemiology of open globe eye injuries: analysis of 1026 cases in 18 years. Klin Monatsbl Augenheilk 221: 629–635

[67] Serrano J, Chalela P, Arias J (2003) Epidemiology of childhood ocular trauma in a northeastern Colombian region. Arch Ophthalmol 121: 1439–1445

[68] Simoni P, Ostendorf R, Cox AR (2003) Effect of air bags and restraining devices on the pattern of facial fractures in motor vehicle crashes. Arch Fac Plast Surg 5: 113–115

[69] Sinclair S, Smith G, Xiang H (2006) Eyeglasses-related injuries treated in U.S. emergency departments in 2002–2003. Ophthal Epidemiol 13: 23–30

[70] Singh D, Sharma Y, Azad R (2005) Visual outcome after fireworks injuries. J Trauma 59: 109–111

[71] Smith R, O'Hagan S, Gole G (2006) Epidemiology of open- and closed-globe trauma presenting to Cairns Base Hospital, Queensland. Clin Exp Ophthalmol 34: 252–259

[72] Thach A, Ward T, Hollifield R, Dugel P, Sipperley J, Marx J, Abrams D, Wroblewski K, Sonkin P, Birdsong R, Dunlap W (1999) Ocular injuries from paintball pellets. Ophthalmology 106: 533–537

[73] Tielsch J, Parver L, Shankar B (1989) Time trends in the incidence of hospitalized ocular trauma. Arch Ophthalmol 107: 519–523

[74] Vinger PF (2002) The need for standardization for protective eyewear in sports. In: Kuhn F, Pieramici D (eds) Ocular trauma: principles and practice. Thieme, New York, pp 455–460

[75] Voon L, See J, Wong T (2001) The epidemiology of ocular trauma in Singapore: perspective from the emergency service of a large tertiary hospital. Eye 15: 75–81

[76] Weitgasser U, Wackernagel W, Oetsch K (2004) Visual outcome and ocular survival after sports related ocular trauma in playing golf. J Trauma 56: 648–650

[77] White M, Morris R, Feist R, Witherspoon C, Helms H, John G (1989) Eye injury: prevalence and prognosis by setting. South Med J 82: 151–158

[78] Wong T, Tielsch J (1999) A population-based study on the incidence of severe ocular trauma in Singapore. Am J Ophthalmol 128: 345–351

1.8 Strategic Thinking in Ocular Traumatology

Ferenc Kuhn

1.8.1 Introduction

What does a car driver do when given the task of driving from home to an unknown destination through unknown territory?

He consults a map, various "driving directions" Internet services, seeks advice from people who already drove between those two endpoints, or may even purchase a Global Positioning System device. One thing he certainly will not do is start the journey without planning. Getting lost can get the driver into trouble ranging from the inconvenient to the dangerous.

If a pilot needs a plan of how to drive from point A to point B, should not an ophthalmologist treating a patient with a serious injury also design a management plan first? This chapter discusses the elements of a systematic thought process. This planning has two levels: the strategy and the tactics.

- *Strategy* involves the grand plan such as indication for or against surgery, timing, type of intervention, and completeness (vs staging) of the surgery.[1] Strategy can be further stratified (Table 1.8.1).
- *Tactics* involve dealing with individual pathologies and tissues.

Just as drivers need *specific* directions, in addition to a general map, for a specific trip,[2] there is no *single* blueprint the ophthalmologist can apply for

1 This chapter addresses the strategic issues; the tactics are discussed in Sections 2 through 4.

2 Indeed, all trips are unique and must have a specific plan developed solely for that trip, but use of a general map is necessary to be able to design that specific plan.

Table 1.8.1 The different components of surgical planning to treat the patient with a serious eye injury

Component	Comment
Overall strategy (general management)	Some of the questions that the surgeon needs to answer before treatment can be started: – Is the patient in good enough general health to survive surgery? – Is it possible to reconstruct the eye at all? If not, and primary enucleation is truly the only option, will the patient agree to it before surgery is started? – Am I able to do it (Do I have the expertise, experience, equipment, personnel, OR facility, time, etc.[a])? – If I cannot do it, to whom should the patient be referred?
Specific strategy (surgical planning)	Are the management's ultimate goals easier to achieve via a staged approach or via a single, comprehensive surgery? How urgent is the initial surgery, what is its optimal timing? What type of intervention offers the best hope to restore the eye's anatomy (i.e., pars plana vitrectomy, endoscopy, TKP)?
Tactics (how to execute the surgical plan)	How to deal with tissue-specific issues (see Chaps. 2.1–3.3

Many of these questions also need to be addressed during counseling (see Chap. 1.4)

[a]Details are provided in Table 1.8.3

each injury. There are no two trauma cases absolutely alike; therefore, all need an individualized treatment plan.[3] Based on the basic building blocks of strategic thinking, the ophthalmologist can develop his own approach to the management of eyes with serious trauma.

A severely injured eye is often a "surprise package"[4]: the surgeon may not know all tissue lesions that have occurred or to what extent, how the injury to one tissue effects the behavior and thus treatment of another, and what problems he will face that he has never experienced before. Nevertheless, a comprehensive management plan should be designed *before* actual treatment is initiated. Conversely, this plan should never be "written in stone": it must be changed according to patient requests (see Chap. 1.4), specific pre- or intraoperative findings, and from noticing how tissues react to his maneuvers.[5] This chapter is dedicated to issues that reflect strategy or general thinking ("what, when, why"),[6] not to tactics such as dealing with specific tissue conditions ("how");[7] these are found in the appropriate chapters in this book (Table 1.8.2).

Pearl

A car driver must know where he is and where he needs to go; he can then figure out how to get there. Similarly, an ocular traumatologist must know the condition of the eye and to what extent the normal anatomy can be restored; a plan must be designed as to how this reconstruction can be achieved.

3 This plan, however, is based on a knowledge of the general rules, on possessing extensive knowledge of the elements of strategic thinking.

4 A very appropriate term coined in this context by R. Morris, Birmingham, Alabama.

5 One example: A healthy retina is able to withstand much more surgical trauma than one in a patient with advanced diabetes. Peeling of PVR membranes is therefore done very differently in eyes with unhealthy retina.

6 To use the driver example: This chapter discusses the need for using maps, how to select the map, and what the rules of choosing the roads to be driven are.

7 Actual driving of the car (when and how to steer or shift, use the turning signal, etc.: this, in our example, is on the same level as the tissue tactics chapters.

Table 1.8.2 Comparison of strategy vs tactics in the management of a patient with serious eye injury

Case summary	An 18-year-old male presents with a 5-h injury; he was chopping wood when a branch hit his eye. His visual acuity dropped to 20/200; he has a 5-mm long corneal laceration with fibrin in the AC. The lens appears intact and the retina can be inspected
Selected strategic questions	Does this eye need to be sutured immediately?
	Is the risk of endophthalmitis high, are prophylactic intravitreal antibiotics necessary?
	Does the patient have to be hospitalized?
Selected tactical questions	Interrupted or running sutures should be used?
	How many sutures are necessary?
	Is there sufficient amount fibrin in the AC to warrant removal?
	Is the anterior lens capsule indeed intact?

1.8.2 Steps/Elements in Designing the Management Plan

1.8.2.1 Triaging

A process needs to be in place to determine the urgency of the intervention. Triaging has two components: a *systemic* one (concerning the patient's systemic condition), and an *ocular* one. Systemic triaging is not discussed here; in this process the ophthalmologist cooperates with ER physicians, internists, general surgeons, neurosurgeons, etc. to determine the order in which the conditions/injuries need to be treated (Fig. 1.8.1).

If an eye requires immediate intervention (chemical[8] injury, level-1 case), evaluation and treatment go "hand in hand". In all other cases, de-

8 "Splash" injury is how laypeople often describe it.

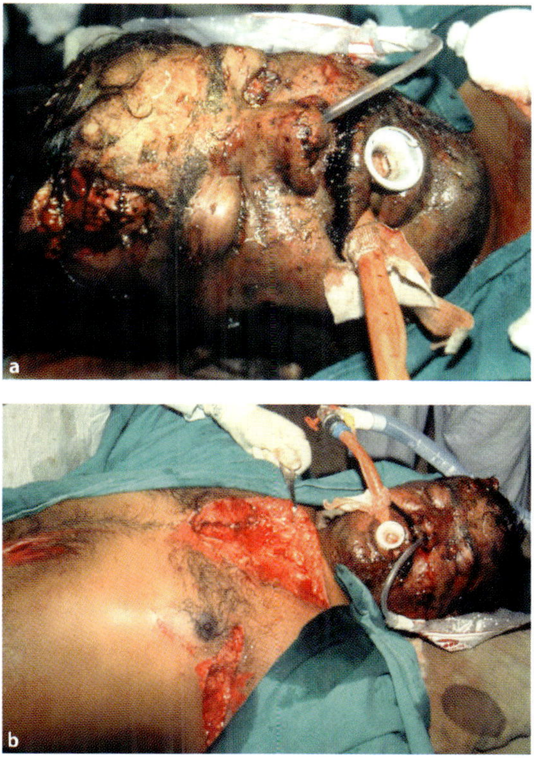

Fig. 1.8.1 The need for systemic triaging in people injured by a blast.[1] **a** While injury to the left is eye is obvious and to the right eye likely, management of the visible brain damage obviously must take precedence. **b** The patient also has chest injuries: the general surgeon and the ophthalmologist must discuss which of them should treat the patient first (Photographs courtesy of D. Kalra, Panchkula, India)

[1] Caused by IED (improvised explosive device), planted by terrorists and exploded by remote control. The IEDs are packed with metal splinters, ball bearings, and nails to increase the carnage.

Fig. 1.8.2 Flowchart showing the triaging of the patient with serious eye injury. If multiple cases are received in the ER simultaneously (e.g., due to a large-scale accident or a terrorist attack), the same rules apply to determine which patients receives attention first

termination of the triage level is done during the evaluation. Figure 1.8.2 shows the basic concepts of the triaging system; further details are presented in Chap. 1.10.

1.8.2.2 Evaluation[9]

The first element in the management process is to determine the type and extent of the injury. Unless a chemical injury has occurred (see Chap. 3.1), history is taken, and the patient and the eye are examined according to information gleaned from history (see Chap. 1.9).

As the results of the evaluation process become available, the ophthalmologist reviews the condition of the patient and of the eye, and develops a treatment plan. The factors to be considered are listed below.

1.8.2.3 Is the Injury Open Globe?

Closed globe trauma rarely warrants emergency surgery; there is time to consider and reconsider what to do (see Chap. 2.10). If the injury is open globe (see Chaps. 2.11–2.14), the decision regarding when to operate becomes urgent.

1.8.2.4 Is a Devastating Complication Likely to Occur If Surgery Is Delayed By a Few Hours?

If ECH threatens (see Chap. 2.8), surgery is an absolute emergency. In almost all other cases, its deferral by a few hours to optimize conditions is not only acceptable but recommended. If the risk of endophthalmitis is

9 Further details on strategy and tactics are given in Chap. 2.11.

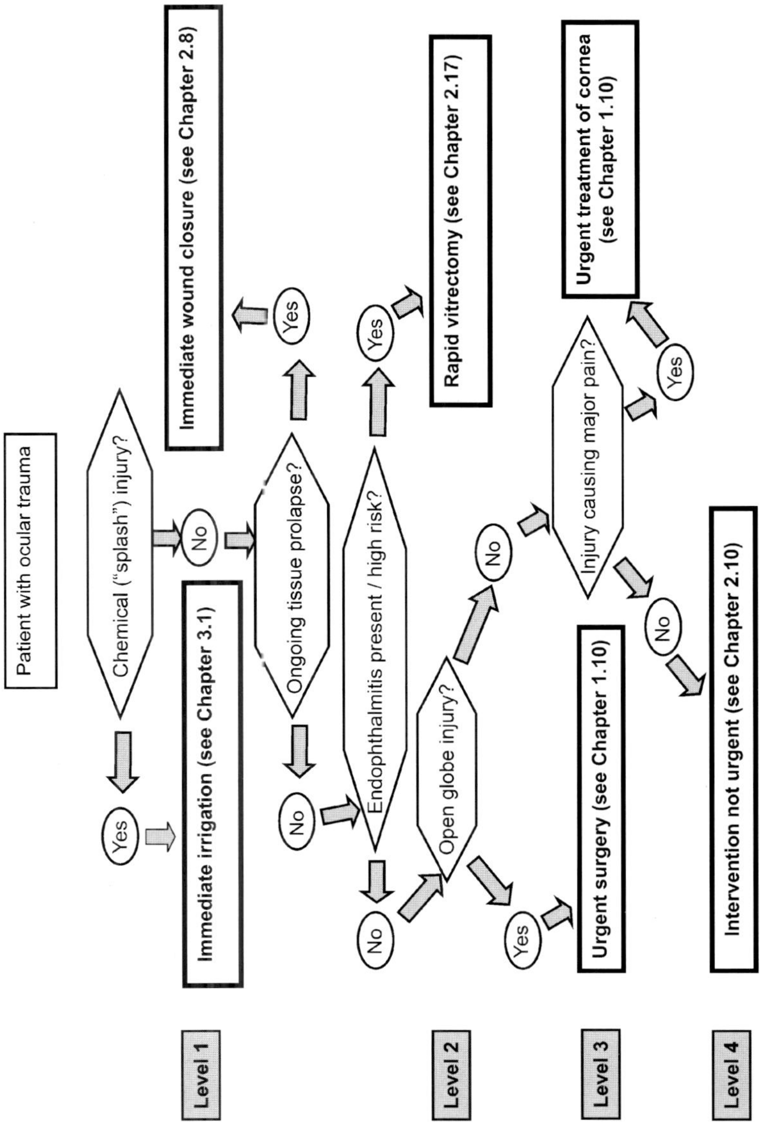
Patient with ocular trauma
Chemical ("splash") injury?
Yes
Immediate irrigation (see Chapter 3.1)
No
Ongoing tissue prolapse?
Yes
Immediate wound closure (see Chapter 2.8)
No
Endophthalmitis present / high risk?
Yes
Rapid vitrectomy (see Chapter 2.17)
No
Open globe injury?
Yes
Urgent surgery (see Chapter 1.10)
No
Injury causing major pain?
Yes
Urgent treatment of cornea (see Chapter 1.10)
No
Intervention not urgent (see Chapter 2.10)
Level 1
Level 2
Level 3
Level 4

very high (see Chap. 2.17), and especially if *Bacillus* is suspected as the organism, surgery is very urgent.

1.8.2.5 Who Should Intervene (Surgery or Referral to Be Chosen)?

Pearl

Before the ophthalmologist decides to treat the consequences of the injury, he must answer the three "*E*" questions: Does he have the *E-xpertise, E-xperience, and E-quipment* to do an optimal job? If the answer to any of these fundamental questions is "no," the patient should be referred to a colleague.

The "nil nocere" rule means much more than not creating an iatrogenic retinal tear or causing an ECH. If the attending ophthalmologist cannot offer optimal treatment (Table 1.8.3), referral is preferred to performing suboptimal or incomplete surgery. Intervention vs referral should never be an "ego" issue or one of ill-perceived "bravery." Both patient and ophthalmologist will suffer the consequences otherwise: the former because the eye will not regain as much vision as it should have, the latter because of the legal implications.

Cave

If the surgeon is inexperienced in dealing with posterior segment trauma and a difficult retinal pathology is unexpectedly encountered, surgery should be stopped and the patient referred. Preferably, the ophthalmologist learns about the retinal pathology preoperatively and chooses referral instead of surgery. The golden rule is: "*If you can't, don't.*"

1.8.2.6 Referral: the Rules of Transportation

Referral must not be defined as applying a patch or shield and organizing transportation:

- Limit manipulations to the absolute minimum.

Table 1.8.3 Selected issues arguing against the attending ophthalmologist undertaking surgery

Issue	Comment
Expertise	The surgeon may be an accomplished anterior segment expert but has never performed vitreoretinal surgery, and the eye has a posterior scleral rupture, possibly with retinal prolapse
Experience	The surgeon may have performed thousands of cataract extractions, but dealing with a disrupted lens that is mixed with blood and vitreous prolapse requires additional skills
Surgeon's readiness	The surgeon may have performed several difficult vitreoretinal cases during the day, was also called in last night, and is now very tired
Equipment	The surgeon may be familiar with, and ready to use, the vitrectomy machine for removal of a dislocated lens, but the machine is unavailable beyond "regular OR hours"
Personnel	The OR nurse available at midnight is not specialized in ophthalmology; she is able to offer some, but not all, the assistance that may become necessary. An assistant surgeon may also be needed but none is at hand
OR facility	Only a general OR is available, the one specifically equipped for intraocular surgery is not
Materials	Silicone oil or heavy liquids are unavailable at night
Time	The surgeon has a plane to catch in 2 h when his duty shift ends, and surgery may not be finished by then

- Do not pull out protruding FBs unless there is a danger that the patient will do so (see Chap. 2.16).
- Do not suture the wound unless transportation is expected to take a long time.[10]
- With rare exceptions, do not employ topical medications (see below).
- Apply a firm shield; if a medical grade, standard shield is unavailable or unfeasible (e.g., because of the size of the protruding IOFB), one can easily be shaped from a Styrofoam cup.
- The patient's attention must be called to avoid touching the shield. A child may have to be restrained.
- Use an ambulance or some type of medical transport company if possible: should something go wrong along the way, there is proper help available, and the risk of legal action is also reduced.
- Send all test results[11] along with the patient, describe in detail the medications used or any intervention you may have performed.
- Give the patient systemic medication[12] as needed to alleviate pain, nausea, high blood pressure, and anxiety.

1.8.2.7 Eyes with NLP Vision

Losing the eye's ability to detect light creates an emergency if caused by an arterial occlusion or an intraorbital hemorrhage from a retrobulbar hemorrhage; paradoxically, in the context of globe trauma it typically does not [14]. Figure 1.8.3 shows the enucleation rates, based on a review of several U.S. studies, of eyes with NLP, LP, or HM vision. Instead of evoking the need for emergency reconstruction, NLP vision all too often prompts the ophthalmologist to do nothing or to remove the globe.

In a fairly high proportion of the cases the loss of LP is temporary – provided that intervention is timely *and* appropriate. If an orbit- or optic canal-related condition (see Chap. 1.10) is the cause, treatment should be

---

10 Alternatively, discuss the issue over the phone with the colleague to whom you are referring the patient, and do as he recommends.

11 The actual CT films or ultrasound printouts are preferred to test readings.

12 *Not* oral: general anesthesia may be desired in the next few hours.

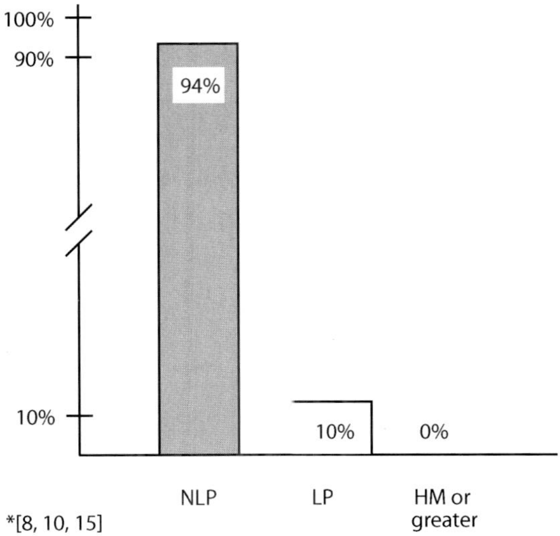

Fig. 1.8.3 Enucleation rates and the initial visual acuity as reported in the U.S. literature. *LP* light perception, *NLP* no light perception, *HM* hand motion

initiated within hours; if – and this is by far the most common – the cause is globe injury, the window of opportunity to intervene is appr. 2 weeks, but earlier surgery has definite advantages. Vitreous hemorrhage alone is able to block (via scattering and absorption) 97% of incoming light. Should pathologies such as corneal edema, hyphema, cataract, retinal detachment, and submacular hemorrhage also be present, it is easy to understand that the loss of LP is not necessarily due to irreversible damage. This explains the high rate of improvement following reconstructive surgery: in a large series of eyes undergoing TKP vitrectomy for NLP vision, 40% of eyes improved to at least LP vision and 10% reached visual acuities ranging from 20/100 to 20/40 [25].

Based on the history and the findings during evaluation, the ophthalmologist should have a rather clear idea of the chance for success of intraocular reconstruction. Technology is available today to preserve most eyes even with severe trauma: it is the mentality toward the fatefulness of NLP that needs to be changed.

Pitfall

If the wound lips can be brought together with sutures, the eyeball can probably be saved. If the posterior retina is not destroyed and the optic nerve has not been severely damaged, there is hope for at least some functional improvement. The only absolute death sentence for the eye comes from enucleation.[13]

Even if the eye is unlikely to regain vision, it makes clinical sense not to abandon the eye; if anatomical reconstruction is not performed, the chance of subsequent enucleation is as high as 34%, and 70% of the remaining eyes eventually becomes phthisical [4]. It is possible that such reconstruction, which reduces the postinjury inflammation, also reduces the risk of sympathetic ophthalmia.

1.8.2.7.1 Sympathetic Ophthalmia

A serious, granulomatous, sterile inflammation, most likely as a result of an autoimmune reaction, may threaten the fellow eye within a few days or even after several decades following trauma or surgery [24]. The incidence and thus risk after open globe trauma is very low (see below). Occasionally, the condition can develop after contusion [1] or laser treatment [20].

- Only a single case has been reported in the entire literature among the many, many thousands of people with war-related eyes injuries following World War II [11].
- Prompt enucleation/evisceration within 2 weeks of the trauma has been suggested as the only absolute method to prevent the threat of sympathetic ophthalmia; however, the condition can occur even if evisceration is very early [11].
- If the patient received detailed information about the early symptoms of sympathetic ophthalmia, it is possible to recognize and treat the pa-

13 The same principles apply for eyes with chronic injury. Reconstruction of such eyes is not the topic of this book, but it must be emphasized that phthisis is not a contraindication to a reconstruction attempt even if the injury is months or even years old. If this eye has at least LP vision, even functional improvement is possible (see Chap. 2.19).

thology immediately, and the prognosis is not as poor as it was in the pre-corticosteroid era (see below).

Complaints include:

- Mild pain
- Light sensitivity
- Accommodation inability
- Decreased visual acuity

Findings include:

- Anterior uveitis with keratitic precipitates
- Iris nodules
- Vitritis
- Optic disc and retinal edema
- Perivasculitis
- Deep yellowish (Dalen–Fuchs) nodules in the retinal periphery
- Retinal detachment

Treatment [9] includes:

- Antiinflammatory (oral and topical corticosteroids, intravitreal TA) [16].
- Immunosuppressive[14] (azathioprine, chlorambucil, cyclophosphamide, cyclosporine, mycophenolate mofetil).

With proper treatment, the *prognosis* is good, with at least half of the eyes having 20/40 or greater final vision [6].

Controversial

It is not known whether the inciting eye should be removed once sympathetic ophthalmia has developed. It appears reasonable to retain an eye with some vision but enucleate/eviscerate those that have become NLP.

14 It is best to leave the use of these drugs in the hands of an internist or immunologist.

- If receiving unbiased, uncoached, truthful (see Chap. 1.4) information about the risk and the early symptoms of sympathetic ophthalmia, it is exceptional that a patient would want to undergo the psychological trauma attached to eye removal. If proper informed consent has been obtained, the ophthalmologist cannot be held liable even if sympathetic ophthalmia does later develop.
- In one study on enucleated eyes, sympathetic ophthalmia was the indication in 108 cases; on histopathology, signs of the disease were found only in 2 eyes [5].

Pearl

The threat of sympathetic ophthalmia alone is no justification for recommending removal of an injured eye with NLP vision.

Primary enucleation/evisceration should be performed only if the eye has been damaged so extensively that it simply cannot be sutured back together (Fig. 1.8.4). The enucleation rate is especially high in war injuries, having reached 16% among U.S. soldiers fighting in Iraq [13]. *Secondary enucleation/evisceration* can be performed if the blind eye becomes painful and the other management options are ineffective or the cosmetic appearance is unacceptable to the patient.

Pearl

If the eye is painful and blind, medical treatment (corticosteroids, antiglaucoma medications), retrobulbar injection (alcohol, chlorpromazine [7] or phenol [2]), or cyclocryopexy may be attempted before enucleation is performed.

The decision to remove the eye must be repeatedly discussed with the patient; those patients whose eye was not removed usually prefer eye retention even many years later [17].

It appears that there is no scientific basis for preferring enucleation over evisceration, or vice versa [15].

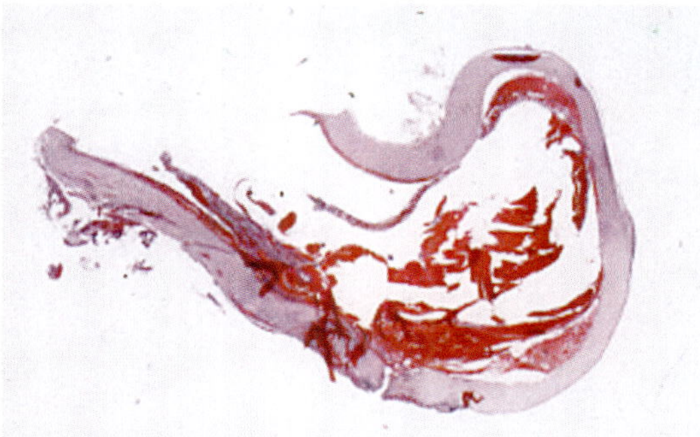

Fig. 1.8.4 Extensive damage justifying enucleation. This eye sustained a rupture and most intraocular contents were lost. There is no hope for functional improvement or even for maintaining a cosmetically acceptable appearance, and (even primary) enucleation is justified

1.8.2.8 General vs Local Anesthesia

General anesthesia is the preferred option; the anesthesiologist must avoid elevating the IOP during induction [21–23]. If the patient ate/drank recently, and the ophthalmologist is convinced that a delay in surgery is unacceptable and that surgery must be performed under general anesthesia, the anesthesiologist should make every effort to comply. If general anesthesia is used, it is strongly recommended that the nose be tamponaded to prevent reflux onto the operative field (Fig. 1.8.5).

If *local anesthesia* is selected, the following needs to be kept in mind:

- Judicious topical application of the drug (lidocaine 2%) provides sufficient analgesia to allow temporary closure of anterior wounds.

Cave

Lidocain applied onto an eye that has an open wound has the risk of allowing the drug to penetrate into the eye. If the retina is "anesthetized," temporary blindness ensues; this a very scary phenomenon, and both patient and ophthalmologist need to be aware of it. Vision should return within an hour.

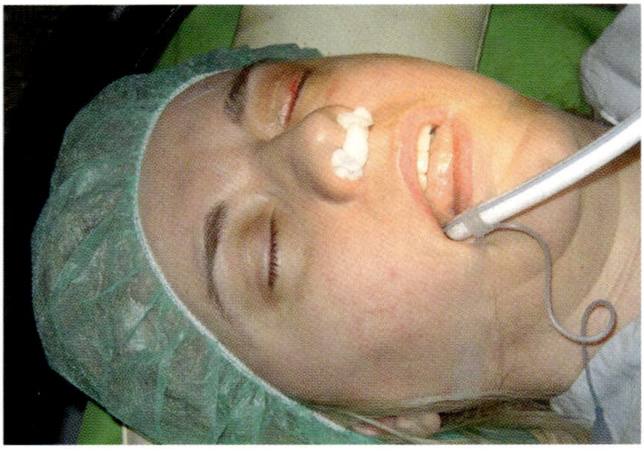

Fig. 1.8.5 Tamponading the nose during general anesthesia. Endophthalmitis can occur because of nasal fluid getting onto the operative field. This can easily be prevented by placing tampons into the nose once the intratracheal tube has been secured

- Topical anesthesia results in pain relief but not immobility. The patient must be constantly reminded not to move his eyes, preferably keeping them *loosely* shot.
- Once the wound is closed with a few temporary sutures, careful peribulbar injection of a combination of short- and long-acting anesthetics[15], such as lidocaine and bupivacaine [8], achieves both anesthesia and immobility.
- Very cautious peribulbar (Fig. 1.8.6) or retrobulbar injection of a small amount of anesthetic can also be attempted [19].
- If surgery on a severely injured eye is performed under local anesthesia, the surgeon may have to compromise in his goals and maneuvers, and defer certain procedures until a second operation under optimal conditions can be arranged.

15 Similar to that used for elective cases

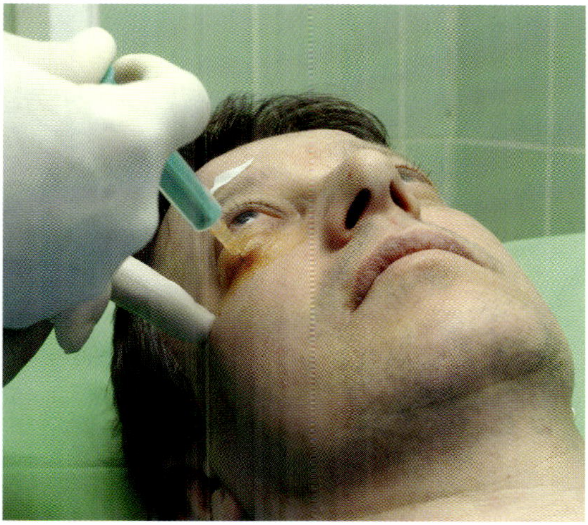

Fig. 1.8.6 Peribulbar anesthesia for an eye with open globe injury. The high risk of endophthalmitis required emergency surgery in this case but the patient had eaten just 1 h before. An anesthesiologist had been consulted, and the conclusion was that inducing general anesthesia would have represented greater risk of an ECH than a peribulbar injection and also would have increased the delay

- The patient's systemic condition (e.g., blood pressure, blood sugar) may be more difficult to monitor, and intervention to correct an abnormality may be more difficult.

1.8.2.9 Staged vs Comprehensive Surgery

Most surgeons in most cases prefer a *staged* approach: wound toilette and closure, occasionally accompanied by additional procedures such as hyphema removal, are performed during the first[16] surgery, followed by a second[17] surgery (typically vitrectomy) a week or so later. Unless extraor-

16 Synonyms are primary, emergency, acute, initial
17 Synonyms are secondary, follow-up, reconstructive

dinary conditions force a longer delay, the second surgery should be performed no later than within 2 weeks.

A *comprehensive* first surgery means that all tissue pathologies are addressed in a single surgical setting.

Table 1.8.4 shows the benefits and disadvantages of the two approaches.

Pearl

For most cases, a staged approach is recommended. Comprehensive primary surgery should not be considered if the surgeon is inexperienced in both anterior and posterior segment techniques in general *and* in trauma surgery in particular. A large scleral wound that has not been surgically closed because it is too posterior is a strong argument against primary vitrectomy.

Regardless of whether reconstruction is performed in a staged or comprehensive fashion, the surgeon must plan the entire management process as a whole[18]: Instead of simply reacting to the individual tissue pathologies as they become known, he has to be *proactive*, i.e., anticipate and incorporate into the management plan the consequences of the pathologies that are:

- Already present
- Likely to develop because of the nature of the injury
- Possible to develop due to the surgical intervention itself (Table 1.8.5)

1.8.2.10 Supplementary Pharmaceutical Therapy

Intravitreal antibiotics and corticosteroids may be given if the risk of endophthalmitis is high (see Chap. 2.17). If the patient is referred, topical antibiotics may be considered.[19] If the threat of tetanus infection warrants it, a booster shot may be given.[20]

18 This is what the concept of strategic thinking is aimed at.

19 This is almost never necessary; if, however, topical antibiotics are instilled, these must be in the form of drops, not ointment.

20 The rules of immunization differ from country to country. A booster shot's effect lasts approximately 10 years.

Table 1.8.4 The advantages and disadvantages of staged vs comprehensive surgery for serious eye injury

Staged	Comprehensive
An unsutured wound is much less likely to reopen during vitrectomy performed a few days after the trauma	Patient has to endure one, instead of two, procedures
Detailed evaluation of the eye can be delayed until after wound closure	Endophthalmitis prevention
Primary surgery can be minimized during after hours. With proper postoperative corticosteroid therapy, the threat of intraoperative ECH is dramatically reduced by the time posterior segment surgery is performed	Dangerous secondary complications (e.g., inflammation, acute retinal detachment, acute metallosis) can be prevented
Certain types of media opacity (e.g., corneal edema surrounding a freshly closed wound) may be limited enough to allow what needs to be performed during the primary procedure and improve by the time secondary reconstruction is performed. It may be easier to determine whether a traumatic cataract is present	Certain types of media opacity (e.g., diffuse corneal edema, lens opacity) may worsen with time
Help can be obtained from various sources to increase the chance of success of the secondary surgery or the patient can be referred	Reduced cost
Timing (e.g., related to elective cases) and circumstances (e.g., determining the IOL's power) of secondary surgery can be optimized	PVR may be prevented

Note that spontaneous PVD is not listed since it rarely occurs by the time of secondary surgery.

The advantages are listed here; the disadvantages are implied

Table 1.8.5 A case example to illustrate the difference between a "reactive" and a "proactive" surgical plan

Case report	A 16-year-old boy injured 10 h earlier by a screwdriver as he was trying to pry open a wooden box at home. He felt a little pain, and his vision was immediately lost. Upon presentation, he has LP vision and a 5-mm corneal wound just adjacent to the visual axis without iris prolapse and an almost total hyphema. The lens is not visible because of the blood, and the IOP is judged normal. No IOFB is found on CT, but there is vitreous hemorrhage on ultrasonography; the retina is attached. The boy is not taking any medications and has not eaten or drank since the injury
Reactive approach	Under general anesthesia, closure of the corneal wound, possibly evacuation of the hyphema; injection of prophylactic antibiotics intravitreally; secondary surgery planned for a week later with hyphema removal, cataract extraction (probably) using phacoemulsification, IOL implantation (possibly), and vitrectomy. Antiinflammatory therapy and objective determination of the IOL power after the initial surgery
Proactive approach	The size of the corneal wound and the presumed momentum of the screwdriver suggest that both of the lens capsules are injured. The shape of a screwdriver and its length as well as the severe vitreous hemorrhage raise the possibility of direct retinal injury or even an exit wound. The plan is, under general anesthesia, to close the corneal wound, remove the hyphema, remove the lens using vitrectomy instrumentation, and not leave the posterior capsule behind since the risk of PVR is significant. Pars plana vitrectomy is then performed with special attention paid to keeping the IOP under 35 mmHg in case there is an exit wound that has not closed. The anesthesiologist is asked to closely monitor the boy's blood pressure, keeping it as low as possible to reduce the risk of ECH. If a deep retinal impact site is found, prophylactic chorioretinectomy is performed, and silicone oil is implanted. If an exit wound is present and it leaks intraoperatively, it may have to be sutured ab interno. Intravitreal antibiotics are not used, but very heavy topical corticosteroid therapy is applied postoperatively, and the eye is closely followed for PVR development. IOL implantation is deferred until the condition of the retina is deemed final and vision will improve with restoration of the lost refractive power.

1.8.2.11 Timing of Secondary Surgery

The optimal time of secondary intervention has never been determined in a scientific study. Clinical experience indicates that earlier (around day 4) intervention may be advantageous in preventing PVR via removing the inflammatory debris and diminishing its inciting effect, although this also has not been confirmed in a scientific study. It is, however, generally accepted that delaying vitreous surgery in eyes with open globe surgery should not exceed 2 weeks. Even for eyes with vitreous hemorrhage after contusion, *early* vitrectomy is beneficial (see Chaps. 2.10, 2.11).

1.8.2.12 Hospitalization vs Outpatient Surgery

Elective surgery in the industrialized countries is increasingly performed on an outpatient basis.[21] A patient with an eye injury requiring surgery or extensive nonsurgical therapy (see Chap. 3.1), however, represents a complex issue. Hospitalization is often advantageous to allow early recognition and treatment of the complications of the injury or of the initial intervention.

In underdeveloped countries, the question often becomes even more complex. There are social issues to consider, logistical and financial difficulties, the unavailability of adequate care at the patient's home place, a hostile or unsanitary home environment, etc.[22] These issues must be carefully considered before the patient is discharged to be treated on an outpatient basis.

1.8.2.13 Postoperative Treatment

The mainstay of the therapy is characterized as the "3 I-s rule":

- (Anti)*infectious*: topical, occasionally intravitreal and systemic, antibiotics – this is especially important if the injury is open globe
- (Anti)*inflammatory*: topical, occasionally intravitreal and systemic, corticosteroids

21 The patient spends less than 24 h in the hospital.

22 All of these may exist in an industrialized country as well.

- (Anti)*IOP elevation*: topical, occasionally oral, glaucoma medications.

These medications greatly improve the prognosis of the injury as well as the comfort of the patient.

1.8.2.14 Medicolegal Considerations

The legal system changes from country to country; certain general rules, however, are applicable everywhere. A brief summary is provided here; the reader is referred to other sources [3] for more detailed information.

Injury is a major source for litigation against the:

- Ophthalmologist by claiming that the care rendered was inappropriate[23]; and/or
- employers, manufacturers of the medical equipment used, makers of the tool that caused the injury, etc. In these cases the ophthalmologist is not the defendant but an expert *witness*.
- Before treatment is performed,[24] informed consent must be obtained. This is done in the context of counseling. The patient must have understood the condition of the eye, the "natural course" of the injury, the risks and benefits of each treatment option, and must agree to the treatment.[25]
- A detailed account of the counseling process should be recorded in the patient's chart, preferably by a health care professional other than the ophthalmologist himself (witness).
- If possible, pretreatment as well as follow-up photographs should be taken.

23 i.e., negligence: the ophthalmologist did not adhere to the standard of care in that particular environment, and the eye's condition worsened because of the ophthalmologist's failure to adhere to that standard of care.

24 An obvious exception is chemical injury (see Chap. 3.1).

25 Preferably, it is the patient who selects the type of treatment to be performed (see Chap. 1.4).

Controversial

Videotaping the surgery is a double-edged sword. On one hand, it can prove that the eye was unsalvageable and that the ophthalmologist went beyond what would have been expected of him in trying to improve the eye's condition; on the other hand no surgery is perfect: an "expert witness" speaking on behalf of the plaintiff can always find details with which he disagrees.

1.8.2.15 Recording of the Injury in a Database

Reporting to a standardized registry (see Chap. 1.7) is of immense help for future research, which in turn is the basis of evaluating the efficacy of current treatment techniques and the development of improved ones. Analysis of information on a large number of cases stored in the database forces the ophthalmologist to rethink existing approaches and design new ones.

Pearl

The treatment of eyes with serious injury does not tolerate dogmas (see Chap. 1.6); an individualized approach is necessary. This, however, does not imply that undue experimentation is allowed. Prior approval for a radically new therapy may have to be obtained from the institution's Ethical Committee (Institutional Review Board).

1.8.2.16 Counseling

Typically, more than a single management option is available for a patient with serious injury. As the last step before actual treatment begins, the ophthalmologist should discuss all reasonable options with the patient and the family. The option chosen should be one with which the patient/family are comfortable (see Chap. 1.4). Since the injured patient is rarely brought to that particular ophthalmologist by his conscious decision, it is of crucial importance that the ophthalmologist show an attitude that gains the patient's confidence.

1.8.3 Trauma Expert or Trauma Center?

What is preferable: If the patient is treated at a major facility where all subspecialists and all equipment are available 24 h a day, 7 days a week – or by a single dedicated individual who is uniquely interested in trauma management and is also willing to offer his services 24/7?

In principle, the *trauma center* is preferred; the patient at such a facility can reasonably expect to receive the best available treatment. On the other hand, such centers are expensive to organize and operate, and their location may be unacceptably distant to allow all patients to be transported there.

Pearl

"Many by few," rather than "few by many," yields the best results: fewer ophthalmologists performing a lot of trauma cases each, instead of many ophthalmologists doing a few.

DO:

- develop a management plan before treatment is initiated
- consciously consider the elements of strategic thinking as they apply to your own practice
- understand and accept your own limitations. Preoperatively: do not indicate and initiate surgery with which you are inexperienced. Intraoperatively: should unexpected difficulties arise, it is wiser to stop surgery and seek help than to "experiment"
- do what is best for the eye, not what your best is

DON'T:

- start surgery if you are not convinced that you can properly deal with complications that can be reasonably expected to occur
- follow and act upon advice from a colleague or recommendation from the literature if you are absolutely convinced that your own approach is superior, and your results prove this to be the case
- act with emotion if an intraoperative complication arises: use cool-headed thinking instead

Summary

Treatment of a patient with a serious eye injury should not be undertaken unless a plan has been designed. This plan is based on certain general rules and on the specifics of the case. Such planning helps achieve the basic principle of any treatment: the intervention should be dictated by what is best for the eye, not by what is possible by the attending ophthalmologist.

References

[1] Bakri SJ, Peters GB III (2005) Sympathetic ophthalmia after a hyphema due to nonpenetrating trauma. Ocul Immunol Inflamm 13: 85–86

[2] Birch M, Strong N, Brittain P, Sandford-Smith J (1993) Retrobulbar phenol injection in blind painful eyes. Ann Ophthalmol 25: 267–270

[3] Blakeslee W (2002) Medicolegal issues. In: Kuhn F, Pieramici D (eds) Ocular trauma: principles and practice. Thieme, New York, pp 33–37

[4] Brackup AB, Carter KD, Nerad JA, Folk JC, Pulido JS (1991) Long-term follow-up of severely injured eyes following globe rupture. Ophthal Plast Reconstr Surg 7: 194–197

[5] Canavan YM, Archer DB (1982) The traumatized eye. Trans Ophthalmol Soc U K 102 (Pt 1): 79–84

[6] Chan C, Roberge F, Withcup S (1995) 32 cases of sympathetic ophthalmia. Arch Ophthalmol 113: 597–600

[7] Chen TC, Ahn Yuen SJ, Sangalang MA, Fernando RE, Leuenberger EU (2002) Retrobulbar chlorpromazine injections for the management of blind and seeing painful eyes. J Glaucoma 11: 209–213

[8] Chin GN, Almquist HT (1983) Bupivacaine and lidocaine retrobulbar anesthesia. A double-blind clinical study. Ophthalmology 90: 369–372

[9] Damico FM, Kiss S, Young LH (2005) Sympathetic ophthalmia. Semin Ophthalmol 20: 191–197

[10] Eide N, Syrdalen P (1987) Contusion rupture of the globe. Acta Ophthalmol 182S: 169–171

[11] Freidlin J, Pak J, Tessler HH, Putterman AM, Goldstein DA (2006) Sympathetic ophthalmia after injury in the Iraq war. Ophthal Plast Reconstr Surg 22: 133–134

[12] Gilbert CM, Soong HK, Hirst LW (1987) A two-year prospective study of penetrating ocular trauma at the Wilmer Ophthalmological Institute. Ann Ophthalmol 19: 104–106

[13] Mader T, Carroll R, Slade C, George R, Ritchey J, Neville S (2006) Ocular war injuries of the Iraqi insurgency. Ophthalmology 113: 97–104

[14] Morris R, Kuhn F, Witherspoon CD (1998) Management of the recently injured eye with no light perception vision. In: Alfaro V, Liggett P (eds) Vitrectomy in the management of the injured globe. Lippincott Raven, Philadelphia, pp 113–125

[15] Nakra T, Simon GJ, Douglas RS, Schwarcz RM, McCann JD, Goldberg RA (2006) Comparing outcomes of enucleation and evisceration. Ophthalmology 113: 2270–2275

[16] Ozdemir H, Karacorlu M, Karacorlu S (2005) Intravitreal triamcinolone acetonide in sympathetic ophthalmia. Graefe's Arch Clin Exp Ophthalmol 243: 734–736

[17] Rofail M, Lee GA, O'Rourke P (2006) Quality of life after open-globe injury. Ophthalmology 113: 1057 e1051–1053

[18] Russell S, Olsen K, Folk J (1988) Predictors of scleral rupture and the role of vitrectomy in severe blunt ocular trauma. Am J Ophthalmol 105: 253–257

[19] Simonson D (1992) Retrobulbar block for open-eye injuries: a report of 19 cases. Cornea 3: 35–37

[20] Su DH, Chee SP (2006) Sympathetic ophthalmia in Singapore: new trends in an old disease. Graefe's Arch Clin Exp Ophthalmol 244: 243–247

[21] Vinik H (1999) Intraocular pressure changes during rapid sequence induction and intubation: a comparison of rocuronium, atracurium, and succinylcholine. J Clin Anesth 11: 95–100

[22] Vinik HR (1995) Rapid sequence induction of general anesthesia in open globe injuries without increasing the intraocular pressure. J Eye Trauma 5: 24

[23] Vinik HR (1999) Intraocular pressure changes during rapid sequence induction and intubation: a comparison of rocuronium, atracurium, and succinylcholine. J Clin Anesth 11: 95–100

[24] Vote BJ, Hall A, Cairns J, Buttery R (2004) Changing trends in sympathetic ophthalmia. Clin Experiment Ophthalmol 32: 542–545

[25] Witherspoon C, Morris R, Phillips R, Kuhn F, Nelson S, Witherspoon R (2002) Severe combined anterior and posterior segment trauma. In: Kuhn F, Pieramici D (eds) Ocular trauma: principles and practice. Thieme, New York, pp 264–272

1.9 Evaluation

Ferenc Kuhn

1.9.1 Introduction

Unless emergency intervention is indicated (chemical injury; see Chaps. 1.10, 3.1), the patient's systemic condition as well as the eye's injury-related pathologies must be properly evaluated. The primary goal of the evaluation process is to obtain all the necessary information from/of the patient to allow:

- Systemic triaging: which of the patient's systemic conditions require primary intervention (brain or thoracic trauma, gastrointestinal bleeding, etc.). Teamwork, including neurosurgeons, trauma specialists, ER and ICU physicians, among others, may be required to make intervention decisions.
- Ocular triaging: this includes the determination of the sequence of interventions (e.g., treatment of an open globe injury must precede reconstruction of a lid laceration) as well as the nature and timing of the intervention (e.g., staged or comprehensive, immediate or delayed; see Chap. 1.8).

The evaluation should be sufficiently thorough so that appropriate management decisions can be based on it, yet it must be limited so that only relevant information is sought and treatment is not needlessly delayed.

Pearl

Diagnostic tests that would have no management implications or that would unnecessarily delay the treatment should not be ordered.

This chapter is dedicated to the evaluation of the acutely injured eye; the treatment of chronic trauma-related conditions is beyond the scope of this book.

1.9.2 Systemic Evaluation

Based on the patient's systemic condition, the ophthalmologist may have to check the vital signs and initiate proper intervention as necessary. If the patient is conscious and mentally stable/reliable, a brief history should be taken to determine whether systemic injuries are present. The patient may also have systemic conditions or take medications that need to be accounted for when treatment decisions concerning the eye are contemplated. Proper evaluation by an anesthesiologist of the patient undergoing surgery is an absolute must. Additional issues that should be addressed include:

- Drug allergies
- Currently taken medications[1]
- The hour the patient last ate or drank[2]
- Whether a tetanus booster shot is indicated

1.9.3 Ophthalmological Evaluation[3]

- The primary goal of evaluation is to establish the most important pathologies caused by the injury so that the intervention can be optimally planned (e.g., type, timing).
- The initial (preoperative) examination also serves as a recording of the eye's baseline condition to which the final outcome will be compared.

1 e.g., those that may increase the risk of intraoperative bleeding

2 The intervention may be urgent enough to warrant surgery without general anesthesia (see Chap. 1.8).

3 Not all of these tests are ordered routinely; every case requires an individualized decision. Further details concerning the evaluation of the injured eye are given in Chap. 2.11.

- The written record and the test results are important evidence if a legal claim is subsequently filed; this is as important for the ophthalmologist (to protect himself) as for the patient (insurance, workman's compensation; see Chap. 1.8).
- It is *not* a goal of the evaluation to try to meticulously list every minor tissue lesion. Even significant pathologies, ones whose presence would have no bearing on the decision-making process, need not be identified if in the process of obtaining them further injury to the eye may threaten. These pathologies will be recognized and addressed later when the risk of iatrogenic damage has already passed.[4]

1.9.3.1 History[5]

Since intervention may urgently be necessary, history-taking in trauma cases is somewhat different than in non-injury-related diseases. Table 1.9.1 summarizes the most important questions. Knowledge of the injury's circumstances can yield important information for the experienced ophthalmologist:

- If a hammer has been used, the ophthalmologist immediately suspects that an IOFB is present and that prophylactic chorioretinectomy may be needed.
- If an explosion occurred, multiple IOFBs may be present.
- If the object is long and sharp, there is a high probability of retinal injury.
- If a blunt object caused the injury, occult rupture may have occurred, and lens extrusion is always a possibility.

4 One example is a contact lens examination of an eye with hyphema: the evaluation of the angle should be deferred until the risk of secondary bleeding has subsided.

5 An eye injury is a mentally, not only physically, traumatic event; much like being in the "fog of war," the injury's circumstances may be difficult for the person to discern. This is the reason why the ophthalmologist should not be a passive listener when taking history but an active "interrogator", why taking history is as much an art as much as it is science, and why being able to also question an eyewitness is so valuable.

Table 1.9.1 The basic questions in taking the history after a mechanical eye injury

Question[1]	Comment
What happened?	General circumstances are sought
Have other body parts also been injured?	A negative answer does not necessarily imply that such an injury has not occurred
What object caused the injury?	Only blunt objects can cause occult ruptures; conversely, an IOFB must always be suspected if a sharp object is the culprit
Is the object available?	Examination of the object can yield important additional information[2]
Was the injury self-inflicted?[3]	The injured person may be a bystander, or a victim of assault or domestic violence
When did the injury occur?	This has significant implications for management
Where did injury take place?	The possibility of soil contamination has utmost importance
	An injury at the workplace has legal implications
What were the initial symptoms?	Loss of vision is the most crucial information
Have the symptoms changed since?	An increase of pain may signal severe intraocular hemorrhage; in children, the lens may become cataractous within hours
What treatment has been applied so far?	Information on topical (e.g., irrigation, foreign body removal) as well as systemic (oral, intravenous) medications is equally important

[1] The line of questions must be adopted to the demands of the individual case.

[2] e.g., the IOFB is often a splinter from the hammer itself, rather than from the object that was hit with the hammer

[3] Caution is always advised with the answer, especially in children.

In *children*, the art of history taking requires even more special skills than usual [7]. The child may be unable (e.g., because of young age, pain, fright) or unwilling to describe what happened. Children even lie (Munchausen's syndrome [16]) about the event to "cover up" an activity perceived as impermissible or to hide the presence/responsibility of another person[6] (see Chap. 2.16 for further details).

In *elderly* patients, difficulties may arise if the person's memory is poor and they are unable to recall exactly what happened.

If it is possible, questioning a *witness* about the event is extremely useful.

1.9.3.2 Subjective Testing of Visual Functions

1.9.3.2.1 Visual Acuity

Unless the patient is unconscious or very uncooperative, or the injury is caused by a chemical agent, it is imperative that the ophthalmologist determines the visual acuity[7] in both the injured and the fellow eye[8] (see Table 1.7.4).

- Care must be taken that the uninjured eye is properly covered during the test.
- Whenever possible, standard charts (Snellen, ETDRS) should be used; for illiterate persons or preliterate children the E or C charts should substitute.
- In infants, fixation and pursuit should be tested.
- In immobilized patients the near card can be used or a gross measurement be taken (e.g., LP, HM/CF at a given distance; there should be proper contrast between finger and background).

6 This is of special importance if child abuse is suspected (see Chap. 3.3).

7 The goal is not to obtain the "best-corrected" visual acuity value but one that serves as an acceptable basis to compare the post-treatment visual acuity with. The pinhole, if the patient can utilize it, is of great help.

8 The fellow eye's *major* findings should also be recorded during the evaluation; however, a detailed examination of the fellow eye should be postponed until after the acute treatment phase.

Testing for NLP must be done with the strongest light of the slit lamp *and* of the indirect ophthalmoscope. The test should be conducted so that no "click" is audible, and both tests should be done in "two directions": changing from darkness to light, and vice versa.

Pearl

Careful testing to determine whether the eye has NLP or LP vision is performed not to justify choosing reconstruction or enucleation but primarily for prognostic purposes (see Chap. 1.8).

Especially if worker's compensation issues are at stake, malingering may have to be ruled out [5].

1.9.3.2.2 Confrontational Visual Field

This simple test may reveal severe retinal injury or optic nerve damage.[9]

1.9.3.2.3 Color Vision

Color vision testing is rarely used in the setting of acute trauma, even though the red saturation phenomenon[10] is a useful indicator of optic nerve damage [6].

1.9.3.3 Objective Testing of Visual Functions

1.9.3.3.1 Pupils

- The *shape* and *position* of the pupil in the injured eye are noted: a drawn or asymmetrical pupil may signal presence of an open wound and iris prolapse.
- The *diameter* of both pupils should be recorded; dilation can be caused by iris trauma (sphincter damage), scattering of incoming light (e.g., vitreous hemorrhage), or by eye's inability to properly perceive light

9 The examiner's hand or a strong light source is used as the target.

10 Compared with the intact other side, the redness of the object appears diminished with time if the optic nerve is damaged.

(retinal or optic nerve damage). Anisocoria can also be caused by damage to the sympathetic fibers (causing miosis); this is characterized by greater anisocoria under scotopic than under photopic conditions.[11]

- Testing the pupils' *reaction* to direct and consensual light.
- If the pupil is nonreactive, it should be determined whether the afferentation (APD) or efferentation is responsible (Fig. 1.9.1).

1.9.3.3.2 Electrophysiology

The test is virtually never used in the acute setting. Contrary to the wildly held belief, the predictive value of ERG [4] is limited; even the *bright flash ERG* may be nonrecordable in the presence of massive vitreous hemorrhage [14]. This test, just as the loss of LP, should not never serve as justification to forgo reconstructive surgery (see Chap. 1.8).

Conversely, the ERG is useful in determining the need for intervention with chronic, otherwise symptomless IOFBs (see Chap. 2.13) [18].

The *VEP* is able to monitor the changes after optic nerve trauma [13].

1.9.3.4 Miscellaneous Other Tests

1.9.3.4.1 Motility

The most important indication of motility testing is a suspected orbital injury [11]. Direct muscle or cranial nerve trauma is rare, and if the ophthalmoplegia cannot be explained by adnexal or orbital injury, a neurosurgeon should be consulted to rule out a central origin. Severe lid edema or orbital hemorrhage, or the lack of patient cooperation, makes the motility test impossible to conduct. If orbital wall fracture with muscle entrapment is suspected and open globe injury can be ruled out, the forced duction test [8, 17] should be performed to distinguish nerve/muscle trauma from entrapment (see Chap. 4.4).

---

11 Traumatic Horner's syndrome

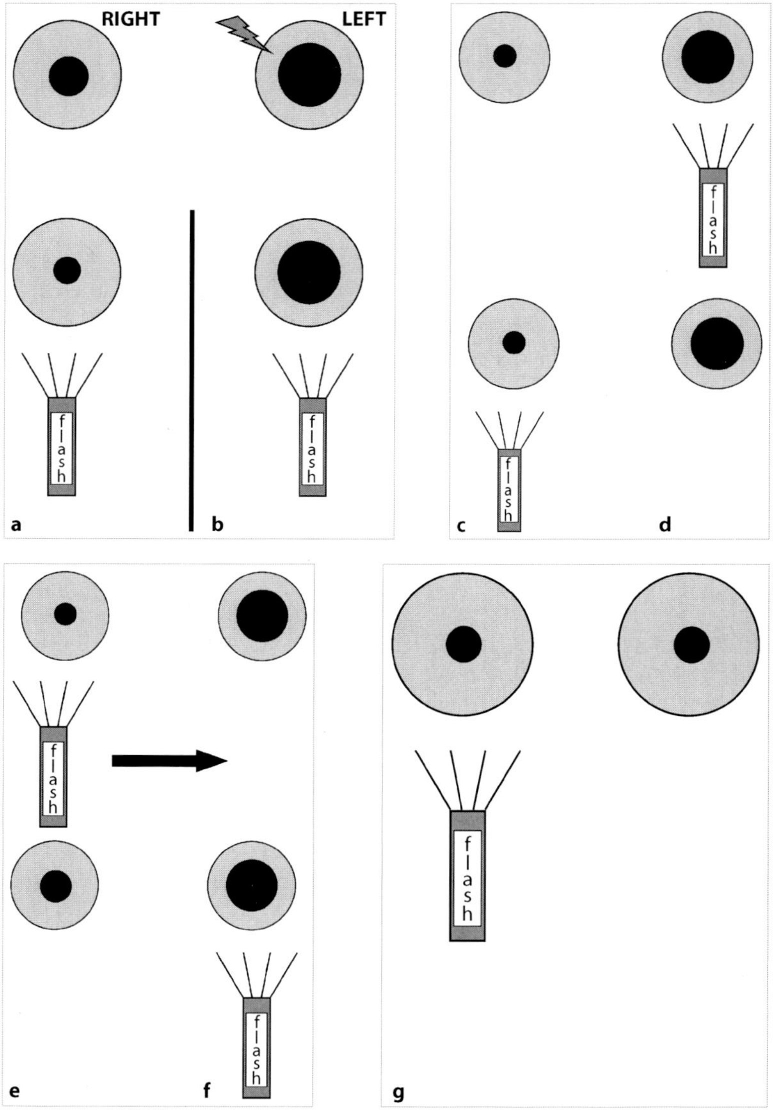
RIGHT
LEFT
flash
a
b
c
d
e
f
g

Fig. 1.9.1 Differential diagnostics in case of a dilated pupil.[1] **a** The left eye is injured and has a dilated pupil; the right eye is not injured. **b** The left pupil does not react to light shone *separately* into the two eyes. **c** If the *afferentation* in the left eye is intact, the right eye's pupil will react to the light shone into the left eye (consensual reaction). **d** If the light is shone into the right eye and the left pupil remains dilated, *efferentation* or a local pathology is the problem (see Table 2.6.1). **e,f** Diagnosis of an APD. By swinging the flashlight between the two eyes and observing the right eye from which the light is moved over to the left eye, the right pupil's dilation is noticed since it now does not receive consensual signal from the left eye. **g** If in the left the *efferentation* is unaffected (and there is no local pathology, see above) and the light is shone into the right eye, the left pupil also reacts via the consensual reaction

[1] Inthe scenario shown here, normal conditions are present in the right eye.

1.9.3.4.2 IOP[12]

- In case of an *acute* injury, a low IOP (or palpation estimate) may be found, suggestive of an occult rupture; however, a normal or even higher value does not rule out the presence of an open wound: the wound can spontaneously close and an intraocular hemorrhage can actually elevate the IOP.

Pearl

Treatment decisions should therefore not be based on whether the IOP is normal, low, or high.

In *chronic* cases, IOP elevation can be caused by many factors. Its proper treatment is one of the more neglected aspects of ocular traumatology (see Chap. 2.18).

1.9.3.5 External Inspection

First under bright diffuse illumination, then with a penlight, the periocular regions as well as the globes should be meticulously evaluated. The exami-

12 Tonometry should be performed only in eyes without a visible open wound.

nation is made much easier if the fellow eye/periocular regions are normal and can be used for comparison.

- Inspect the periocular region for wounds, hemorrhages, edema, ptosis, FBs, and any bony asymmetry or step-off deformity.
- Examine the eye's position (eso/exo/hypo/hyperphoria) and location (sideways dislocation, enophthalmos, or exophthalmos). Looking at the patient's forehead from above is a good indication of whether the eye is pushed inward or outward, but the Hertel prism yields an accurate and reproducible measurement. The globe may also luxate in front of the lids.
- Inspect the globe for wounds, tissue prolapse, chemosis, hemorrhage, and FBs, both superficial and protruding. If the lids are swollen, careful exploration using a speculum/lid retractor[13] may be performed if the patient cooperates. If the swelling is very severe, it may be impossible to open them without exerting major pressure on the globe. In such cases ice packs and corticosteroid ointment should be applied to reduce the swelling as rapidly as possible.

Cave

If the lids are swollen, an assistant should help to hold the lids apart. The pressure must be exerted over the bone, never over the globe (Fig. 1.9.2).

- Periocular subcutaneous hemorrhage, especially if it is fairly symmetrical and bilateral, should always raise the possibility of skull basis fracture.
- Liquorrhea may also be found and should be treated as an emergency.

The lids may have to everted to allow gross examination of the tarsal conjunctiva (see Chap. 2.1).

13 See Chap. 2.1 for retractor use.

Gentle *palpation* of the periocular region is an often neglected part of the examination. Palpation can help finding bone dislocation and subcutaneous foreign bodies and air. It can also elicit pain, which signifies an underlying pathology. Estimating the IOP may also be an indication for palpation if the traditional methods of pressure-taking are not feasible (see above).

- If bone asymmetry is found, testing for infraorbital hypo/anesthesia is recommended.
- If the lids are swollen without a proportional hemorrhage being present, palpate for crepitus. If crepitation is found, forbid nose-blowing, and ask for ear–nose–throat consultation.

1.9.3.6 Slit Lamp

The slit lamp is able to provide crucial information on the periocular soft tissues and the anterior segment of the globe (Fig. 1.9.3) [9],[14] even the anterior vitreous.

When examining the cornea, it may be necessary to determine whether a recent wound is self-sealing or it leaks. The Seidel test is performed by momentarily inserting a wet fluorescein strip into the conjunctival cul-de-sac, and examining the ocular surface under blue light. If there is aqueous leak,[15] the fairly stagnant yellowish dye cover is broken by a green stream originating from the wound.

Chapter 2.2 provides additional details on how to use the slit lamp to examine the cornea and how to utilize certain vital stains. Retroillumination is a very useful technique to show pathologies such as pigment deposits on the lens surface, loss of iris pigmentation, occluded iridectomy, or lens subluxation.

If the lids can be separated and the media are clear, the vitreous and the retina can be examined with a 90-diopter lens. The image is erect and has

---

14 Virtually all conditions listed in Chaps. 2.1–2.7, and many in Chaps. 2.11–2.15 are diagnosed using the slit lamp; see these chapters for further information.

15 Mild pressure on the globe may be necessary to "provoke" the leak.

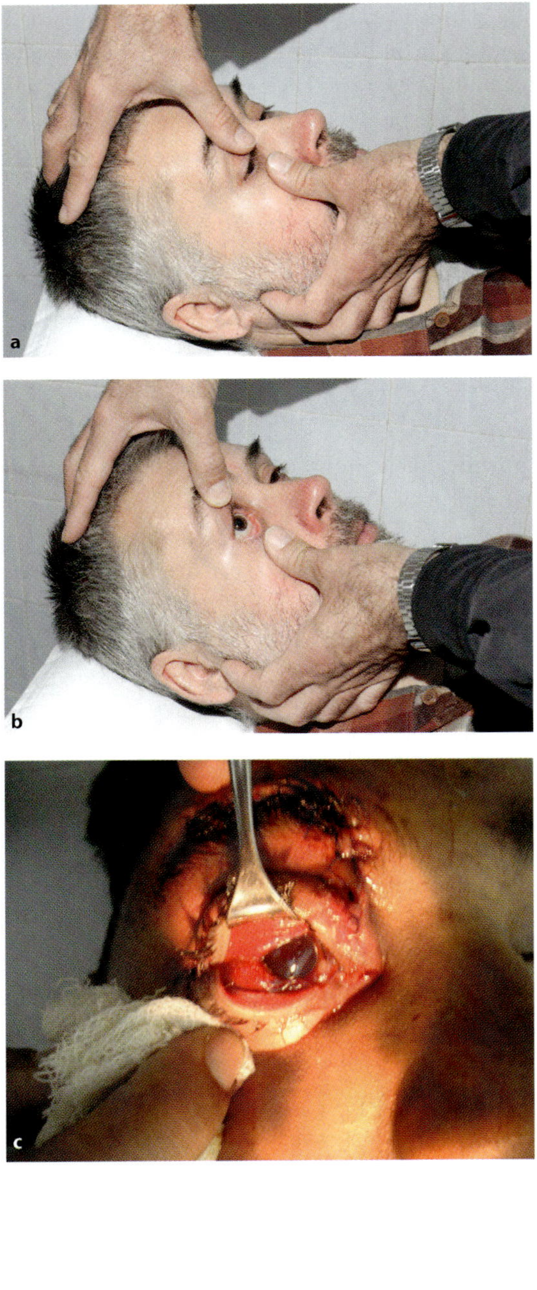

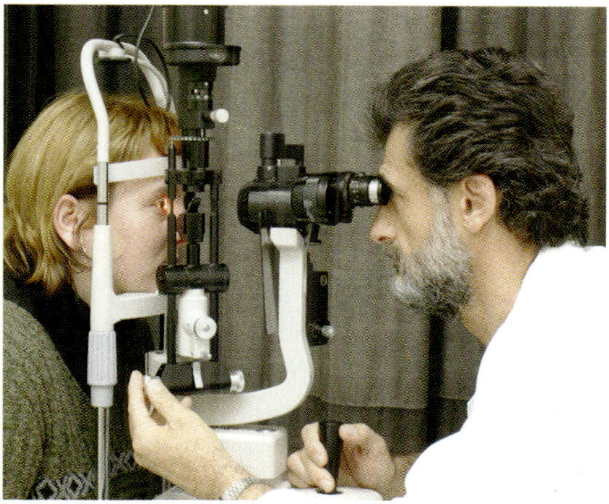

Fig. 1.9.3 Slit-lamp evaluation of the cornea A superficial corneal FB is being identified. The angle and power of illumination are adjusted by the examiner's left hand

Fig. 1.9.2 Spreading the lids for inspection.[1] **a** The assistant's fingers are gently placed over the lids; the patient is asked not to squeeze; the lids are carefully pulled apart. **b** Now that the fissure is open, pressure can be applied to keep the lids in this position. Notice that this pressure is over the orbital bones, not over the globe.[2] **c** A combination of using a finger and a Desmarres lid retractor may also be utilized (Photograph courtesy of D. Kalra, Panchkula, India)

[1] Gloves must be worn if blood is present; the use of gauze is helpful if the lids are slippery.

[2] Even if an open globe injury were present, the intraocular contents are unlikely to be extruded due to the lack of external pressure on the eye itself.

a higher magnification than ophthalmoscopy, allowing evaluation of finer details. The angle and the retinal periphery can be examined with a three-mirror contact lens, although this examination should not be performed if the injury is open globe.

1.9.3.7 Ophthalmoscopy

Unless media opacity interfere, the indirect ophthalmoscope[16] is able to provide a wealth of information on the vitreous and retina. The image is inverted but 3D and a large area[17] of the vitreous and retina can simultaneously be observed. By directing the patient to move the eye side to side and up and down, the dynamic components of certain vitreoretinal pathologies can be observed. The test is ideally performed with the patient in a supine position (Fig. 1.9.4) to spare the ophthalmologist of uncomfortable body postures.

Scleral indentation should be used only if the examiner is first able to rule out the presence of an open wound.

1.9.3.8 Imaging Studies

Whether and which type of imaging test to use is not always an easy decision. The indication is primarily for diagnostic but also for medicolegal purposes. It is important to realize that no test is 100% reliable; therefore, the test results must always be interpreted within the context of the entirety of the specific situation. The inability to identify an IOFB does not necessarily mean that none is present (see below); conversely, a test may be false positive. If the test is negative but history is strongly suggestive, the surgeon should presume that history is correct.

16 Obviously, a binocular ophthalmoscope is used.

17 The size of the area and the magnification also depend on the power (20 or 28 D) of the double aspheric lens used.

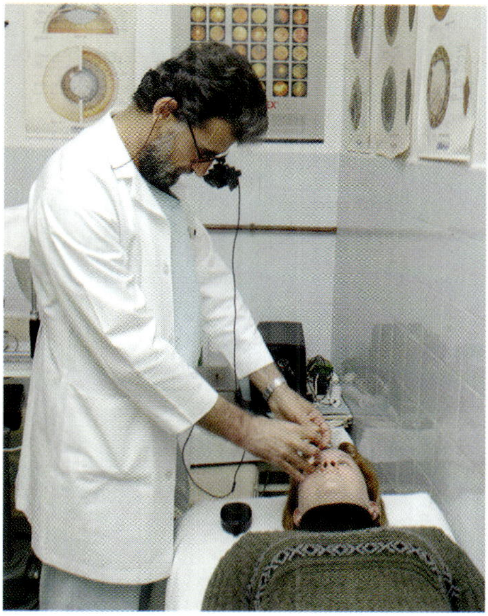

Fig. 1.9.4 The proper technique of indirect ophthalmoscopy. The ophthalmologist is standing with a straight back. The patient is in a supine position, and his head is slightly elevated

1.9.3.8.1 Ultrasonography

In the hands of an experienced examiner, the B-scan is a reliable method to demonstrate both static and dynamic pathologies of the eye. A series of tests conducted over time allows observing how the condition progresses.

Pearl

Ultrasonography should be performed by the surgeon who is in the best position to correlate the test's results with the clinical findings.

With improving technology (20-MHz transducer), high-resolution images can be obtained [2], revealing information about the presence/absence of:

- Eye wall wounds
- IOFBs (whether these are radiolucent or opaque)
- Lens/IOL dislocation

- Condition of the posterior lens capsule
- Vitreous hemorrhage and other opacities (e.g., due to endophthalmitis)
- PVD[18]
- Vitreous incarceration into a wound
- Vitreous mobility and vitreoretinal adhesions
- Retinal breaks
- Retinal detachment, distinguishing between serous, tractional, and hemorrhagic
- Choroidal thickening/detachment

Cave

Even an experienced trauma surgeon may not be able to differentiate on the B scan between a PVD and a detached retina in an eye with dense hemorrhage (Fig. 1.9.5); other diagnostic traps also exist in ultrasonography of the injured eye (Fig. 1.9.6).

A contact method, ultrasonography is risky if the eye has an open globe injury. Although under sterile conditions and with great care it is possible to conduct the test, tissue extrusion and contamination remain a concern.[19]

1.9.3.8.1.1 Ultrasound Biomicroscopy

This test may be the sole method[20] of identifying distinct anterior segment pathologies such as IOL haptic dislocation, presence of an IOFB at the iris root, ciliary epithelium detachment, or trabecular meshwork tearing [3]. It is also the best method to diagnose a cyclodialysis (see Chap. 2.8). The test is not recommended if the injury is open globe, and, to prevent an iat-

18 The usefulness of ultrasonography is highly questionable (see Chap. 2.9 and Fig. 1.9.5).

19 A safer alternative is to utilize it in the OR under sterile conditions after the wound has been sutured.

20 Noninvasive; endoscopy (see Chap. 2.20) is an invasive alternative.

rogenic hemorrhage, pressure on the eye should not be exerted even if the injury is a contusion.

1.9.3.8.2 X-ray

Once a mainstay of detecting otherwise invisible pathologies, such as an IOFB in eyes with vitreous hemorrhage, the test is rarely used today because of a high false-negative reading rate [15].

1.9.3.8.3 Computed Tomography

Modern (helical) CTs constitute the most accurate and thus most often used radiological method in evaluating the injured eye and especially the orbit [10, 12]. The noncontact test is able to determine the presence/absence of:

- Optic nerve damage
- Orbital and facial fractures
- Orbital pathologies such as hemorrhage, abscess, air
- Extraocular muscle damage

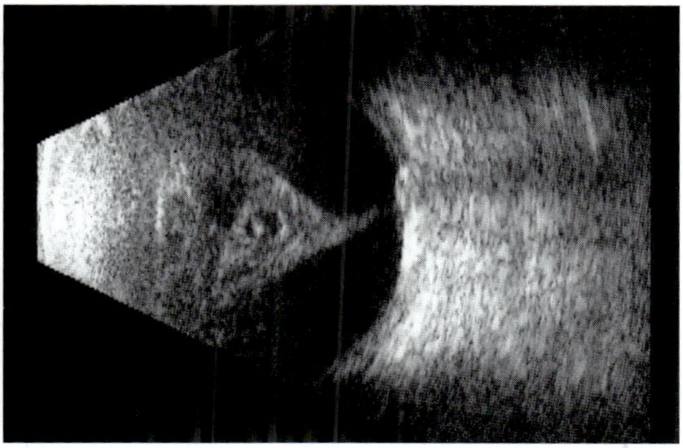

Fig. 1.9.5 Ultrasonography of a severely injured eye: PVD or a retinal detachment? The interpretation of the test in this 9-year-old boy who sustained a rupture was "total retinal detachment inserting on the optic nerve; retina very thin at insertion." During surgery, no retinal detachment was found after the vitreous hemorrhage had been removed

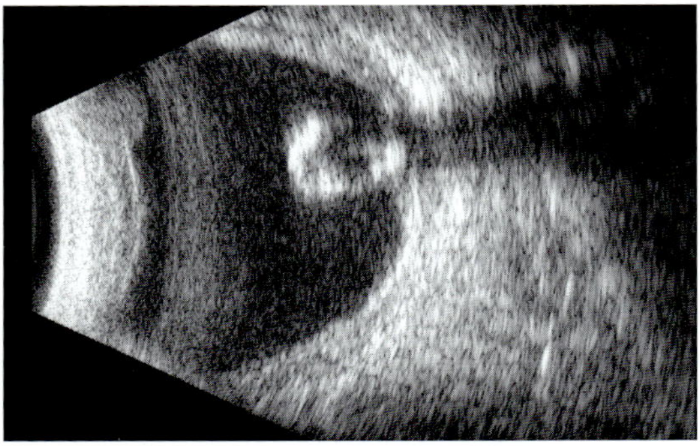

Fig. 1.9.6 Ultrasound image of an "IOFB." The patient had a chronic IOFB injury. The eye was aphakic but vitreous hemorrhage prevented direct inspection of the posterior pole. The mass suspected to be the IOFB on the ultrasonogram proved to be the calcified crystalline lens. The IOFB has dissolved over time and was not found during surgery

- Intraorbital and intraocular FBs[21]
- Occult scleral wounds
- Certain additional intraocular pathologies (e.g., intraocular air, lens damage, vitreous hemorrhage, retinal detachment)

The radiologist should always be consulted about the expected pathology so that he can set the parameters (thickness of cuts or, occasionally, the use of contrast materials if vascular trauma is suspected) of the test accordingly. Figures 1.9.7–1.9.9 show various pathologies detected on CT.

Cave

Although CT is a very sensitive method for detecting a wide variety of pathologies, a negative test reading should not be considered as an absolute indicator that a pathology (i.e., an IOFB) is not present.

21 The surgeon must be careful when interpreting the CT measurements of an IOFB: the test overestimates the real IOFB size by 17–129%; the enlargement factor depends on the composition of the IOFB (D. Briscoe et al., in press).

1.9.3.8.4 Magnetic Resonance Imaging

Pearl

The test provides superior images of all soft tissues (Fig. 1.9.10), and can detect very small nonmetallic[22] IOFBs [20]. It is expensive, though, and some patients may object to it for feeling claustrophobic "in the tube."

1.9.3.8.5 OCT

While an increasingly important diagnostic tool, the use of OCT in acute trauma cases is extremely limited. The method is exceptionally effective, however, in identifying several pathologies (e.g., macular hole, EMP) that can be surgically treated or in showing the spontaneous resolution of such pathologies [1]. High-speed, ultra-high-resolution OCT offers to delineate details never captured before [19].

1.9.3.9 Exploratory Surgery

- In the *acute* phase following the injury, even advanced diagnostic testing may not allow determining whether an occult scleral rupture is present (see Chap. 2.12).
- In such cases the patient should be taken to the OR to verify whether the sclera is intact. Topical anesthesia is usually sufficient[23] to allow opening of the conjunctiva, and draining the blood or removing the clot. Inspection of the sclera far posterior to the equator is dangerous and should not be attempted (see Chap. 2.3).
- In the *subacute* phase (a few days postinjury), the severity of the intraocular damage needs to be determined.

22 It is contraindicated to use MRI in cases of magnetic IOFBs since they can easily be mobilized, risking severe additional injury. Metallic object elsewhere in the body (e.g., pacemakers) are also prohibitive.

23 If extensive manipulations are deemed necessary, other forms of anesthesia are available (see Chap. 1.8).

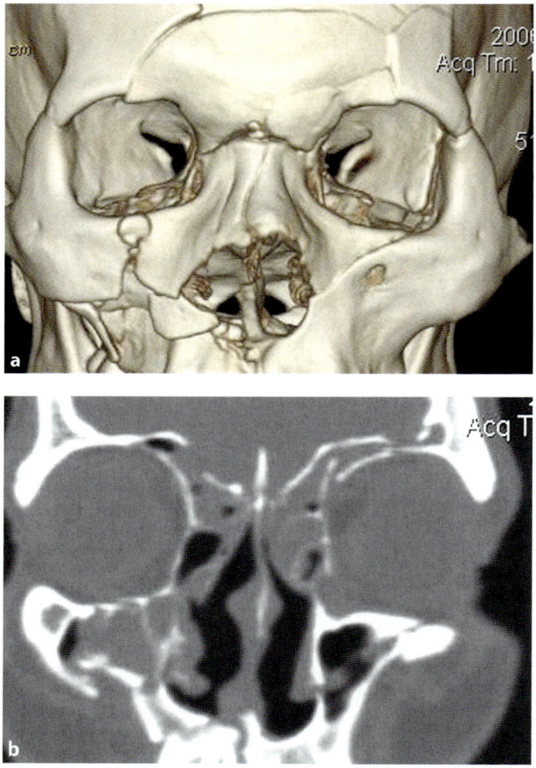

Fig. 1.9.7 CT imaging of multiple cranial fractures (Lefort III). A young male was involved in an MVC. Several fractures are visible, involving, among others, the orbital rim. **a** Coronal image; **b** three-dimensional reconstruction (Courtesy of A. Palkó, Szeged, Hungary)

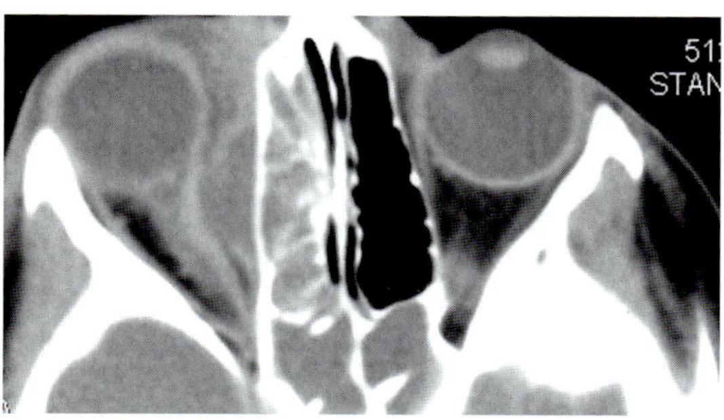

Fig. 1.9.8 CT image of an orbital abscess. An abscess is seen nasally in the right orbit, originating from a fracture of the lamina papiracea (not visible) (Courtesy of A. Palkó, Szeged, Hungary)

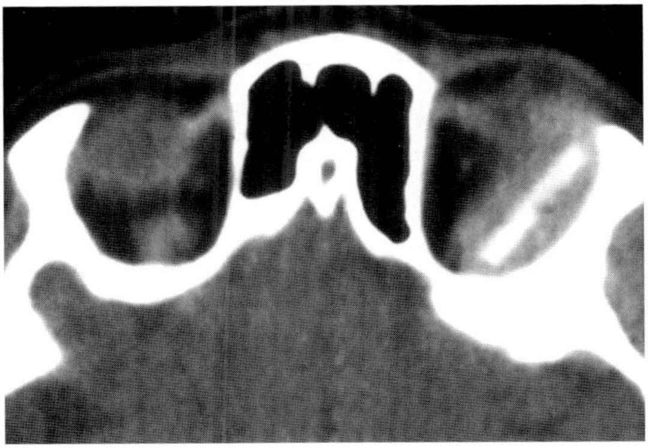

Fig. 1.9.9 CT image of an orbita FB. The hyperdense object (windshield glass fragment) in the left orbit measures 2×2×20 mm on the scan (Courtesy of A. Palkó, Szeged, Hungary)

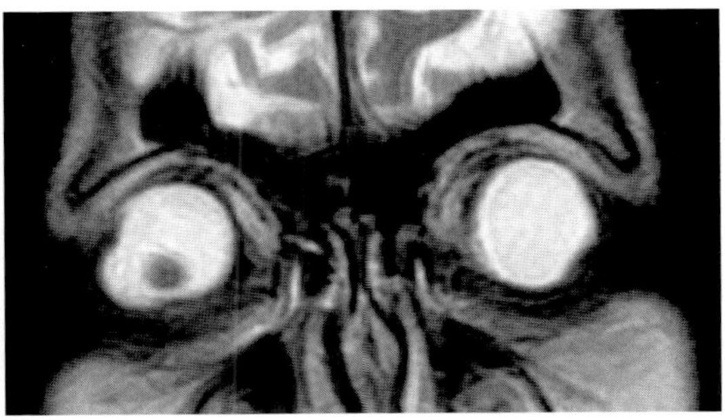

Fig. 1.9.10 An MRI of lens luxation. The accidental discovery[1] of luxation of the right lens; there is no accompanying vitreous hemorrhage. T2 coronal image (Courtesy of A. Palkó, Szeged, Hungary)

[1] The test was conducted for a different disease.

- *Exploratory vitrectomy* can be performed to visualize the postequatorial retina and the optic disc; this alone is a somewhat curative effort since the vitreous hemorrhage must be removed first. The technique is described in Chaps 1.9 and 2.12.

- The *endoscope* may be utilized to in eyes with opaque cornea to allow making an informed decision regarding management (see Chaps. 2.15, 2.20).

Based on the type and extent of the damage found during exploratory surgery, and on the patient's preferences[24], the diagnostic procedure can be extended to become a therapeutic one.

1.9.4 Documentation

As mentioned previously, for both medical and legal purposes it is necessary to meticulously document the information gained during history-taking and examination. In addition to the narrative and the attached test readings, drawings should be made and photographs taken.

To aid in (self-)training and research, both the initial and final outcome data should be reported to a standardized database (www.weironline.org; see Chap. 1.7). Data gathering and analysis of such large data sets are the prerequisite to improve the management of the injured patient.

Further details on evaluation are provided in Chap. 2.11.

DO:

- find the right balance between a patient wanting to describe all minor, often irrelevant, details of the injury vs only letting him answer your questions
- be wary of the possibility of an open globe injury when opening swollen lids
- weigh the usefulness and cost of a diagnostic test before ordering it
- consult with the radiologist before a test is conducted so that he knows exactly what question needs to be answered

24 A detailed discussion of "what to do if we find such and such a pathology" should precede the onset of the procedure (see Chap. 1.4).

DON'T:

- be on "autopilot" when ordering a diagnostic test but tailor it according to the individual case
- neglect entering the case into a standardized eye injury surveillance database

Summary

The purposes of evaluation are to take account of the eye's (patient's) condition as a result of the injury and to gather sufficient information to guide treatment, but also to offer legal protection to the ophthalmologist. The entering of nonidentified data into a surveillance system is crucial for research.

References

[1] Carpineto P, Ciancaglini M, Aharrh-Gnama A, Agnifili L, Cerulli AM, Cirone D, Mastropasqua L (2005) Optical coherence tomography and fundus microperimetry imaging of spontaneous closure of traumatic macular hole: a case report. Eur J Ophthalmol 15: 165–169

[2] Coleman DJ, Silverman RH, Chabi A, Rondeau MJ, Shung KK, Cannata J, Lincoff H (2004) High-resolution ultrasonic imaging of the posterior segment. Ophthalmology 111: 1344–1351

[3] Endo S, Ishida N, Yamaguchi T (2001) Tear in the trabecular meshwork caused by an airsoft gun. Am J Ophthalmol 131: 656–657

[4] Fuller DG, Hutton WL (1990) Prediction of postoperative vision in eyes with severe trauma. Retina 10 (Suppl 1): S20–S34

[5] Harlan J Jr, Ng E, Pieramici D (2002) Evaluation. Thieme, Stuttgart, pp 53–69

[6] Hart WM Jr, Burde RM (1985) Color contrast perimetry. The spatial distribution of color defects in optic nerve and retinal diseases. Ophthalmology 92: 768–776

[7] Jandeck C, Kellner U, Bornfeld N, Foerster M (2000) Open globe injuries in children. Graefe's Arch Ophthalmol 238: 420–426

[8] Kakizaki H, Zako M, Iwaki M, Mito H, Katori N (2005) Incarceration of the inferior oblique muscle branch of the oculomotor nerve in two cases of orbital floor trapdoor fracture. Jpn J Ophthalmol 49: 246–252

[9] Knoop K, Trott A (1995) Ophthalmologic procedures in the emergency department: Part III: Slit lamp use and foreign bodies. Acad Emerg Med 2: 224–230

[10] Lee HJ, Jilani M, Frohman L, Baker S (2004) CT of orbital trauma. Emerg Radiol 10: 168–172

[11] Ludwig IH, Brown MS (2001) Strabismus due to flap tear of a rectus muscle. Trans Am Ophthalmol Soc 99: 53–62

[12] Mafee MF, Mafee RF, Malik M, Pierce J (2003) Medical imaging in pediatric ophthalmology. Pediatr Clin North Am 50: 259–286

[13] Mahapatra A (1992) Optic nerve injury in children. A prospective study of 35 patients. J Neurosurg Sci 36: 79–84

[14] Mandelbaum S, Cleary PE, Ryan SJ, Ogden TE (1980) Bright-flash electroretinography and vitreous hemorrhage. Arch. Ophthalmol. 98: 1823–1828

[15] McElvanney AM, Fielder AR (1993) Intraocular foreign body missed by radiography. Br Med J 306: 1060–1061

[16] Olver J, Hague S (1989) Children presenting to an ophthalmic casualty department. Eye 3: 415–419

[17] Van Eeckhoutte L, De Clippeleir L, Apers R, Van Lammeren M, Janssens H, Baekeland L (1998) A protocol for extraocular muscle surgery after orbital floor fracture ("blow-out"). Binocul Vis Strabismus Q 13: 29–36

[18] Weiss MJ, Hofeldt AJ, Behrens M, Fisher K (1997) Ocular siderosis. Diagnosis and management. Retina 17: 105–108

[19] Wojtkowski M, Srinivasan V, Fujimoto JG, Ko T, Schuman JS, Kowalczyk A, Duker JS (2005) Three-dimensional retinal imaging with high-speed ultrahigh-resolution optical coherence tomography. Ophthalmology 112: 1734–1746

[20] Yoshii M, Enoki T, Mizukawa A, Okisaka S (2004) Intraorbital wooden foreign body. Acta Ophthalmol Scand 82: 492–493

1.10 Emergency Management

Ferenc Kuhn

1.10.1 Introduction and Definition

While the definition of an injury-related ophthalmic emergency may appear straightforward, in reality it is not so unambiguous:

- A *chemical* insult is a clear case of emergency to both patient and ophthalmologist.
- A welder's *photokeratitis* is an absolute emergency to the patient, yet it may cause nothing but aggravation to an ophthalmologist who is awakened at night after a full day of work for such a non-sight-threatening and easily avoidable condition.
- A full-thickness corneal *wound* with iris prolapse leads the ophthalmologist to at least consider an emergency intervention, although the patient does not necessarily understand the acute need for surgery.
- Even ophthalmologists disagree among themselves whether conditions such as an IOFB or a retinal detachment truly require immediate surgery.

The definition of "emergency" depends on the severity of the pathology and on the projected loss of function that would be preventable or reversible with urgent therapy.

In this chapter we include conditions that forces the ophthalmologist and/or the patient to perform or at least consider immediate intervention. The urgency may be due to pain and/or for the fear of irreversible anatomical and/or functional damage. Since all conditions are addressed in other chapters in this book, only a brief summary is provided here, and the reader is referred to the relevant chapters for further information. The conditions are presented in alphabetical order, but their acuteness[1] is indicated by a scale where *** represents an absolute emergency and * represents one that is a relative urgency.

1.10.2 Specific Conditions

1.10.2.1 Chemical Injury***

This is the insult that requires the most urgent intervention, especially if an alkali agent is involved. Alkali agents cause colliquative necrosis: the destruction of tissue continues as long as the agent is present. The agent can penetrate intraocularly, resulting in severe late complications such as secondary glaucoma. Conversely, acid agents cause coagulative necrosis: the process slows down and eventually stops tissue destruction beyond the original insult.[2]

1.10.2.1.1 Recognition

Recognition of the condition is usually easy as the victim immediately seeks medical attention and describes what happened; however, in unconscious patients the ophthalmologist must take a more proactive role.

1.10.2.1.2 Management

As mentioned previously, management must be immediate:[3]

- *Irrigation* is what can arrest the destruction and prevent loss of vision or even the eye. Neutral fluids are preferred, although virtually any fluid suffices if a neutral fluid, such as water, is unavailable. A litmus paper must be used to check the pH in the conjunctival fornix to determine

1 From the ophthalmologist's, not from the patient's, viewpoint
2 This must not be interpreted as if acids could not lead to fatal ocular consequences.
3 "Intervene first and ask later."

when irrigation can be stopped, but the pH must periodically be rechecked to assure that the equilibration is maintained.

- *Mechanical cleansing/debridement*[4] must follow, removing agent remnants and/or necrotic tissue from all surfaces, including the upper fornix. This requires double eversion of the lid, for which a Desmarres lid retractor may be necessary (see Chap 2.1).
- *Complementary treatment* (Table 1.10.1; see Chap. 3.1 for further details).

1.10.2.2 Corneal Erosion*

The erosion can be caused by an object still present (FB on the tarsal conjunctiva) or already withdrawn (e.g., a fingernail), or by noncontact mechanism (e.g., welding). In this condition the patient demands intervention; the urgency is determined by the pain, not by the condition's significance as it relates to vision.

1.10.2.2.1 Recognition

Recognition represents no difficulty because of the excruciating pain. Vital stains can be used to delineate the area of epithelial loss.

1.10.2.2.2 Management

Management is aimed at reepithelialization, preferably without the use of anesthetic drops. (See Chap. 2.2 for further details.)

1.10.2.3 ECH***

In this under-recognized condition,[5] bleeding from a severed ciliary artery rapidly leads to the extrusion of intraocular tissues. Progression is

4 Topical anesthesia may be necessary to alleviate the pain, without which even the irrigation may be difficult to complete. Since all anesthetics are toxic, their application should be kept to a minimum.

5 The author has reviewed 30 eyes removed after severe rupture. All pathological specimens showed significant amounts of suprachoroidal blood, and none were described clinically.

Table 1.10.1 Secondary elements in the acute treatment of patients with chemical injury

Medication (route)	Dosage	Comment
Cycloplegics (topical)	As needed	To keep the pupil wide; avoid vasoconstrictors such as phenylephrin
Corticosteroids (topical)	Hourly or at least several times a day	Discontinue after the first week
Antibiotics (topical)	As needed	To lessen the risk of suprainfection
Antibiotics (oral)	Tetracycline 4×250 mg or doxycycline 2×100 mg daily	To lessen the risk of suprainfection
Sodium citrate (10%) and ascorbate (10%; topical)	Hourly	
Sodium ascorbate	2–4×2 g daily	
Artificial tears (topical)	As needed	
Antiglaucoma (topical, oral)	As needed	
Antipain medication	As needed	
Patching	As needed	To maintain high oxygen supply to cornea, it is preferred not to patch; however, most patients prefer it

halted only when the extruded tissue tamponades the wound or the surgeon closes it.[6]

6 If the condition is caught intraoperatively, the surgeon has at least a chance to arrest it; if it occurs outside the OR, the only chance is literally put a finger on it, trying to tamponade the wound and stop the bleeding.

1.10.2.3.1 Recognition

Recognition is easy when the tissue extrusion is in progress but more difficult once a natural tamponade has stopped it. It is therefore important to always keep in mind the ECH potential when dealing with tissue prolapse.

1.10.2.3.2 Management

Management is straightforward: if an ECH is occurring, the wound must be closed immediately, irrespective of whether tissue gets incarcerated in the wound. This and other complications must be addressed in a subsequent surgery. If the ECH has been tamponaded by prolapsed tissue, cautious intervention is still urgent[7] by an experienced surgeon under proper circumstances in the OR. (See Chaps. 2.4 and 2.8 for additional details.)

1.10.2.4 Endophthalmitis**/***

Since the proportion of eyes having the purulent infection caused by *Bacillus* species is much higher in the context of trauma than following surgery, the presence (or even the risk) of infection constitutes an emergency. Unlike in cases of a chemical injury or ECH, however, minutes do not count; there is a little more time for planning the intervention. One exception is *Bacillus* infection, which can destroy any hope for retaining vision in a matter of hours, making vitrectomy a uniquely urgent indication.

1.10.2.4.1 Recognition

Recognition is much more difficult in the injured eye than in those with a postoperative infection. Even if a hypopyon is not visible, the presence of undue pain may be a helpful hint, as is a stronger than expected periocular reaction (edema, erythema, proptosis).

7 To prevent reopening of the wound by the patient somehow exerting pressure on the eye (even strong squeezing may be enough) or by elevation of the systemic the blood pressure.

1.10.2.4.2 Management

Management is immediate surgery, typically vitrectomy, with intravitreal and systemic antibiotics or antifungal agents. (See Chap. 2.17 for additional details.)

1.10.2.5 High IOP*/***

Although rarely requiring immediate surgical intervention, occasionally the IOP may be very high and difficult to control with medications. The condition is most commonly seen in eyes with severe intraocular hemorrhage or a disrupted crystalline lens, especially in children.

1.10.2.5.1 Recognition

Recognition is easy because of the pain and the high tonometry reading.

1.10.2.5.2 Management

Management is determined by the underlying condition (e.g., removal of the blood or the injured lens). If the IOP is very high, however rare, the case does constitute an emergency. (See Chaps. 2.5, 2.7, and 2.18 for further details.)

1.10.2.6 NLP vision**/***

Although this is a functional finding, not a pathology, loss of the eye's ability to recognize light is – and should be – a condition that the ophthalmologist appreciates as an emergency. The direct cause for the loss of LP may be intraocular (bleeding, retinal detachment) or intraorbital (see below).

1.10.2.6.1 Recognition

Recognition is straightforward; as opposed to common practice, a candle or a penlight projects insufficient light to determine whether vision is truly NLP.

1.10.2.6.2 Management

Management is immediate: orbital decompression if the cause is orbital; if an intraocular etiology is responsible, which is the majority of the cases, early surgery is to be performed, after extensive counseling. (See Chap. 1.8 for further details.)

1.10.2.7 Open Wound**

Deferring closure for a few hours has no adverse impact on the outcome; however, urgent closure is necessary if the risk of ECH or infection is high.

1.10.2.7.1 Recognition

Recognition is usually easy at the slit lamp, although occult ruptures can pose a significant diagnostic dilemma (see Chaps. 1.9, 2.12).

1.10.2.7.2 Management

Management is proper wound closure unless the wound is securely self-sealing or too posterior. (See Chaps. 1.8, 2.2–2.4, 2.11–2.14 for additional details.)

1.10.2.8 Orbital Cellulitis**/***

Prior to the antibiotic age, blindness and death from orbital cellulitis were common. The prognosis is much better today, but the condition is still serious enough to warrant immediate and appropriate therapy.

1.10.2.8.1 Recognition

Recognition is relatively easy with proptosis and ophthalmoplegia being the lead symptoms. Pain, especially on eye movement, is also present. The lids are livid and swollen, as is the conjunctiva, and there may be purulent discharge.

1.10.2.8.2 Management

Management primarily consists of intravenous, broad-spectrum antibiotics, although surgical drainage may also become necessary. If an ophthalmologist specialized in the orbit is unavailable, an ear–nose–throat specialist or a neurosurgeon should be consulted.

1.10.2.9 Orbital Hemorrhage*/***

Bleeding into the orbit can occur both in the context of penetrating trauma[8] or a contusion. The condition is benign if the amount of blood is small, but it may warrant instant intervention if it results in the loss of LP and the intraorbital and intraocular pressures are highly elevated so that the central retinal artery becomes occluded.

1.10.2.9.1 Recognition

Recognition is relatively straightforward, as there are signs of a elevated intraorbital pressure (e.g., pain, decreased motility, proptosis, swollen lids).

1.10.2.9.2 Management

Management is medical in mild cases, but canthotomy or cantholysis has to also be considered if the retinal perfusion is seriously affected. Lateral orbitotomy is necessary if the central retinal artery does not reopen. If an ophthalmologist specialized in the orbit is unavailable, an ear–nose–throat specialist or a neurosurgeon should be consulted.

1.10.2.10 Retinal Detachment*/**

For many ophthalmologists a nontraumatic retinal detachment represents an emergency condition.[9] Conversely, a traumatic retinal detachment often does not invoke the same sense of urgency. Closing the wound during the first intervention and deferring retinal reattachment surgery for a few days is not uncommon, even though common sense does argue for very early intervention.

Within the retinal detachment category, a hemorrhagic macular detachment, especially if the subretinal blood is thick, constitutes a real emer-

8 Can be the consequence of a retro- or even peribulbar injection

9 For many ophthalmologists, a retinal detachment calls for a Saturday night operation if need be, and deferral of the case until the regular Monday morning shift is unacceptable, for medical and legal reasons.

gency since photoreceptor death can occur within a very short period of time.

1.10.2.10.1 Recognition

Recognition is much more difficult than in a nontraumatic setting since the visual acuity may be poor for other reasons (e.g., vitreous hemorrhage) and ultrasonography may not be performed acutely or its interpretation can be misleading (see Fig. 1.9.5).

1.10.2.10.2 Management

Management depends on the type and extent of the retinal detachment and on the coexisting tissue injuries. (See Chap. 2.9 for additional details.)

1.10.2.11 TON**

A variety of conditions can cause TON, and some of the consequences may be reversible with proper intervention.

1.10.2.11.1 Recognition

Recognition is difficult and may require advanced radiological testing; an APD is always present.

1.10.2.11.2 Management

Management is usually medical (high-dose intravenous methylprednisolone therapy), although surgical intervention (optic canal/sheath decompression) may also become necessary.

DO:

- be mentally prepared to deal with ophthalmic emergencies and also have the facility ready (materials, personnel); in cases of chemical trauma, irrigation should not be delayed for the sake of taking a detailed history

DON'T:

- forget that pain caused by, and the severity of, the condition are usually inversely proportional
- delay vitrectomy if a Bacillus infection can be suspected
- rush to close an injury-associated open wound, nor defer it beyond a few hours

Summary

There are relatively few diseases in ophthalmology where treatment delay can be catastrophic. In traumatology, a disproportionally high number of such conditions exist. Since there may be no time available to consult a colleague or a textbook, extensive knowledge of how to recognize and act in such conditions is mandatory for all practicing ophthalmologists.

SECTION II

2.1 Conjunctiva

Ferenc Kuhn

2.1.1 Introduction

The conjunctiva's role is neither visual nor structural, but it does offer protection against chemical agents and FBs with low momentum. It is highly vascularized and therefore its wounds heal rapidly.

2.1.2 Evaluation

The procedure for evaluation is as follows:

- The bulbar conjunctiva is easy to examine with the naked eye, a penlight, or, preferably, the slit lamp.
- The lower fornix is examined by pulling the lid down and having the patient look up. This also allows inspection of the lower palpebral conjunctiva.
- The upper (tarsal) palpebral conjunctiva is more difficult to visualize and requires patient cooperation throughout the entire process.
  - Explain to the patient, especially if it is a child, that no pain will be experienced but that the lack of cooperation may cause discomfort and loss of a few eyelashes.
  - Throughout the process, repeatedly remind the patient to keep looking down with both eyes *open* and that looking up is counterproductive.
  - A long, narrow, rigid object (e.g., instrument handle, match stick, glass rod, or even the finger of an experienced examiner) is necessary (Figs. 2.1.1).

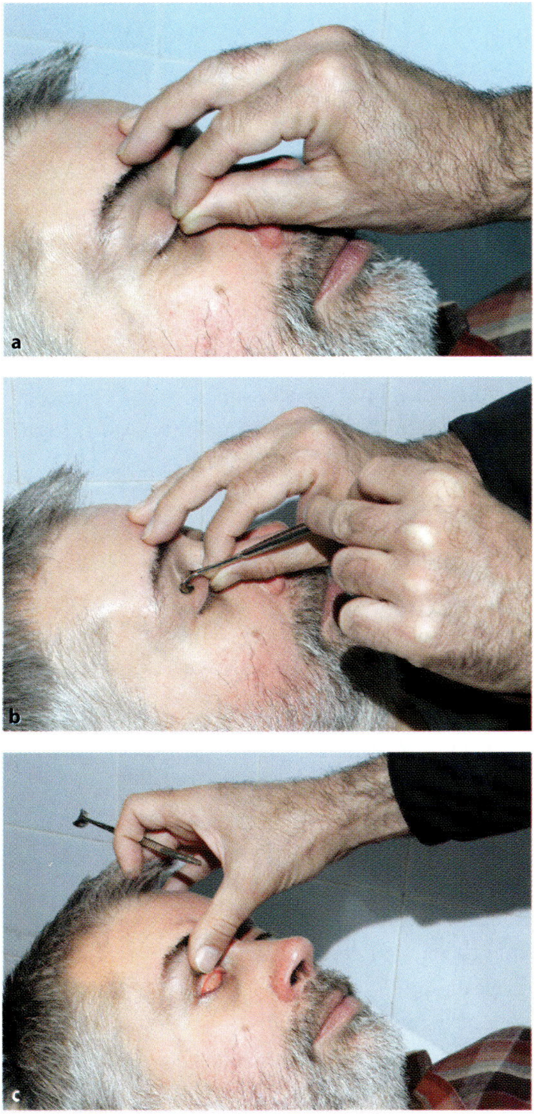

Fig. 2.1.1 Eversion of the upper eyelid. **a** The upper lid is grabbed by the eyelashes; the patient is asked to keep the eye open and look down. **b** The lid is gently pulled downward, a rigid tool (e.g., Desmarres retractor) is used to push down on the upper edge of the tarsus; the lid is then turned upwards until the tarsus "flips," revealing the tarsal conjunctiva. **c** The everted tarsus can easily be held in this position for inspection and intervention unless the patient looks up or wants to close the eye

- The superior fornix is much more difficult to bring into view; it requires double eversion of the lid using a Desmarres lid retractor[1] (see Fig. 3.1.2) and a light source to that can be directed so as to illuminate this hard-to-access area.
- Vital stains can also be used, but their significance is less important for conjunctival than for corneal trauma (see Chap. 2.2).

2.1.3 Specific Injuries

2.1.3.1 Erosion

Loss of the conjunctival epithelium is much less painful than that of the cornea, and healing is fast. When de-epithelization occurs in the context of a chemical injury and is accompanied by ischemia, the condition is extremely serious and requires immediate treatment (see Chaps. 1.10, 3.1). Stains can be useful in showing the defect in the epithelium (Table 2.2.3).

If there is pain associated with an erosion, antibiotic ointment can be applied as a lubricant.

1 Once the lid is everted, the Desmarres everter is inserted between the lid and the globe. The maneuver is not easy, requires close patient cooperation, and access to this narrow space is still limited and difficult.

2.1.3.2 Chemosis

Conjunctival edema is a pathology that may accompany virtually any type of eye trauma. While itself insignificant, it may point toward severe conditions such as chemical injury, endophthalmitis, orbital hemorrhage, or carotid–cavernous fistula. The severity of the underlying pathology and the degree of chemosis are not necessarily proportional.

There is no specific treatment: the causative condition must be addressed. Corticosteroids may help reduce the edema.

2.1.3.3 Emphysema

Intra- or subconjunctival air can originate from external sources such as a ruptured pressurized air hose. More commonly, however, the source is a paranasal sinus in the presence of an orbital fracture [3]. Blowing the nose exacerbates the emphysema and should strongly be discouraged until the etiology is treated (see Chap. 1.9).

Removal of the air is not necessary; once the resupply is cut off, the air quickly absorbs.

2.1.3.4 Hemorrhage

Being a richly vascularized tissue that quickly responds to virtually any noxa by dilatation of the blood vessels, intra- and subconjunctival hemorrhages commonly occur in trauma (Fig. 2.1.2). The etiology and significance varies and includes:

- Spontaneous ("idiopathic")
- Systemic conditions (e.g., physical strain;[2] hypertension [1]; amyloidosis)
- Minor trauma such as (inadvertent) rubbing of the eye
- Major injury

2 Especially in the context of a Valsalva maneuver (see Chapter 3.3).

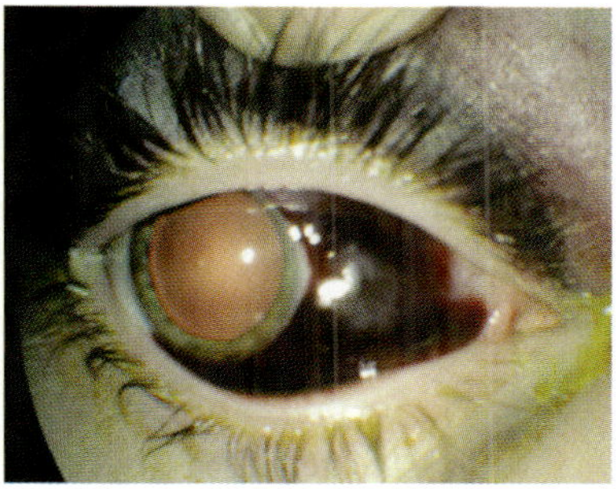

Fig. 2.1.2 Thick subconjunctival hemorrhage. The patient sustained a fist injury. The appearance of the blood raises suspicion that a scleral rupture may also have occurred, especially because the IOP is 7 mmHg; however, the lid hemorrhage is a telling sign that at least some of the force was blocked by the orbital bones. The visual acuity is good, there is excellent red reflex, and the subconjunctival hemorrhage itself affects a limited area. All of these indications point to a closed globe injury. In this case a detailed fundus examination is possible to conduct and will determine whether an occult rupture is present

The significance of the condition lies not in the presence of blood, which absorbs spontaneously and without adverse consequences.[3] The real danger is a thick layer of blood concealing an underlying wound (occult scleral rupture; see Chaps. 2.3, 2.12).

The condition itself does not require treatment.

2.1.3.5 Foreign Body

Superficial objects are usually easy to recognize and remove.[4] Virtually any tool can be used, including the tip of finger or the edge of a preferably wet-

3 Even if the conspicuous discoloration, which can persist for weeks and change color with time, may be disturbing to some people.

4 If superglue is the object, it generally does not stick to a wet surface. If it did stick, it is impossible to remove nonsurgically but the glue patch will spontaneously detach in a few days. Whether surgical removal is indicated depends on how rough its surface is and how much complaint it causes.

ted, clean napkin. The FBs embedded deeper require some type of a sharp instrument and often topical anesthesia as well.

Pearl

Anesthetizing a small area of the conjunctiva is best done not with drops but a moisturized cotton-tipped applicator held over the area for a minute.

- If the FB is lodged in the upper fornix, recognition may be delayed[5] and removal difficult. The most common object to be involved is the wing of an insect.
- Sharp objects on the upper tarsal conjunctiva cause the most pain since they scratch the cornea with each blink; their removal brings tremendous relief to the patient.
- The FB may be subconjunctival and thus harder to find. If it is inert and does not cause symptoms, it can be left in situ. Spontaneously FB delivery can also occur with time.

2.1.3.6 Wound

Regardless of the type of agent, the conjunctival wound is always a laceration.[6] The conjunctiva is elastic and mobile and therefore very resistant to trauma from blunt objects [6]. The wound has important management implications related to the entire globe (Chap. 2.11), and it may warn the ophthalmologist of an underlying pathology such as a clear wound with or without the presence of an IOFB (see Fig. 2.13.1).

- Small conjunctival wounds need not be closed. Cleansing, disinfection, and short-term antibiotic treatment suffice.

---

5 The symptoms may not present early; even a granuloma may develop before the patient seeks medical help.

6 I.e., even if the eye sustained a rupture, the conjunctiva itself is not ruptured but torn due a shearing force.

- Larger wounds require closure. Suturing of the conjunctiva is easy, but *proper* suturing requires recognition of certain characteristics that are unique to the conjunctiva. This is especially important if the wound is at or near the limbus.
- In most cases, the conjunctiva remains attached to the underlying Tenon' capsule and the two are treated as if being a single layer.
- The conjunctiva is anchored at the limbus and to a much lesser degree over the extraocular muscles, but the tissue is extremely mobile everywhere else.[7]
- The conjunctiva does not offer resistance against manipulation or needle introduction.[8] Advancing the tissue edge to where it needs to be and threading it with the needle are easily accomplished.
- In elderly patients, the conjunctiva is often thin and very fragile. Extreme caution must be exercised to avoid tearing it, which makes closure increasingly all the more difficult.

Pearl

If the conjunctival dissection is done with a blunt instrument, it is the tissue itself that determines where the cleavage plane of the dissection occurs; if a sharp instrument is used, the surgeon determines the cleavage plane. Blunt dissection is convenient if no subconjunctival scarring is present; in eyes that have undergone previous surgery, such as vitrectomy or especially scleral buckling, sharp dissection may be advantageous to avoid scleral or muscle injury.

- Because the tissue is so mobile, care must be taken to avoid overtightening the knot: if the knot is made too tight,[9] it will fold the conjunctiva

---

7 Except in areas of previous injury or surgery where scar tissue has formed.

8 Except in areas of previous injury or surgery where scar tissue has formed.

9 One method to prevent overtightening is to make the initial throw a triple one and leave it relatively loosely tightened to avoid tissue flip; the second and third, single throws are made tight (see Chapter 2.2 for further details on knot preparation) to lock the knot.

over. Although this does not interfere with the success of the "water-tightness" of wound, it does result in a change of the overall configuration of the conjunctiva. The surface will never be even and smooth: a small prominence will remain there unless this "bump" is later excised.

- Thin (9 or 8/0) absorbable sutures[10] are sufficient; *vicryl* is the most widely used material today.
- It makes clinical sense to use numerous sutures: the relatively loose, absorbable sutures may fall out prematurely or get accidentally removed by the patient who rubs his eye. Extra sutures are especially beneficial if the wound is at the limbus; this is the area most important to properly cover (see above).
- Prior to closure, the sclera must be thoroughly inspected (see Chaps. 2.11, 2.12).

Cave

The scleral wound may be located at a significant distance from the conjunctival tear.

- Other methods are also available to close the conjunctival wound: a bipolar diathermy probe or fibrin glue [7].

Pearl

The conjunctiva is able to properly heal even if left unsutured. If torn at the limbus in a phakic eye's rupture and the patient goes untreated for a few days, the conjunctiva spontaneously reattaches at the limbus. The conjunctival scar is not conspicuous, and the disappearance of the crystalline lens (found neither inside the eye nor subconjunctivally) appears as a mystery to the unsuspecting ophthalmologist.

10 e.g., chromic or plain gut, vicryl.

2.1.3.7 Ischemia and Necrosis

This is the most significant pathology of the conjunctiva: a stoppage in the perilimbal blood flow eliminates the major nutrient supply to the cornea [5]. Immediate rinsing is crucial in the management [2]. (See Chap. 3.1 for a complete list of to-do's.)

Recent data give new support to the old clinical observation that subconjunctival injection of the patient's own blood has therapeutic benefit [4].

DO:

- learn the unique characteristics of conjunctival behavior to aid in properly closing its wounds
- irrigate the ocular surface immediately after a chemical injury

DON'T:

- fail to open the conjunctiva with thick hemorrhage if presence of an occult rupture cannot otherwise be excluded

Summary

Most conjunctival injuries are not significant, and only those that are caused by a chemical agent have long-term consequences. It is critical to determine whether a scleral rupture is present underneath a subconjunctival hemorrhage.

References

[1] Fukuyama J, Hayasaka S, Yamada K, Setogawa T (1990) Causes of subconjunctival hemorrhage. Ophthalmologica 200: 63–67

[2] Ikeda N, Hayasaka S, Hayasaka Y, Watanabe K (2006) Alkali burns of the eye: effect of immediate copious irrigation with tap water on their severity. Ophthalmologica 220: 225–228

[3] Kaiserman I (2003) Large subconjunctival emphysema causing diplopia and lagophthalmos. Eur J Ophthalmol 13: 86–87

[4] Nakamura T, Inatomi T, Sotozono C, Ang L P, Koizumi N, Yokoi N, Kinoshita S (2006) Transplantation of autologous serum-derived cultivated corneal epithelial equivalents for the treatment of severe ocular surface disease. Ophthalmology 113: 1765–1772

[5] Reim M (1992) The results of ischaemia in chemical injuries. Eye 6: 376–380

[6] Wenzel M, Aral H (2003) Indirect traumatic rupture of the globe without conjunctival injury. Klin Monatsbl Augenheilkd 220: 35–38 [in German]

[7] Zauberman H, Hemo I (1988) Use of fibrin glue in ocular surgery. Ophthalmic Surg 19: 132–133

2.2 Cornea

Ferenc Kuhn

2.2.1 Introduction

Injury to the cornea is very common: 10% of all new patient visits to an eye casualty clinic in one study were due to corneal trauma [8]. The cornea is involved in over half of all *serious* ocular trauma cases in the USEIR [20]. The typical injury occurs at home and is caused by a sharp object. Associated injuries are fairly common (Table 2.2.1).

Corneal trauma can be extremely painful: the epithelium, only 50 μm thick, has a large number of unmyelinated nerve endings. Trauma deeper than the epithelium[1] causes scar formation, which:

- Reduces the cornea's transparency by absorbing or scattering light
- Causes halo formation
- Alters the cornea's unique shape,[2] causing hyperopic[3] astigmia
- Makes the normally smooth surface[4] uneven
- Leads to significant and permanent [12] structural weakness

An injured cornea's initial functional loss is caused by a dysfunctional endothelial pump, resulting in corneal edema. The ophthalmologist should treat the corneal injury so as to minimizes the undesirable consequences of both the trauma and the treatment itself.

1 The cornea is approximately 1.0 mm thick in the periphery but only 0.5 mm in the center.

2 A dome, similar to the glass on a classic wristwatch

3 Two-thirds of eye's refractive power comes from the cornea.

4 The tear film contributes to the smoothness.

Table 2.2.1 Selected associated pathologies in eyes with full-thickness corneal wound in the USEIR database

Pathology	Laceration (%)	Rupture (%)
Hyphema	28	35
Cataract	39	27
IOFB	19	0
Endophthalmitis	3	2
Vitreous hemorrhage	26	29
Retinal break	7	7
Retinal detachment	10	12
Total	4030 (28%)	575 (4%)

Based on 14,523 injuries involving the globe

2.2.2 Evaluation

If the injury is caused by a chemical agent, history-taking must be limited to asking a few crucial questions before treatment is started: type of the agent; time of the incident; and the therapy already applied (see Chap. 1.10, 3.1). In all other cases, history should be detailed[5] to learn about the circumstances and consequences of the injury, the risk factors, etc. (see Chap. 1.9).

Especially if a blunt object caused the injury, it is important to determine whether refractive or open globe surgery had ever been performed on the cornea, and if yes, what type and when[6] (Table 2.2.2). Wound healing may take months, and even a completely healed wound has less tensile strength then uncut corneal fibrils [14, 23]. At a given impact, the vulnerability primarily depends on wound construction: length and steepness. A

5 How detailed is directly related to injury severity and the threat posed by treatment delay.

6 If available, it is always preferable to rely on the official discharge summary, not on the patient's recalling.

Table 2.2.2 Various surgical incisions in the cornea and their effect on tissue resistance. (Based on [44])

Type of corneal surgery	Consequence
Paracentesis (MVR blade, oblique)	Negligible effect [44]
Radial keratotomy (standard and hexagonal)	Reduces the corneal resistance to rupture by one-half [5]
Radial keratotomy (mini)	Reduces the corneal resistance to rupture by one-third to one-half [31]
PRK	Can reduce the corneal resistance to rupture [43]
LASIK	Shearing of the flap can occur [7]; the cohesive tensile strength of the cornea is permanently weaker [36]
PK	2.5–5.7% lifetime risk of corneal rupture [4, 41]
Clear corneal cataract incision	May offer similar corneal resistance to rupture as scleral tunnel incisions [25]
Corneoscleral incision with internal lip	Offers more corneal resistance to rupture than rectangular clear corneal cataract incisions [13]

surgical incision on the cornea thus represents a long-term risk factor for injury:[7] in the USEIR database, incidents were found to have occurred as late as 75 years after surgery [44].

Cave

In a USEIR study on ruptured eyes, 47% of those without prior eye surgery reached 20/200 or better final vision, as opposed to only 21% of eyes that had undergone surgery prior to the injury.

---

7 It does not, obviously, imply that elective surgery (including refractive procedures) should not be performed, only that the patients must be informed about the risk *before* consenting to surgery.

Inspection should be performed after the eyelids have been carefully pulled apart (see Chap. 1.9) to allow viewing the cornea in its entirety. Utilizing focal, rather than diffuse, illumination[8] may reveal erosions, blood vessels, scars, edema, infiltration, foreign bodies, and lamellar or full-thickness wounds. Changing the angle of illumination increases the chance of detecting the abnormality.

The *slit lamp* is the most valuable tool in identifying corneal pathologies. Figure 2.2.1 shows several techniques for recognizing past or current corneal trauma. Application of certain vital stains helps identify epithelial lesions (Table 2.2.3). Topical anesthesia (e.g., proparacaine 0.5%) may be necessary if the pain is intense,[9] especially if treatment is otherwise impossible to provide (e.g., irrigation for chemical injury; see Chaps. 1.10, 3.1). All topical anesthetics are toxic, however, and their longer-term use is contraindicated.

Table 2.2.3 Diagnostic staining of the corneal surface

Dye	Purpose	Technique
Fluorescein sodium[1,a]	Staining signals loss of integrity of the tight junctions of epithelial cells in the cornea and conjunctiva (pooling within intracellular defects) or denudation of the epithelial basement membrane	Use *blue* light (cobalt filter) and wide beam illumination; examine cornea rapidly, before the dye diffuses into the tissue
Rose bengal	Stains damaged epithelial cells	Use *white* light (no filter)

[a] Application using a sterile strip, rather than the 25% solution, is preferred (see Chap. 1.9). The strip should be placed over the conjunctiva, never over the cornea

[1] Fluorescein is also useful to show aqueous leakage from the anterior chamber in eyes with open globe injury: Seidel's test (see Chap. 1.9).

8 Such as that projected by a *penlight*
9 Such as that associated with erosion

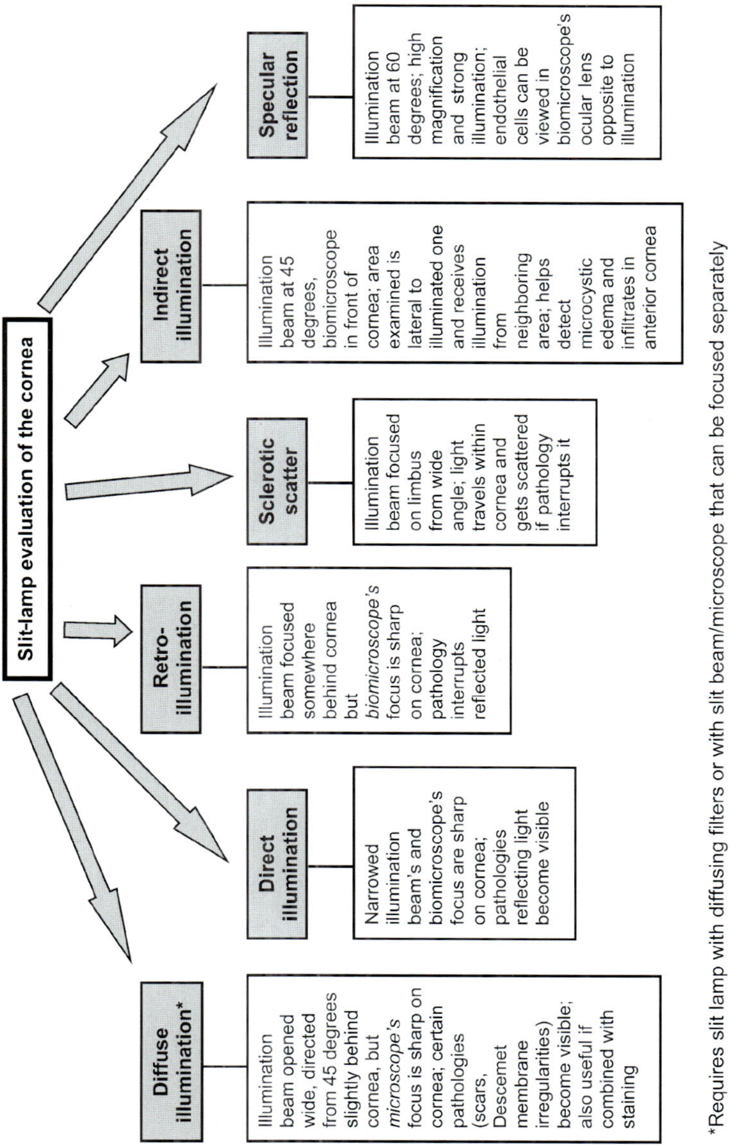

Fig. 2.2.1 Various illumination techniques used to examine the injured cornea

2.2.3 Specific Injuries

2.2.3.1 Erosion[10]

In this condition, the epithelial-cell cover over the basement membrane is partially or totally lost. The denuded area heals by peripheral cells migrating onto, and proliferating on, the denuded basement membrane; finally, hemidesmosomal attachments for strong anchorage develop. Limbal stem cells play an important role in the process, and their injury can lead to significant healing difficulties.

2.2.3.1.1 Symptoms

The symptoms are as follows:

- Severe and usually instantaneous[11] *pain* (in milder cases *foreign body sensation, irritation,* or *dryness* may also be reported by the patient)

Pearl

Injury severity and consequent pain in the cornea is typically inversely proportional: a tiny, fast-healing erosion is dramatically more painful than a sight-threatening laceration.

- *Blurred* vision (especially if the epithelial defect is in the visual axis)
- Significant *photophobia*
- *Lacrimation*

2.2.3.1.2 Evaluation

Fluorescein staining can reveal even small epithelial defects (Table 2.2.3). If the underlying corneal stroma has a granular appearance or edema is present, the injury is at least a few hours old.

---

10 Abrasion is another term used for the same condition.

11 A notable exception is welder's photokeratitis, caused by UV light; this is typically seen in those who perform/watch welding and do not wear proper eye protection. Symptoms take 6–10 h to develop.

Pitfall

Finding one pathology (e.g., erosion) does not mean that another one (e.g., occult scleral rupture) is not present; do not terminate the evaluation prematurely.

2.2.3.1.3 Treatment

- *Antibiotic ointment*[12] to cover the sensitive surface and to prevent infection.
- *Corticosteroid*[13] *drops* to counter the consequences of inflammation[14] and to positively influence corneal metabolism [11].
- *Cycloplegic drops* to alleviate the pain resulting from reactive spasm of the sphincter muscle. The drug should be short-acting (cyclopentolate 0.5%) or mid-range (scopolamine hydrobromide[15] [3] 0.25%) to keep the pupil mobile, rather than long-acting (atropine 1%).
- *Bandage soft contact lens* may also be used; this does not interfere with the external oxygen supply or the patient's ability to use the eye during the healing process.
- The use of *tight pressure-patching* is not recommended as it interferes with the external oxygen supply, raises the surface temperature, and prolongs healing [18].

---

12 Topical antibiotics are toxic [30, 38]. Their use is nevertheless recommended because of the risk of infection via the denuded cornea, but the antibiotics should be discontinued as soon as possible.

13 These should be used for a few days but not past the first week if the erosion persists. The negligibly increased risk of infection due to local immunosupression is more than offset by the benefits from reduction of the inflammation, especially if antibiotics prophylaxis is used (see above).

14 Excessive edema in the short- and extensive scarring in the long term

15 Cave: may cause psychosis in elderly patients

Controversial

Many patients prefer the eye to be patched for a corneal erosion; others want the patch removed. An individual decision should be made regarding patch use.

Most erosions heal rapidly, especially in younger patients. Conversely, the process is much slower in diabetics.[16] The healing line appears similar to a dendrite; history helps in the differential diagnosis, and sensitivity is maintained in the injured eye.

2.2.3.1.4 Recurrent Erosion

Up to 8% of erosions recur [46]. The original agent is most often a fingernail, a sheet of paper, or vegetable matter. Typically, the recurrence presents in the morning[17] upon opening the eyelids, and heals by midday. Large erosions may persist for several days.

2.2.3.1.5 Treatment[18]

- Topical hyperosmotics (e.g., 2.5 or 5% sodium chloride drops during the day and ointment at bedtime), applied for 2 months[19]: this reduces the epithelial edema and helps the epithelium to adhere to Bowman's layer.
- Autologous serum applied topically [42].
- Extended-wear bandage contact lens, changed weekly and worn day and night for up to 6 months.
- Surgical debridement to remove the loose epithelium and scrub the basement membrane without damaging Bowman's layer. Remove any hypertrophy using a cotton-tip applicator, a blade, or a diamond burr [35].

16 For this reason, the epithelium should be removed during vitrectomy only as a last resort in diabetic patients (see Chap. 2.9).

17 Due to a lack of evaporation during sleep, the tear film becomes hypotonic, making the corneal epithelium edematous; it is wiped off with the first blinks of the day.

18 If one therapy fails, turn to the next option.

19 Recurrence of the erosion should start a new treatment cycle.

- Stromal micropunctures to create anchors for the epithelium by using a small hypodermic needle to penetrate into the anterior corneal stroma[20] [35].
- YAG laser treatment of Bowman's layer [17].
- PTK: excimer laser to ablate the basement membrane/Bowman's layer [16].

2.2.3.2 Foreign Bodies

Corneal FBs are the second most common form of eye trauma [28]; they represented 17% of all ocular injuries in a recent war [15] and 1.8% of all injuries seen in an ER in one study [1]. Although the spectrum is wide from superficial FBs to those penetrating the cornea deeply (see Fig. 1.1.2a), most FBs do not reach Bowman's layer.

2.2.3.2.1 Evaluation

The symptoms usually present acutely and are similar to those seen with erosion, but the pain is less intense. Unless the FB is completely transparent or nonreflective,[21] it is easily recognized with a penlight or – especially – at the slit lamp. Multiple FBs are occasionally present, especially if the etiology is explosion.

Pearl

It may appear paradoxical that an FB lying on the hypersensitive corneal surface causes less pain than an FB lodged in the much less sensitive tarsal conjunctiva; however, the latter scratches the corneal epithelium with every blink, causing multiple vertical lines of erosion.

---

20 Be careful not to penetrate *too* deeply.

21 Changing the slit lamp's angle of illumination is helpful to detect reflection (e.g., in case of a glass fragment).

2.2.3.2.2 Treatment

- The cornea must be properly anesthetized with drops.[22]
- *Superficial* FBs are best removed using a cotton-tip applicator; outside the office, even the tip of a clean handkerchief or paper tissue will suffice. Rust rings, which can develop as early as within a few hours [47], should also be removed, using a diamond burr or a sharp needle. Once the FB has been extracted, the condition is treated as an erosion.
- *Deep* FBs, whether or not protruding into the AC, require considerable skill to remove.[23] The patient should be seated at the slit lamp, and his head must be secured by an assistant and/or a tight strap. This is especially important if the patient is less likely to cooperate (e.g., a young child or a mentally challenged adult).[24] The potential complications of pushing the FB into the AC are severe. If the risk is high,[25] FB removal may have to be done in the OR. A fine-tipped forceps, a small probe, or a strong IOM [19] if the FB is ferrous, can be used.

Pitfall

If the operating microscope does not have a built-in slit lamp, depth perception is more difficult, and a transparent FB, easily recognizable at the slit lamp, may all of a sudden become invisible. Careful prior mapping (drawing, marking) is highly recommended.

---

22 Anesthesia is not absolutely necessary if the FB is very superficial and no rust ring is present.

23 If the FB is embedded in the cornea so that it does not protrude in either direction, is of inert material (e.g., glass, plastic), and does not cause symptoms, it may be left in situ, especially if the wound is of a shelving type. Organic material that can be irritating (e.g., tarantula hair) should always be removed [6].

24 It is not only the uncooperative patient whose treatment calls for caution; those willing to cooperate may also reflectively move their head away from the slit lamp bar. Asking them to "come back against the bar" can cause the tool in the ophthalmologist's hand to penetrate into an approaching cornea deeper than intended. This is why presence of an assistant is crucial, to assure that the patient's head is always pressed forward.

25 Regardless of whether this happens due to improper maneuvering by the ophthalmologist or forward head movement by the patient

2.2.3.3 Contusion

Direct trauma to the cornea by a blunt object[26] can lead to:

- Fractures in Bowman's layer/stroma, especially in eyes with previous RK surgery.
- Edema due to endothelial damage [22]. The edema can interfere with visualization of the eye's deeper structures during evaluation or surgery.

Treatment varies from observation to DSAEK [40] or even PK (see below). If PK is performed on a recently traumatized eye, it is advisable to leave viscoelastics in the AC to keep the angle open, fight synechia formation, and maintain chamber depth.

2.2.3.4 Endothelium Failure

Whether caused by the original injury or the treatment (i.e., silicone oil touch), the endothelium may fail even if the anterior corneal layers are intact. In addition to PK, several new surgical options are available today to restore the endothelial layer (deep lamellar endothelial keratoplasty [40], Descemet's membrane endothelial keratoplasty [27], and posterior lamellar keratoplasty [24]).

2.2.3.5 Partial-thickness Laceration

Careful slit lamp examination can confirm the presence of this condition; the Seidel test (see Chap. 1.9) may be necessary to rule out the existence of a full-thickness wound. The decision whether closure is necessary is not always straightforward:

- Non-self-sealing wounds should be sutured.
- Small, self-sealing, clean wounds require no intervention other than prophylactic antibiotics and mild cycloplegics for a few days.

26 Concussions are also caused by blunt objects, but the impact is elsewhere and the energy transfer is via shockwaves. Common consequences include cell loss [26, 33].

- Flaps: if undisplaced, prophylactic antibiotics and mild cycloplegics applied for a few days suffice; if displaced, they need to be repositioned and sutured in place. If there is epithelial undergrowth, this must be removed prior to reposition.
- Larger, self-sealing, clean wounds need a bandage contact lens or gluing. Various glues are available (cyanoacrylate [29], fibrin [37])[27] or under investigation (chondroitin sulfate aldehyde [32]) to close partial- or even full-thickness wounds. Cyanoacrylate glue prevents collagenase activity and has bacteriostatic capability. Before applying the glue, the epithelium should be removed and the surface dried. If both suture and glue are used, the two must not come into contact with each other. Proper glue application avoids inadvertent dripping, prevents epithelial downgrowth and endothelial toxicity, and provides a smooth surface [45]. Amniotic membrane and glue use can also be combined [39].

If patient noncompliance is a risk of (e.g., rubbing of the eye likely before complete wound healing), closure with suture and/or glue is recommended.

2.2.3.6 Full-thickness Wound[28]

The slit lamp (occasionally employing the Seidel test) is used to confirm the diagnosis. Unless the wound is firmly self-sealing, surgical closure is recommended.

> **Cave**
>
> Unnecessary suturing of a self-sealing wound may be *inconvenient*; but to forgo suturing and suffer endophthalmitis, tissue prolapse, or ECH as a result is a *disaster*.

---

27 One of the many differences between these two glues is that cyanoacrylate works on the surface while fibrin (e.g., Tisseel, Baxter, Deerfield, Ill.) works between the wound edges as well; the latter is FDA-approved.

28 Laceration or rupture

2.2.3.6.1 Suturing the Cornea[29]

The goal of surgery is not limited to the reestablishment of ocular watertightness. The eye may need additional operations, and proper wound management is aimed at minimizing the interference of the corneal injury with subsequent surgical intervention/s on the posterior segment. The surgeon must understand:

- The effects of the wound and of the sutures on corneal anatomy and function.
- The basic concepts of how sutures work.
- The importance of a conscious planning of suture introduction.

Before actual wound closure, all elements of strategic thinking (see Chap. 1.8) must be considered, as should the implications and requirements of any additional tissue pathology caused by the injury. The variables involved in corneal suturing are discussed in Tables 2.2.4–2.2.6 and Figs. 2.2.2–2.2.10.[30] Clinical examples are shown in Figs. 2.2.11–2.2.15.

Chapter 2.11 provides further details on managing eyes with corneal wounds, and present the similarities and differences between eyes with corneal vs scleral wound.

2.2.3.6.2 Postoperative Treatment

- In addition to the use of full-thickness sutures, intense topical corticosteroid therapy is the other crucial factor in hastening edema resolution.[31]
- Antibiotics should also be used for a few days.

29 The author is greatly indebted to Bowes Hamill, M.D., for his invaluable contributions in developing the approach to suturing full-thickness corneal wounds as presented in this chapter.

30 The use of full-thickness sutures is somewhat controversial; this is discussed in Table 2.2.5.

31 In most cases, the combination of full-thickness sutures and intensive postoperative corticosteroid treatment allows the surgeon to perform vitreoretinal surgery within a few days and without having to compromise in the timing and completeness of vitrectomy due to cornea-related visualization difficulties.

Table 2.2.4 Effects of the wound and wound closure on the cornea; general rules of suturing

Variable	Comment
Wound	Causes change in corneal curvature (i.e., refractive error and possibly AC shallowing): radial wounds flatten the cornea adjacent and 90° away; the flattening effect increases as the visual axis is approached
Suture	Causes change in corneal curvature [flattening of the dome and unevenness (astigmatism)]; loose limbal sutures cause flattening adjacent to the wound and 180° away; tight limbal sutures cause flattening 90° away
Optimal suture	Makes wound watertight
	Minimizes postoperative edema
	Minimizes scar formation
	Minimizes interference with corneal curvature
	Minimizes late complications (e.g., synechia formation)
Scar	Causes change in corneal curvature (flattening and astigmatism)
	Causes reduction in corneal transparency
Closure mechanism	Explained on Fig. 2.2.2
Timing of suturing	As soon as possible: the risk of endophthalmitis increases after 24 h [2] and the threat of ECH is also real [21]; conversely, a short delay is preferred to improper suturing due to lack of expertise/experience, material, etc.[2]
Suturing	Clean wound edges first (Table 2.2.5 provides further details on suture introduction)
	Deal with prolapsed tissue (see Chap. 2.4)
	Preserve edges/flaps: not even small pieces of corneal tissue should be excised since this leads to flattening and astigmatism due to the suture requiring extreme tightness to achieve watertightness; the "missing" piece is commonly found folded under
Suture removal	6–8 weeks in children; 2–6 months in adults[3]

[2] One alternative to permanent suturing is to temporarily cover the corneal wound with conjunctiva; this can reduce the ECH risk, and prevent infection and iatrogenic damage by improper corneal suturing.

[3] Also influenced by other factors: speed of wound healing; length and location of the wound; irritation from the suture

- Whether and how long a patch and/or shield is used depends on wound characteristics, wound healing characteristics, patient compliance, and patient preference.

Table 2.2.5 Basic principles of suture introduction for corneal wounds

Variable	Comment
Type of suture	Running or interrupted (Fig. 2.2.4)
Material of suture	Nylon, 10-0 or 11-0
Bite length	Should be identical on both sides, unless the wound is oblique (shelved; Fig. 2.2.9)
No. of sutures	Determined by the length of the wound and the length of the sutures bites, the spacing, and the tension put on the sutures (Fig. 2.2.2)
Order of sutures placement	If landmarks such as the limbus or an angle in the wound are present, these should be closed first (Figs. 2.2.5b, 2.2.10); if the wound is limbus to limbus and crosses much of the cornea, suturing should start from the outsides and continue inwards; otherwise, the 50% rule is generally applied (Fig. 2.2.5d)
Forceps use	There is no need to grab the cornea with forceps. The spatula needles used today are sharp enough to easily perforate the cornea.[4] If counterforce is needed when the needle engages the cornea (*entry*), the adjacent conjunctiva should be grabbed.[5] If counter pressure is needed when the needle enters the cornea from the AC (*exit*), this can be achieved by pressing down on the corneal surface with the arms[6] of the forceps, which is held slightly opened; the needle should exit the cornea between the two arms of the forceps

[4] A spatula needle of approximately 6 mm in length and 3/8 in. circle is recommended; the wire diameter is approximately 0.15 mm.

[5] Always on the side where the needle enters the cornea, not on the opposite side, even if the conjunctiva in that location appears more convenient to grab

[6] Not by grabbing the cornea with the working tip of the forceps; this eliminates causing additional corneal damage

Table 2.2.5 *(continued)* Basic principles of suture introduction for corneal wounds

Variable	Comment
Depth of sutures	Full thickness (Fig. 2.2.6b)
Angle/direction of the needle	At 90°, unless a single running suture is used (Figs. 2.2.2, and 2.2.4)
Knot creation and handling	The knot should be small enough to be easily buried but strong enough to prevent release or loosening. The ideal knot has three throws: the first is a triple one, tightened after the surgeon crossed his/her hands (Fig. 2.2.7). Tightening is perpendicular to the wound's plane; the second throw is a single one and tightened parallel to the wound's plane (i.e., perpendicular to the initial tightening plane); the third throw is also a single one and tightening is perpendicular to the wound's plane. All knots must be buried since they can cause severe inflammation/irritation. The knot can be turned in either direction as the suture channels are, and their directions should be, identical on the two sides[7]

[7] If the cornea is very edematous, it may be difficult to bury the knot; in such cases, a flat-faced forceps can be used to "compress" the knot first. Such a maneuver usually allows the knot to easily slip into the channel – this extremely useful pearl is the idea of the author's head OR nurse, N. Rudolf.

Table 2.2.6 Pro- and contra arguments regarding the use of full-thickness corneal sutures

Don't use full-thickness sutures because...	Full-thickness sutures can safely be used because...
The risk of endophthalmitis is increased: a channel is established between the extraocular space and the AC	The channel cut by the needle (A) is not much larger than the cross-section of the thread (B); the channel is rapidly closed as the surrounding cornea's edema compresses it (C). As soon as a few minutes after suture introduction, pressure on the eye is unable to produce aqueous leakage from the AC through the suture channel[8] 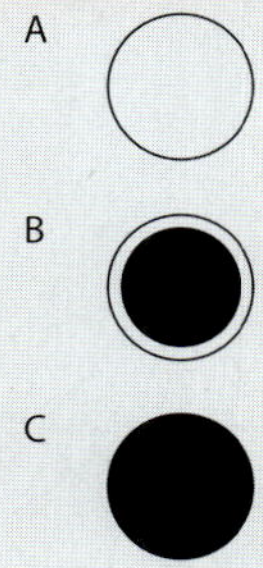
The thread pressed against the endothelium causes cell death and leads to increased edema formation	The thread pressed against the endothelium probably indeed causes cell death in that very tiny area; however, by immediately blocking aqueous access to the stroma and not forcing the endothelial cells to cover such a large area, overall endothelial damage by a full-thickness suture is smaller then it would be if a "90%" depth" suture were used. Clinical experience shows that corneas whose wounds have been closed with full-thickness sutures become clear much faster than those closed with partial-thickness sutures

[8] *Removal* of a full-thickness suture, however, indeed presents increased endophthalmitis risk. As the suture is cut and turned for removal, the part having previously been outside the eye may become intracameral. To prevent introduction of organisms into the AC, the eye has to be prepared with betadine (10% on the skin and 5% on the conjunctiva, applied for one minute) as if intraocular surgery were to be performed, and use of an eyelid speculum is also recommended.

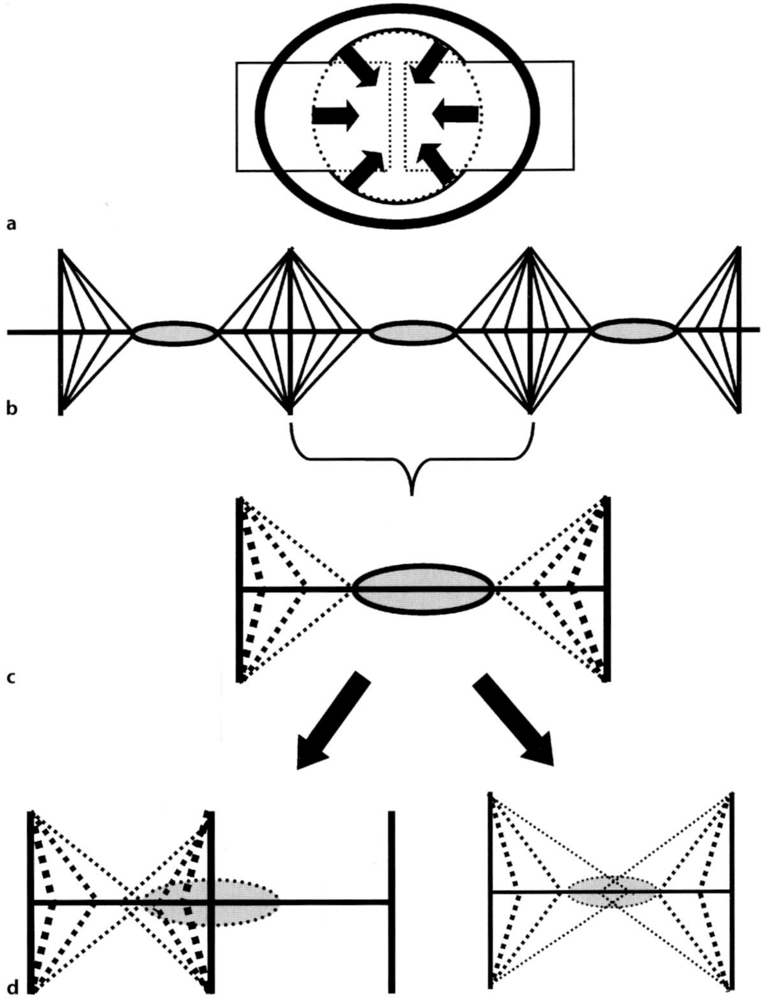
a
b
c
d

Fig. 2.2.2 Sutures work via tissue compression. **a** All sutures, even if they were introduced in a different geometrical formation (*thick, continuous line*), want to form a *circle* (*dotted line*) upon tightening; the tissue it "encircles" is compressed. **b,c** All sutures have a *compression zone*: this is greatest in the plane of the suture itself and gradually decreases with increasing distance from that plane. To create a watertight seal, the compression zones should overlap or at least "touch" each other. If the compression zones do not meet, gaping occurs. **d** The gaping can be eliminated by further tightening of the existing suture(s), but this may cause major tissue distortion. The proper way to create watertightness is either via the introduction of additional suture(s) (*left*) or by using sutures with longer bites (*right*), which have larger compression zones.[1] The effect of tissue compression is reflected on the corneal surface; this is why it is advisable to check the tightness of the sutures at the conclusion of wound closure (Fig. 2.2.3). Upon suture removal, the tissue compression effect disappears[2]

[1] Other techniques are also available if there is gaping: (cyanoacrylate) glue, bandage contact lens, patch graft, PK.

[2] Conversely, misalignment (tissue shift or override) caused by improper suturing is permanent.

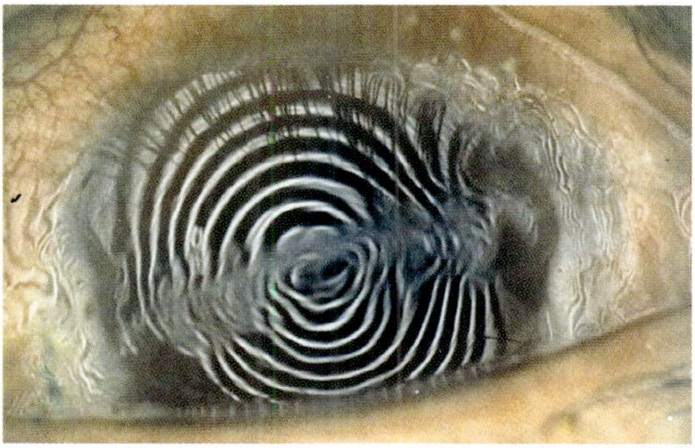

Fig. 2.2.3 Intraoperative keratoscopy following closure of a large corneal wound. Using the keratoscope, a Flieringa ring, or a safety pin allows detection of undesirable irregularities. Alternatively, an adjustable slip knot can also be used [9]. (Courtesy of B. Hamill, Houston, TX)

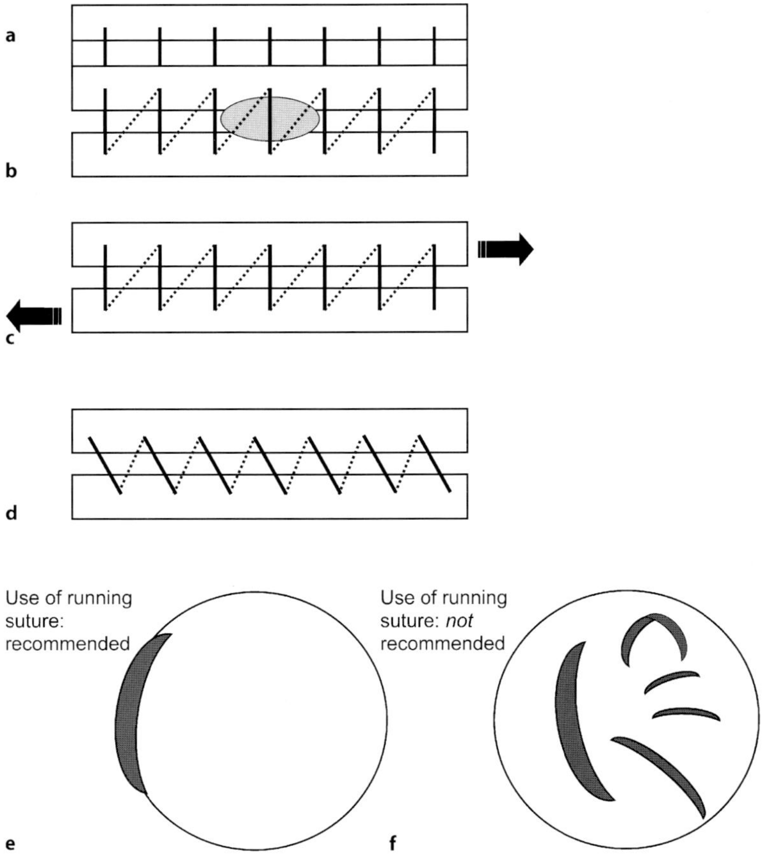
a
b
c
d
Use of running suture: recommended
e
Use of running suture: *not* recommended
f

Fig. 2.2.4 Interrupted vs running sutures. **a** Interrupted sutures provide maximal flexibility (length, tension, number, adjustability) but require more work (e.g., repeated steps of introduction, tying, burying the knot, and adjustment). **b** Running sutures have the advantage of creating an even, continuous zone of compression and require less work,[1] but they cause flattening of the underlying convex structure. Running sutures tend to cause gaping in the wound's midsection (*shaded area*), and the surgeon must counter this by increasing the tension on the suture, which enhances the flattening effect. **c** If a running suture's individual bites are introduced at the traditional 90° angle,[2] the wound lips shift to create equal distribution of the tension. Unlike tissue compression, which disappears upon suture removal, this shift is permanent (see above). **d** To prevent tissue shift (slippage), the bites of a running suture should be introduced at 45°. Alternatively, a bootlace suture (a second, mirroring suture line) can be used. Both running sutures are introduced at 90° in the latter case. **e** Running suture should be used if the wound is: in the periphery; rather long; and limbus-parallel. **f** In all cases other than **e**, interrupted sutures should be used to avoid corneal flattening

[1] Unless, of course, they break as they are being tied or buried

[2] Which is a must with interrupted sutures

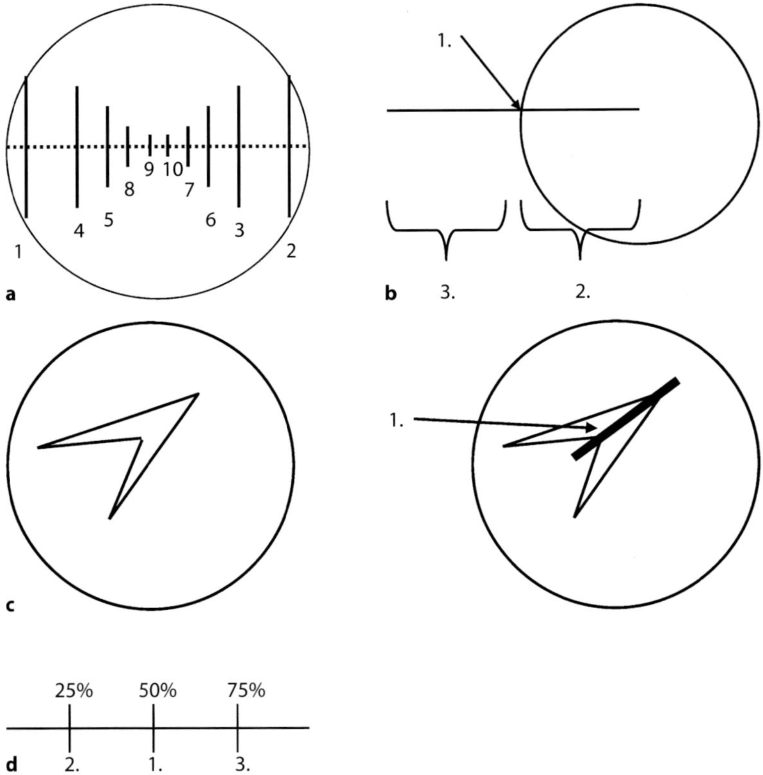

Fig. 2.2.5 The order of suture introduction in the cornea. **a** If the wound is long and transects the cornea, the risk of flattening the corneal dome shape by the scar is significant [34]. To counter this effect, suture introduction should start from the two peripheries and with long bites; the bites get progressively shorter as the center is approached. In the apex of the cornea – the visual center – no suture should be placed unless absolutely necessary. The *numbers* indicate the order of suture placement. **b** If the wound crosses the limbus, the limbus is closed first since this is an absolute indicator of proper apposition; the corneal part is closed second and the scleral part last. **c** An angular wound's (*left*) initial suture must be placed at the angle (*right*). Suturing should proceed from, instead of toward, the angle; otherwise, too much tension needs to be placed on the final suture to achieve watertightness, which would result in major tissue distortion. **d** In most other cases the typical "divide at 50%" rule may be applied

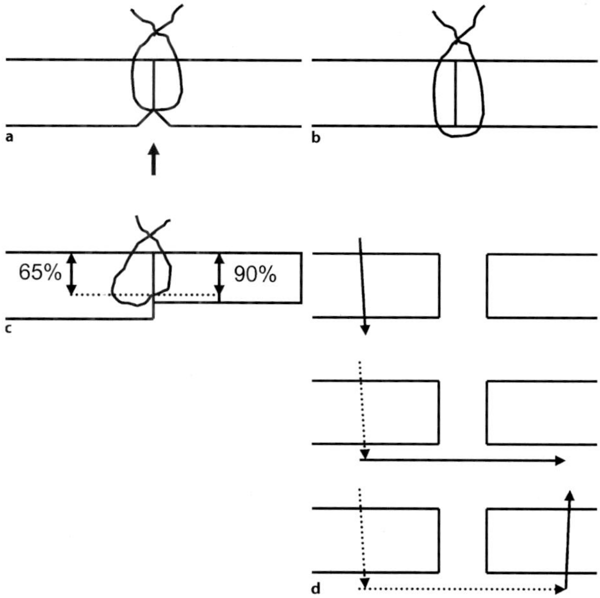

Fig. 2.2.6 The depth of corneal sutures. **a** Traditionally, corneal sutures are recommended to be 90% deep, although this has obvious disadvantages[1]. **b** A full-thickness suture immediately and permanently closes the wound; this effectively blocks the access of aqueous to the stroma. Sutures of 100% depth shorten the time the cornea needs to become dry and clear, hastening visual recovery for the patient and reducing the time until the deeper structures of the eye can be examined. Vitreoretinal surgery can thus be performed when this is *necessary*, not when it is *possible*. **c** A full-thickness suture also prevents tissue misalignment ("override") caused by unequal suture depth. **d** The direction of the needle during the three components of the introduction of a full-thickness suture. Upon entry, the needle's tip[2] is held almost perpendicular to the corneal surface (*top*; in the AC, the vector of needle movement is more or less parallel to the surface; upon exit (*center*), the needle's tip is again turned almost perpendicular to the corneal surface (*bottom*)

[1] *1* It is difficult to determine in a real life situation where that 90% exactly is. *2* Tissue thickness differs on the two sides of the wound, due to different degrees of edema. *3* Manipulation of the wound edges with forceps to "peek" inside the wound to verify needle depth is traumatic to the cornea, increasing edema development and thus interfering with postoperative visualization. *4* The 10% of the wound, which is left unsutured (*arrows*), allows aqueous access to the stroma, extending the duration of edema. *5* The endothelium has a larger area to cover, slowing postoperative recovery.

[2] "Tip" here also represents the shaft or axis of the needle.

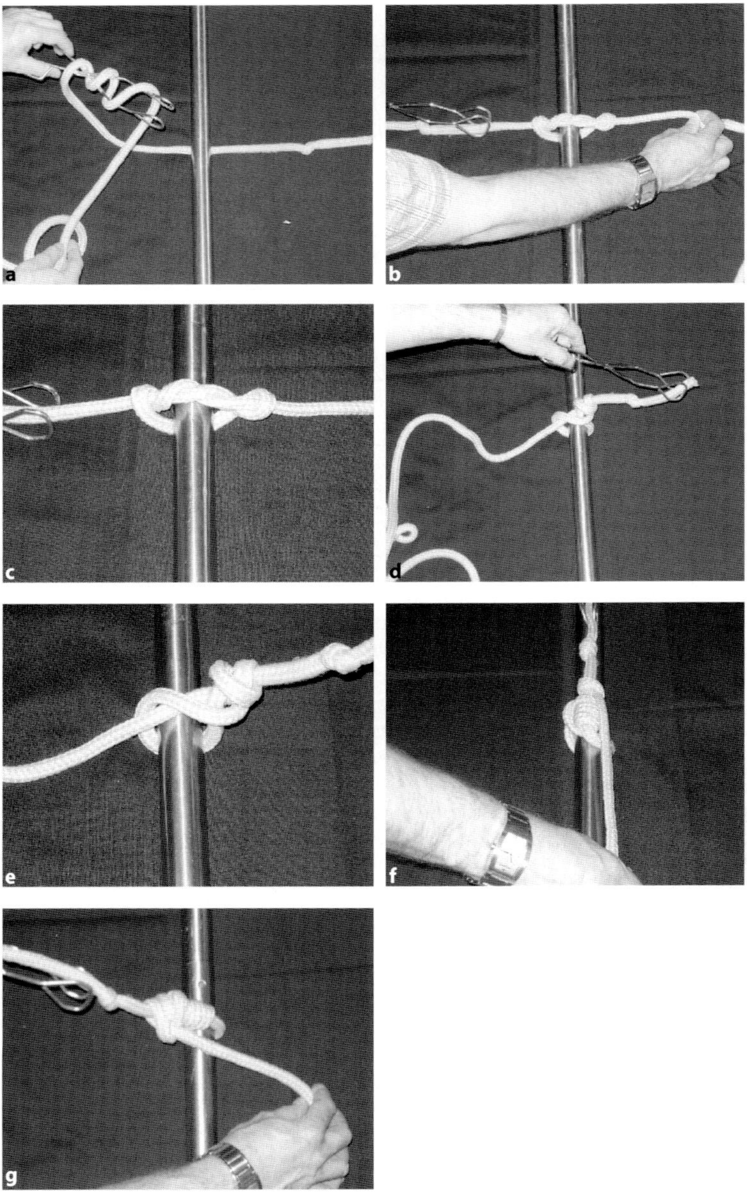
a
b
c
d
e
f
g

Fig. 2.2.7 Details of creating an "ideal" knot. Certain steps of suture management are modeled here to show the creation of a knot that is small enough to allow easy burying while providing sufficient postoperative strength to maintain wound closure. A *string* represents the suture, a *salad server* the needle holder, and a *metal bar* the wound. **a** The first step is a triple throw over the needle holder. Notice that the left-handed surgeon's right hand, which holds the long arm of the suture (the one that has the needle on its end), is on the left side of the wound (close to himself). **b** The first step is being completed. The surgeon has crossed his hands: the right hand is now on the right side of the wound (away from himself). The triple throw is clearly visible and the suture is properly aligned. Notice that the suture is tightened *perpendicular* to the plane of the wound. **c** Close-up of the properly aligned triple throw. **d** If the surgeon does not cross his hands (notice that the left hand with the needle holder is on the right side of the wound), a large tangle is formed as the triple throw is tightened. This tangle makes it more difficult to satisfy the two requirements of the knot: strong yet small. **e** Close-up of the improperly aligned triple throw (compare it with the image in **c**). **f** The second step in creating a proper knot is a single throw, which is tightened *parallel* to the plane of the wound (i.e., perpendicular to the plane of the first, triple throw). This locks the knot: once tightened, it is impossible for the knot to become loose. **g** The final step is another single throw, which is tightened *perpendicular* to the plane of the wound (i.e., parallel to the plane of the first, triple throw). This provides extra reassurance that the know will not loosen with time

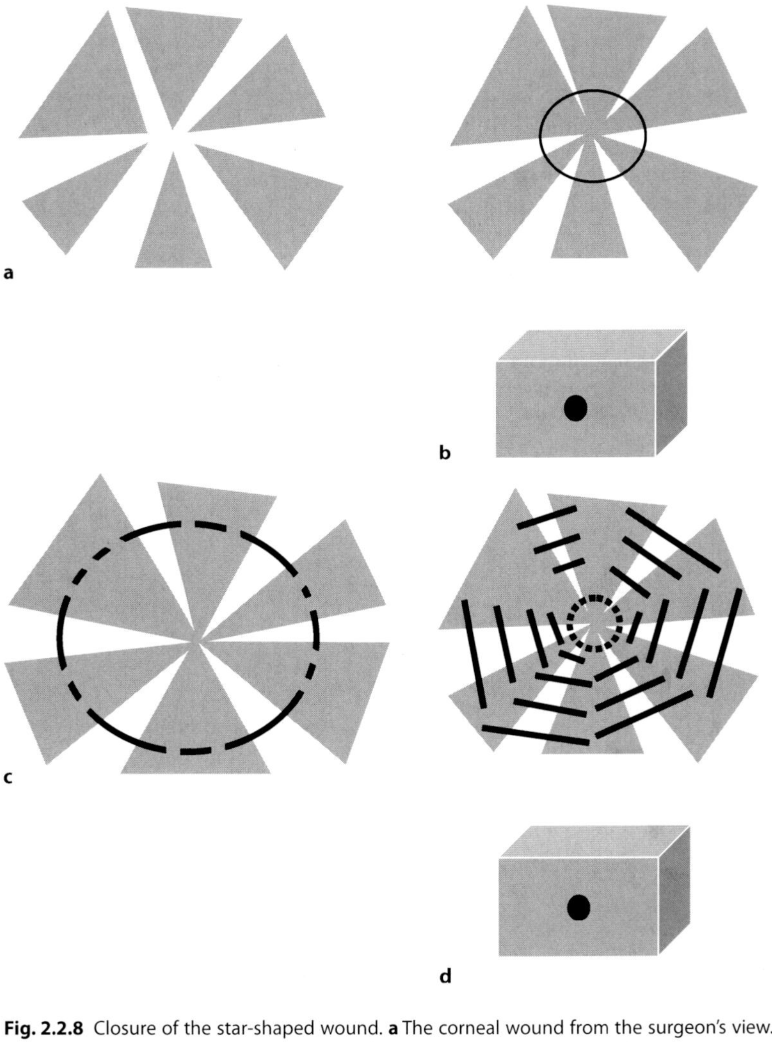

Fig. 2.2.8 Closure of the star-shaped wound. **a** The corneal wound from the surgeon's view. **b** The initial suture is an intrastromal one in the center (*top:* surgeon's view; *bottom:* cross-sectional view). The intrastromal suture is placed roughly at mid-depth. It is a permanent suture (i.e., never to be removed). **c** Enlarged view of **b**, top. **d** The intrastromal suture brought all wound edges together, and have created several individual wounds, which are now dealt with one at a time. This is done in a way determined by the location and length of the individual wounds (see earlier). These sutures are full thickness. *Top:* surgeon's view; *bottom:* cross-sectional view

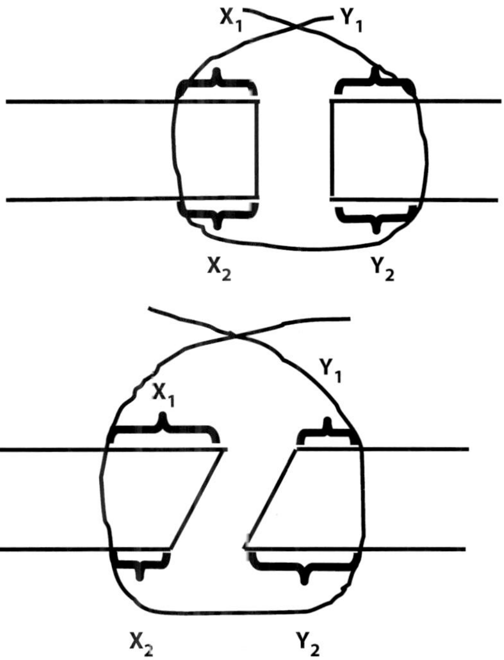

a

b

Fig. 2.2.9 Closure of perpendicular vs oblique (shelved) wounds. **a** If the wound's plane is close to vertical as it relates to the surface[1], the needle's entry and exit points should be at equal distance from the wound on both the epithelial and endothelial corneal surfaces (x_1=y_1) and (x_2=y_2). **b** If the wound's plane is oblique, use of full-thickness sutures becomes especially crucial. The distances as measured for needle entry and exit relative to the edge of the wound need to be modified so as to create the same compression on either side. As shown, the epithelial distance on one side is matched up with the endothelial distance on the other side (x_1=y_2) and (x_1=y_2). This technique prevents tissue override, which is a permanent[2] abnormality

[1] Which is the majority of the cases

[2] i.e., it does not disappear with suture removal

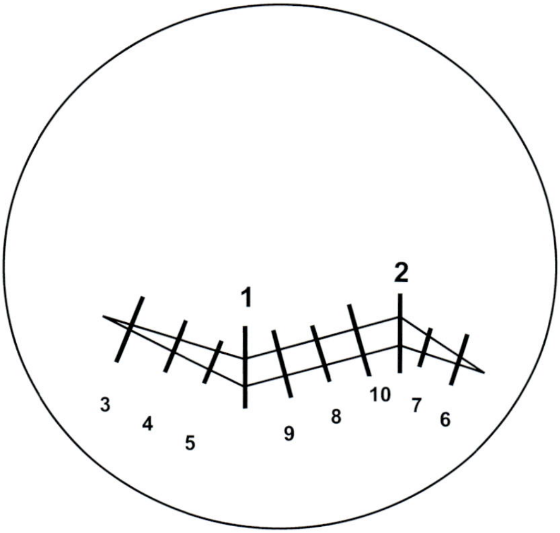

Fig. 2.2.10 Closure of a complex, angled corneal wound. The wound that has two angles should be considered as three separate wounds. To achieve this, the single wound is first divided into three by placing the first two sutures at the angles (as in Fig. 2.2.5c). The two peripheral wounds are closed then, and the central part last. The *numbers* represent the order of suture placement

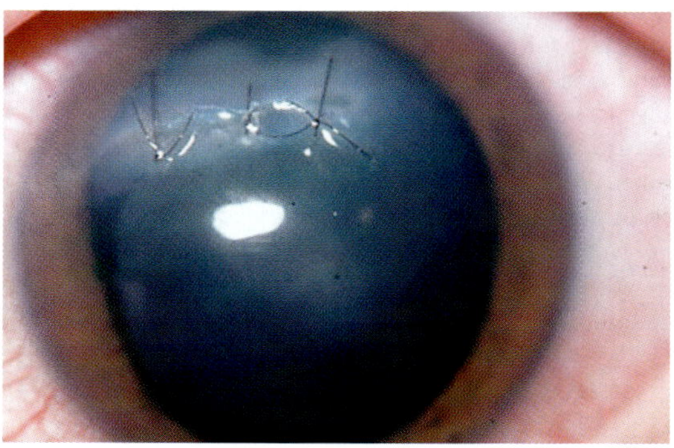

Fig. 2.2.11 Closure of a small corneal wound. Closure is correct here in terms of suture length (longer in the periphery and shorter in the center); however, the knots still need to be buried, and leaving the tags too long makes this difficult. The tags may also cause additional problems once turned into the AC

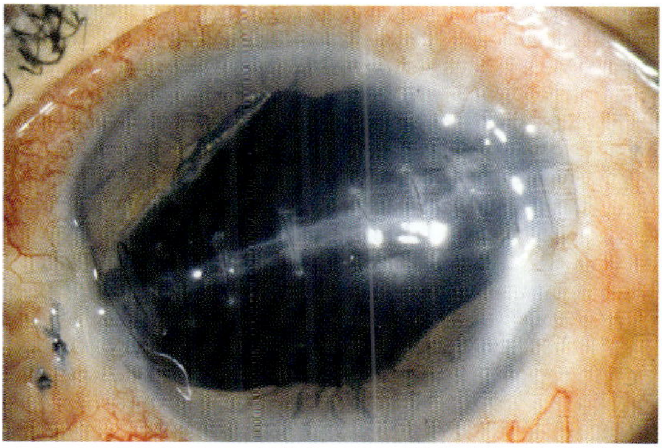

Fig. 2.2.12 Closure of a long corneal wound. A properly closed wound., note that the sutures are longer in the periphery and that scar formation is minimal (Courtesy of B. Hamill)

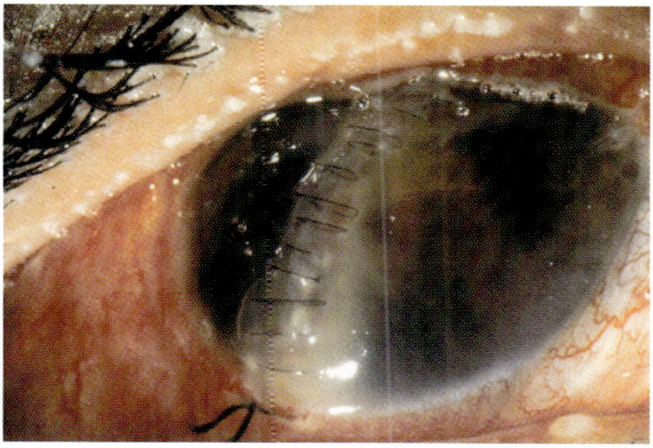

Fig. 2.2.13 Closure of a long corneal wound. A similarly long wound as in Fig. 2.2.11; however, the suture bites are arbitrary in terms of length, and introduction sequence is also presumed to have been haphazard. Suture placement was obviously not based on a carefully designed plan. Furthermore, the sutures are too tight, making the surface uneven (bulging wound edges). It will take a long time for this cornea to clear, and permanent visual impairment is inevitable

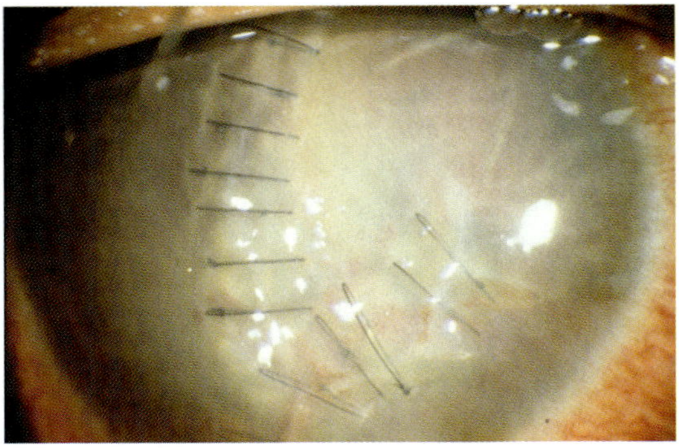

Fig. 2.2.14 Corneal blood staining. This wound was closed with evenly spaced sutures, which appears esthetical but causes flattening. Nonetheless, closure technique in this case has relatively little significance. The cornea has become nontransparent due to blood staining; posterior segment surgery is impossible without using the TKP (see Chap. 2.15), making PK unavoidable[1]

[1] Endoscopy is also an option (see Chap. 2.20), but it is doubtful that this cornea will escape the need for a PK.

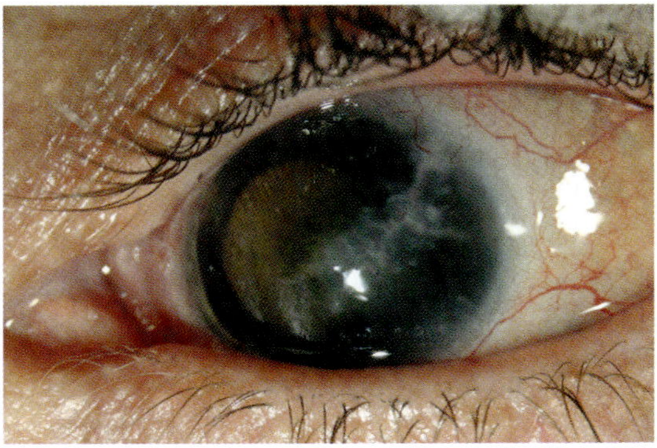

Fig. 2.2.15 Scar formation following closure of a corneal wound. Although scarring cannot be avoided once the wound is deeper than the epithelium, it can be minimized by proper suturing techniques and the judicious use of corticosteroids postoperatively

2.2.3.7 Scar Management

If the scar is in the visual axis or causes major distortion of the cornea's curvature, surgical intervention may be necessary to alleviate the undesirable consequences. Even deep scars may be treated with PTK [10]; otherwise, surgical excision, including PK, may be employed.

2.2.3.8 Suture Removal

If full-thickness sutures have been used (Fig. 2.2.6b), certain precautions must be taken to prevent endophthalmitis development following suture removal.

> **Cave**
>
> Removal of a full-thickness corneal suture should be regarded as if an intravitreal injection were given; proper disinfection of the lids and conjunctiva with betadine (10 and 5%, respectively) and the use of a lid speculum is recommended.

DO:

- master the techniques of examining the cornea at the slit lamp
- have increased concern for injuries with little or no pain
- be careful not to push a deep corneal FB into the AC by inappropriate removal techniques
- plan all aspects of wound closure before introducing any suture into the cornea
- make use of the benefits of full-thickness sutures

DON'T:

- hesitate to start a new therapy if on current management the corneal erosion keeps recurring
- neglect to consider all posttreatment eventualities (such as rubbing of the eye) when deciding whether to suture an apparently self-sealing partial-thickness laceration
- forget the need to prepare the eye as if it were undergoing an intraocular procedure when a full-thickness suture is to be removed

Summary

The cornea is the most commonly injured ocular tissue. In most cases, pain is inversely proportional to significance. Full-thickness wounds are of major concern since they represent increased endophthalmitis and ECH risk. Improper treatment of the corneal injury can result in visual impairment because of several factors ranging from an unnecessarily prominent scar to vitrectomy delayed too long because of undue corneal edema. Scleral and corneal wounds have very different implications; this is discussed in Chap. 2.11.

References

[1] Banerjee A (1990) Effectiveness of eye protection in the metal working industry. Br Med J 301: 645–646

[2] Barr C (1983) Prognostic factors in corneoscleral lacerations. Arch Ophthalmol 101: 919–924

[3] Birkhimer L, Jacobson P, Olson J, Goyette D (1984) Ocular scopolamine-induced psychosis. J Fam Pract 18: 464–466

[4] Bowman R, Yorston D, Aitchison T, McIntyre B, Kirkness C (1999) Traumatic wound rupture after penetrating keratoplasty in Africa. Br J Ophthalmol 83: 530–534

[5] Campos M, Lee M, McDonnell P (1992) Ocular integrity after refractive surgery: effects of photorefractive keratectomy, phototherapeutic keratectomy, and radial keratotomy. Ophthal Surg: 598–602

[6] Chang P, Soong H, Barnett J (1991) Corneal penetrations by tarantula hairs. Br J Ophthalmol 75: 253–254

[7] Chaudhry N, Smiddy W (1998) Displacement of corneal cap during vitrectomy in a post-LASIK eye. Retina 18: 554–555

[8] Chiapella A, Rosenthal A (1985) One year in eye casualty. Br J Ophthalmol 69: 865–870

[9] Dangel M, Kestes R (1980) The adjustable slipknot. An alternative technique. Ophthalmic Surg 12: 843–846

[10] Dogru M, Katakami C, Miyashita M, Hida E, Uenishi M, Tetsumoto K, Kanno S, Nishida T, Yamanaka A (2000) Visual and tear function improvement after superficial phototherapeutic keratectomy (PTK) for mid-stromal corneal scarring. Eye 14: 779–784

[11] Dursun D, Kim MC, Solomon A, Pflugfelder SC (2001) Treatment of recalcitrant recurrent corneal erosions with inhibitors of matrix metalloproteinase-9, doxycycline and corticosteroids. Am J Ophthalmol 132: 8–13

[12] Elder M, Stack R (2004) Globe rupture following penetrating keratoplasty: How often, why, and what can we do to prevent it? Cornea 23: 776–780

[13] Ernest P, Lavery K, Kiessling L (1994) Relative strength of scleral corneal and clear corneal incisions constructed in cadaver eyes. J Cataract Refract Surg 20: 626–629

[14] Gasset A, Dohlman C (1968) The tensile strength of corneal wounds. Arch Ophthalmol 79: 595–602

[15] Heier J, Enzenauer R, Wintermeyer S (1993) Ocular injuries and disease at a combat supported hospital in support of operations Desert Shield and Desert Storm. Arch Ophthalmol 111: 795–798

[16] John M, Van der Karr M, Noblitt R (1984) Excimer laser phototherapeutic keratectomy for treatment of recurrent erosion. J Cataract Refract Surg 20: 179–181

[17] Katz H, Snyder M, Green W (1994) Nd:YAG laser photo-induced adhesion of the corneal epithelium. Am J Ophthalmol 118: 612–612

[18] Kirkpatrick J, Hoh H, Cook S (1993) No eye pad for corneal abrasion. Eye 7: 468–471

[19] Kuhn F, Heimann K (1991) Ein neuer Dauermagnet zur Entfernung intraokularer ferromagnetischer Fremdkoerper. Klin Mbl Augenheilk 198: 301–303

[20] Kuhn F, Mester V, Berta A, Morris R (1998) Epidemiology of serious ocular trauma: The United States Eye Injury Registry (USEIR) and the Hungarian Eye Injury Registry (HEIR). Ophthalmologe 95: 332–343

[21] Kuhn F, Morris R, Mester V (2001) Choroidal detachment and expulsive choroidal hemorrhage. Ophthalmol Clin N Am 14: 639–650

[22] Lesher M, Durrie D, Stiles M (1993) Corneal edema, hyphema, and angle recession after air bag inflation. Arch Ophthalmol 111: 1320–1322

[23] Lindquist T (1992) Complications of corneal refractive surgery. Int Ophthalmol Clin 32: 97–114

[24] Lord RK, Price FW, Price MO, Werner L, Mamalis N (2006) Histology of posterior lamellar keratoplasty. Cornea 25: 1093–1096

[25] Mackool R, Russell R (1996) Strength of clear corneal incisions in cadaver eyes. J Cataract Refract Surg 22: 721–725

[26] Maloney W, Colvard M, Bourne W (1979) Specular microscopy of traumatic posterior annular keratopathy. Arch Ophthalmol 97: 1647–1650

[27] Melles GR, Ong TS, Ververs B, van der Wees J (2006) Descemet's membrane endothelial keratoplasty (DMEK). Cornea 25: 987–990

[28] Mönestam E, Björnstig U (1991) Eye injuries in northern Sweden. Acta Ophthalmol 69: 1–5

[29] Moschos M, Droutsas D, Boussalis P, Tsioulias G (1996) Clinical experience with cyanoacrylate tissue adhesive. Doc Ophthalmol 93: 237–245

[30] Pfister R, Burnstein N (1976) The effects of ophthalmic drugs, vehicles, and preservatives on corneal epithelium: a scanning electron microscope study. Invest Ophthalmol Vis Sci 15: 246–259

[31] Pinheiro MJ, Bryant M, Tayyanipour R, Nassaralla B, Wee W, McDonnell P (1995) Corneal integrity after refractive surgery. Effects of radial keratotomy and mini-radial keratotomy. Ophthalmology 102: 297–301

[32] Reyes JM, Herretes S, Pirouzmanesh A, Wang D, Elisseeff J, Jun A, McDonnell P, Chuck R, Behrens A (2005) A modified chondroitin sulfate aldehyde adhesive for sealing corneal incisions. Invest Ophthalmol Vis Sci 46: 1247–1250

[33] Roberson M, Wicheta W (1985) Endothelial loss in corneal concussion injury. Ann Ophthalmol 17: 457–458

[34] Rowsey J, Hays J (1984) Refractive reconstruction for acute eye injuries. Ophthalmic Surg 15: 569–574

[35] Rubinfeld R, Laibson P, Cohen E (1990) Anterior stromal puncture for recurrent erosion: further experience and new instrumentation. Ophthalmic Surg 21: 318–326

[36] Schmack I, Dawson D, McCarey B, Waring G, Grossniklaus H, Edelhauser H (2005) Cohesive tensile strength of human LASIK wounds with histologic, ultrastructural, and clinical correlations. J Refr Surg 433–445

[37] Sharma A, Kaur R, Kumar S, Gupta P, Pandav S, Patnaik B, Gupta A (2003) Fibrin glue versus N-butyl-2-cyanoacrylate in corneal perforations. Ophthalmology 110: 291–298

[38] Stern G, Schemmer G, Farber R (1983) Effect of topical antibiotic solutions on corneal epithelial wound healing. Arch Ophthalmol 101: 644–647

[39] Su CY, Lin CP (2000) Combined use of an amniotic membrane and tissue adhesive in treating corneal perforation: a case report. Ophthalmic Surg Lasers 31: 151–154

[40] Terry M, Ousley P (2006) Deep lamellar endothelial keratoplasty: early complications and their management. Cornea 25: 37–43

[41] Tseng S, Lin S, Chen F (1999) Traumatic wound dehiscence after penetrating keratoplasty: clinical features and outcome in 21 cases. Cornea 18: 553–558

[42] Tsubota K, Goto E, Shimmura S, Shimazaki J (1999) Treatment of persistent corneal epithelial defect by autologous serum application. Ophthalmology 106: 1984–1989

[43] Uchio E, Watanabe Y, Kadonosono K, Matsuoka Y, Goto S (2003) Simulation of airbag impact on eyes after photorefractive keratectomy by finite element analysis method. Graefe's Arch Clin Exp Ophthalmol 241: 497–504

[44] Vinger PF (2002) Injury to the postsurgical eye. In: Kuhn F, Pieramici D (eds) Ocular trauma: principles and practice. Thieme, New York, pp 280–292

[45] Vote BJ, Elder MJ (2000) Cyanoacrylate glue for corneal perforations: a description of a surgical technique and a review of the literature. Clin Experiment Ophthalmol 28: 437–442

[46] Weene L (1985) Recurrent corneal erosion after trauma: a statistical study. Ann Ophthalmol 17: 521–524

[47] Zuckerman B, Lieberman T (1960) Corneal rust ring. Arch Ophthalmol 63: 254–264

2.3 Sclera and Limbus

Ferenc Kuhn

2.3.1 Introduction

While playing only limited and indirect role in vision,[1] the sclera is responsible for much of the globe's strength and integrity. The proximity of the scleral "shell" to vital tissues such as the choroid, ciliary body, and the retina gives it significant clinical implications. Compared with most ocular tissues, the sclera has few pathologies. The limbus is one of the loci minoris resistantiae of the globe[2], which is further excerbated by the fact that it is often the site of elective surgical incisions.

2.3.2 Evaluation

Through the usually transparent conjunctiva, it is typically possible to directly inspect the limbus and the *anterior* sclera with the naked eye, but especially at the slit lamp. Subconjunctival hemorrhage, among other pathologies, however, can interfere with direct inspection of the sclera, making it necessary to use radiological tests (most importantly, CT), ultrasonography, or even exploratory surgery (see Chap. 1.9).

1 e.g., an improperly sutured anterior scleral or limbal wound can cause significant astigmia

2 As is the area at the insertion of the extraocular muscles (see Chap. 2.12)

Examining the *posterior* sclera is even more difficult. Taking a thorough history may provide some clues as can a detailed inspection using the slit lamp (see Fig. 2.4.1). Ultrasonography and CT may yield information that otherwise cannot be obtained, but if scleral integrity cannot adeqately be confirmed by these diagnostic tests, exploratory surgery becomes necessary.

Areas of thin sclera may be persent as a result of current trauma or surgery, past injury, autoimmune disease, or myopia. Extreme caution is necessary to avoid iatrogenic rupture (see below).

2.3.3 Specific Conditions

2.3.3.1 Intrascleral FB[3]

- If the FB is *anterior*, it should carefully be freed and removed. This is relatively easy because access to it is unhindered. The surgeon should know whether the object's distal end has penetrated the eye (open globe injury; the object is appreciated as an IOFB), and if yes, how deep and what additional injuries may have occurred.
- If the FB is *posterior*, the decision whether and how to remove it becomes more complex.
  - If the FB is relatively easily accessible, a scleral cutdown spares patient and ophthalmologists the risks of intraocular surgery, but if major intraocular damage has also occurred, vitreoretinal surgery, alone or in combination with scleral cutdown, may have to be utilized.
  - If the object is too posterior to allow convenient ab externo access, the object should either be left in situ[4] or removed from the inside.

3 An anteriorly located FB usually penetrates the sclera from the outside (i.e., directly). A posterior FB typically traverses the globe first, and also causes intraocular damage.
4 Vitrectomy may still be indicated to deal with coexisting intraocular pathologies.

Controversial

Forceful attempts to dislodge an IOFB that is "stuck" in the posterior sclera can result in serious intraoperative complications; retention of such an object, if ferrous, threatens with siderosis development. The risks and benefits of removal vs retention must be discussed with the patient/family in detail (see Chap. 1.4).

2.3.3.2 Partial-thickness Laceration

In this rarely diagnosed condition, the surgeon should make an individual decision whether suturing is required. If a suture is felt to be necessary, the same material and basic principles apply as detailed under "full-thickness wound" below.

2.3.3.3 Full-thickness Wound[5]

Although ruptures and lacerations have different implications (see Chaps. 2.11, 2.12), certain rules regarding suture closure apply to both. The human body's response to the injury is scar formation, which starts from the episclera and virtualy immediately. One of the goals of surgical wound closure is to stop the natural healing process before the developing scar tissue reaches the inside of the eye and incarcerates the retina (see Chap. 2.14).

2.3.3.3.1 Principles of Wound Closure

The principles of wound closure are as follows:

- If the wound is corneoscleral, the limbus is closed first[6], followed by closure of the cornea, and finally the sclera (see Chap. 2.2 and Fig. 2.3.1).
- If the wound is limited to the easily accessible anterior sclera, the "50%" rule applies.

5 Rupture or laceration

6 It is here where the apposing tissue edges can most accurately be paired up with each other.

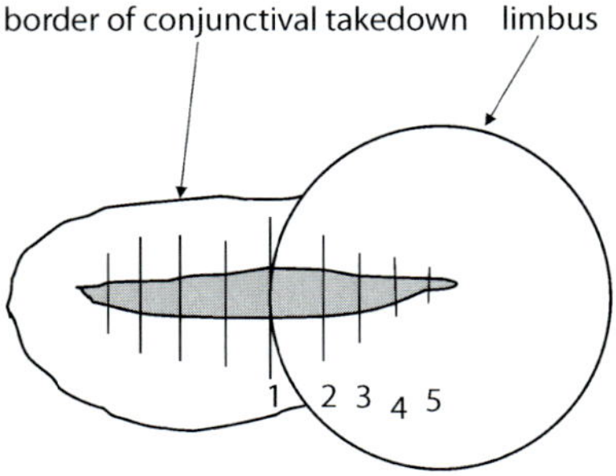

Fig. 2.3.1 Closure strategy for corneoscleral wounds with a short scleral extension. The numbers represent the order of suture placement (as shown in Fig. 2.2.5b). The limbal and the corneal portions of the wound must be closed first. On the scleral side, the surgeon can start at the limbus and continue suture placement away from the limbus. Alternatively, the "50% rule" can be applied: once the distal end of the wound is visualized and the wound is exposed in its entirety, the initial suture is placed at the half point (50%), the next at 25%, then at 75%, etc

- If the wound is partially underneath an extraocular muscle, the easily accessible part is closed first, followed by the difficult-to-access portion (see below).
- If the wound is posterior, the "close-as-you-go" technique is recommended (see below).

2.3.3.3.2 Surgical Technique

The surgical techniques is as follows:

- If possible, general anesthesia should be used, although even topical anesthesia (see Chap. 1.8) is an alternative if necessary [1].
- The first task is to open the conjunctiva anteriorly and establish a clean surgical field.
- Judicious diathermy must be applied to stop any bleeding.
- An orbital retractor may have to carefully be inserted to keep subconjunctival tissues and orbital fat out.[7]

7 This author prefers to insert and position the retractor himself and then hand it over to the nurse.

- The use of traction sutures (see Chap. 2.12) offers advantages but also raises certain risks if too much tension is put on them.
- The episcleral tissue, especially if vitreous prolapse is also present, may be difficult to separate from the sclera. Pressure must never be exerted onto the globe; it is an individual decision whether a sharp instrument or a blunt spatula with proper counterforce[8] is used. A blunt-tipped scissor provides both, allowing blunt tissue separation as well as cutting as necessary.

Pitfall

If the scleral surface is not cleansed properly, the surgeon may end up suturing Tenon's instead of the sclera. This may explain why it is so often necessary for the vitreoretinal surgeon to have to resuture the scleral wound as he prepares for a secondary, intraocular procedure. Before the initial surgery is completed, the surgeon must be convinced that the wound is watertight.

- The surgeon should try to avoid incarcerating tissue in the scleral wound as he closes it with the sutures.

Pearl

The more posterior a scleral wound, the more difficult it is to avoid incarcerating vitreous, choroid, even retina, in the suture track.

- The vitrectomy probe should be used to trim the vitreous at the level of the wound. The probe should not, however, be pushed deep inside the wound to avoid injuring the choroid.
- The assistant plays a crucial role in reducing the incarceration rate. Keeping a spatula over the wound as the surgeon introduces the suture, the assistant should gently push/hold the prolapsing tissues back.
- Interrupted, never running, sutures are to be used (Fig. 2.3.2).

8 i.e., holding the sclera against the movement of the spatula.

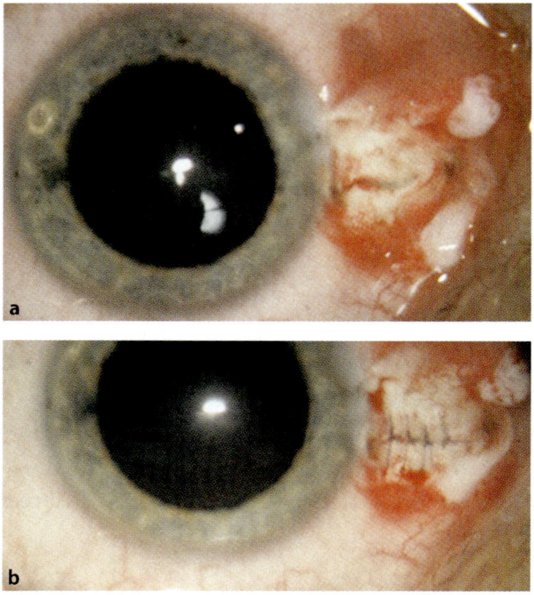

Fig. 2.3.2 Radial wound in the anterior sclera. **a** The conjunctiva has been carefully dissected to expose the scleral wound, which is approximately 4 mm long and makes a slight "S" curve. There is no tissue prolapse, but the dark color of the underlying uvea is visible at the bottom of the wound. **b** Closure is with interrupted, 8-0 vicryl sutures.

- The intended suture depth is ~80%. Unlike in the cornea, tissue edema is rarely an issue. If the suture is a 100% deep, this is not a problem unless the wound is posterior to the ora serrata; hemorrhage from the choroid is extremely rare, but any retinal injury must be avoided. Too shallow a suture track threatens with the suture "cheesewiring" as it is tightened.
- To prevent gaping, it is better to use an increased number of sutures, rather than ones with longer bite (see Chap. 2.2), especially in the anterior sclera, to avoid astigmatism.
- Unlike with corneal wounds, forceps use is mandatory to securely grasp the resistant sclera as the needle passes through; a firm grab also reduces the risk of inadvertent needle movement, which could push the needle holder against the globe and raise the IOP.
- It is often beneficial not to pass the needle through both wound edges with a single sweep, but introduce the needle on one side only, pull the

suture through as far as the tying will later require, then introduce the needle on the other side.

- Even when the wound is underneath an extraocular muscle, closure can often be accomplished without removing the muscle: the assistant should gently hold it away using a muscle hook or a suture.[9]
- If an extraocular muscle needs to be taken down, it should be carefully done so that it does not get "lost into orbit".[10] Two sutures should firmly secure the muscle before it is severed, and two sutures should be used to fixate it back to the sclera.
- The more posterior the wound, the more difficult it is for the assistant to provide access to the operative field, for the surgeon to executive his planned maneuvers – and to do all this while avoiding pressure on the eye. Even minimal pressure can lead to ECH or retinal incarceration. The two key issues are: how to do the closure and when to stop it.
- The "*close-as-you-go*" technique for posterior wounds means that the wound is closed sequentially; the details are explained on Fig. 2.3.3.
- The surgeon needs both of his hands for suturing; the assistant's role is again crucial in providing access without pressure. The assistant's job is twofold: use of a properly sized retractor[11] to keep orbital fat and conjunctival tissues from collapsing onto the surgical field from the *outside*; and use of a spatula to hold back tissues from prolapsing into the wound from the *inside*.

9 The assistant must find the right balance between avoiding pressure on the globe while providing sufficient and convenient access for the surgeon for suture introduction.

10 The surgeon's attention is almost singularly focused on the wound, and there is always the risk of a "silly" mistake when performing tasks that in the "fog of war" appear as of secondary importance.

11 Ideally, the retractor is *large* so that it is able to keep all tissues away from the operative field, but the retractor may have to be "downsized" so that it does not become a physical obstacle interfering with the surgeon's own instruments. The assistant must be alert throughout the procedure and cautiously change the position of the retractor if necessary as the surgeon's tools are moved around.

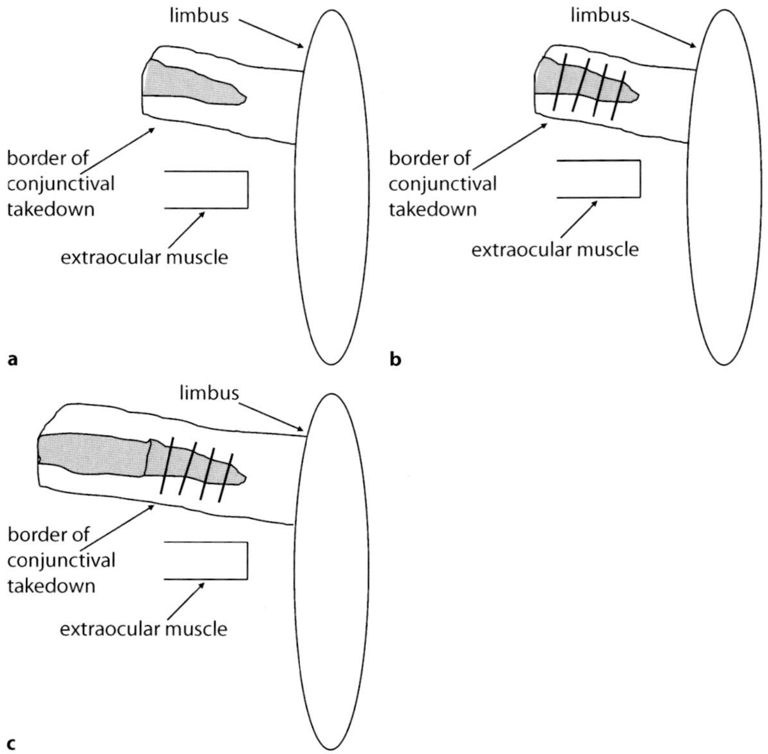

Fig. 2.3.3 Radial wound in the posterior sclera: the "close-as-you-go" technique. **a** The conjunctiva is dissected anteriorly to confirm posterior continuation of the scleral wound. Even if the scleral wound's endpoint is not reached, the conjunctiva is not opened further posteriorly (see the text on details regarding cleaning the scleral surface). **b** The exposed scleral wound is closed with sutures. The direction of suture introduction is anterior to posterior: the "50% rule" does not apply. **c** The conjunctiva is dissected further posteriorly, avoiding any pressure on the sclera.[1] Dissection should be stopped at a convenient point to allow suturing the newly exposed sclera (not shown here). Once the risk of exerting pressure on the globe is high and tissue extrusion becomes unavoidable, suturing of the sclera must stop, and the wound is left to spontaneously scar over (see the text for more details). The conjunctival wound is meticulously closed, and the patient must wear a shield over the eye for a few days

[1]This is the most important warning for the assistant who uses some type of retractor to make the operative field accessible for the surgeon (see text for further details).

- One useful trick to "increase the number of hands without increasing the number of hands"[12] is to put two sutures into the conjunctiva first, and lift the conjunctiva up with these sutures. The sutures can be held against the shaft of the retractor so a single hand is now holding three "tools."
- Another trick is to not cut the proximal, just introduced scleral suture but to use this as a traction suture to gently pull and turn the globe. This suture can be clamped to the drape or be left very long and be held by the OR nurse – hers is now the fifth hand, but it is outside the immediate operative field. This second option is more advantageous than the clamping version since the traction suture is adjustable.
- Regardless of how effective and nontraumatic the assistant is in using the retractor, the wound may extend too far posteriorly to allow closure without increasing the threat of (further) extruding intraocular tissues and ECH.

Selected pathologies in eyes with full-thickness scleral wound, recorded in the USEIR database, are given in Table 2.3.1.

Pitfall

If the scleral wound is very posterior, forcible closure is not simply counterproductive but dangerous. The wound should be left unsutured, and management should shift from an external to an internal approach (prophylactic chorioretinectomy; see below and Chap. 2.14). The conjunctiva over the unsutured scleral wound must be meticulously closed to eliminate the endophthalmitis risk.

12 The actual operative field is too small to conveniently allow access of four hands of two assistants.

Table 2.3.1 Selected pathologies in eyes with full-thickness scleral wound in the USEIR database

Pathology	Laceration (%)	Rupture (%)
Hyphema	45	54
Cataract	18	13
IOFB	16	0
Endophthalmitis	2	1
Vitreous hemorrhage	48	48
Retinal break	12	10
Retinal detachment	21	24
Total	2446 (17%)	877 (6%)

Based on 14,523 injuries involving the globe

2.3.3.3.3 *Material*

- For a *limbal* wound, 8/0 to 10/0 nylon is appropriate. The knot must be buried.
- For *scleral* wounds, 6/0 to 8/0 vicryl gives sufficient strength if used properly (see Chap. 2.2) during the (rather rapid) healing process. The suture is absorbable, but its desintegration will be preceeded by complete wound healing. The same suture material is used for closing the conjunctiva, which is an additional advantage. An alternative is to use polypropylene sutures.

If a surgeon is uncomfortable using absorbable material to suture a scleral wound, nylon (silk, polyester) can also be used.

Chapter 2.11 provides further details on managing eyes with corneal wounds and presents the similarities and differences between eyes with corneal vs scleral wound.

2.3.3.4 Thin or Necrotic Sclera

Occasionally, it is not possible to close the defect with sutures because the sclera is too thin or necrotic. It usually occurs in persons with:

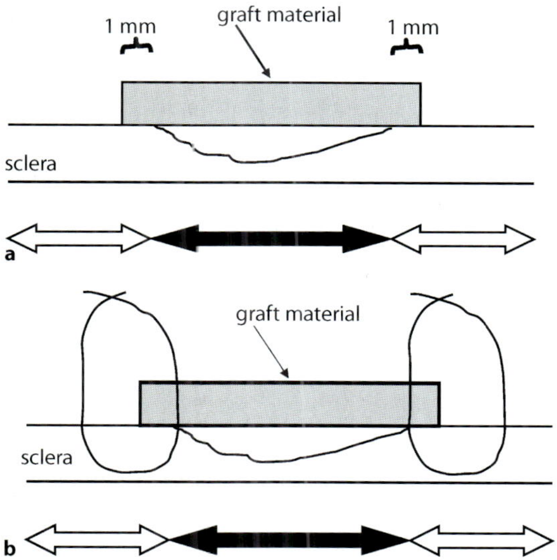

Fig. 2.3.4 Securing a patch over the nonhealthy sclera. **a** The graft is overlayed by 1 mm on all sides (except at the limbus where it is meticulously trimmed). The *dark central arrow* shows the boundary of the pathological sclera, the *blank arrows* represent the healthy sclera. **b** The suture fixating the graft onto the recipient sclera is full-thickness in the graft and ~80% in the underlying sclera. This method helps avoid putting undue tension on the graft

- Long axial length (high myopia)
- Buphthalmus
- Degenerative autoimmune disease (e.g., rheumatoid arthritis)
- Previous injury or surgery (filtration, scleral buckling, vitrectomy)
- Infection

Recognition of an area of thin and weak sclera is very important not only after injury but also if vitrectomy is to be performed. Whenever possible, healthy sclera should be used for sclerotomy placement.

If thin or necrotic sclera is found during postinjury inspection of the sclera and the area is very small,[13] it can be infolded using a mattress suture with long bites.

If the area is large, a scleral patch should be used. It is beyond the scope of this book to detail the various types of materials used as graft or the techiques of grafting [2, 3],[14] but it is important to emphasize that the graft must be meticulously fashioned over the area[15] and be sutured to healthy sclera in an "overlay" fashion (Fig. 2.3.4).

If no suitable graft material is available, the conjunctiva can be temporarily used to cover the damaged area.

DO:

- learn to treat the sclera with respect; although only indirectly, it does have a major impact on the outcome of the injury
- consider an internal approach to scleral wounds not easily accessible from the outside

DON'T:

- start operating on a posterior scleral wound if a knowledgeable assistant is unavailable
- force closure of a scleral wound too posterior for convenient access

13 e.g., it is the result to previous surgery

14 e.g., homologous sclera, autologous sclera, cornea, tarsoconjunctival flap, Tenon's capsule (for small defects), fascia lata, lyophilized dura, periosteum, dermal tissue, cadaver aorta, Gore-Tex

15 Which must first undergo thorough debridement

Summary

Although the number of trauma-related pathologies involving the sclera is low, the significance of a full-thickness scleral wound cannot be overestimated. Retinal involvement in the scleral wound, whether from the injury, improper surgery, or the healing process (scarring) has a decisive impact on the outcome.

Scleral and corneal wounds have very different implications; this is discussed in Chap. 2.11.

References

[1] Auffarth GU, Vargas LG, Klett J, Volcker HE (2004) Repair of a ruptured globe using topical anesthesia. J Cataract Refract Surg 30: 726–729

[2] Lindsey J, Hamill B (2002) Scleral and corneoscleral injuries. In: Kuhn F, Pieramici D (eds) Ocular trauma: principles and practice. Thieme, New York, pp 111–122

[3] Witherspoon CD, Kuhn F, Morris R, Collins P (1995) Scleral staphyloma and dehiscences. In: Roy H (eds) Master techniques in ophthalmic surgery. Williams and Wilkins, Baltimore, pp 1176–1183

2.4 Tissue Prolapse

Ferenc Kuhn

2.4.1 Introduction

Extrusion of intraocular contents[1] commonly occurs when an eye injury is full thickness; Table 2.4.1 shows selected incidence figures with different types of trauma. The tissue extrusion typically occurs at the time of injury as the IOP rises during impact;[2] escape of aqueous and tissues through the wound follows a pressure gradient until the IOP is normalized[3].

Unless an ECH occurs (see Chaps. 1.10, 2.8), the surgeon should deal with the prolapsed tissue before closing the wound.

The incidence and consequences of tissue prolapse with different types of trauma, as recorded in the USEIR database, are given in Table 2.4.2.

2.4.2 Evaluation

If uvea has prolapsed, it is usually easily recognizable; vitreous may be more difficult to identify, especially if there is lens disruption or the wound is

1 In this chapter we do not discuss internal tissue prolapse (i.e., lens in the vitreous cavity/AC, vitreous in the AC), which are described in their respective chapters.

2 Factors that may exacerbate tissue extrusion include, among others, intraorbital and intraocular hemorrhage, contraction of the lid and extraocular muscles, and pressure on the eye by the ophthalmologist during examination or surgery.

3 The IOP and the atmospheric pressure rapidly equalize (i.e., the IOP approaches the atmospheric pressure) unless wound closure halts the process.

Table 2.4.1 The incidence (%) and consequences of tissue prolapse with different types of trauma in the USEIR database

Injury type	Prolapsed tissue		Retinal detachment rate	
	Iris/uvea	Vitreous	With tissue prolapse	Without tissue prolapse
Rupture (2117)	54	5	21	10
Penetrating (4220)	38	2	15	4
IOFB (1235)	24	1	31	11
Perforating (464)	41	3	27	19

Based on 9036 cases

Table 2.4.2 Tissue prolapse: summary of management preferences

Tissue	Excise	Reposit	Comment
Iris	+	+++	As much of the iris as possible should be preserved; if excision cannot be avoided, concurrent or subsequent iridoplasty should be considered (see Chap. 2.6)
Ciliary body and choroid	(+)	+++	Because of the risk of hemorrhage, phthisis, and inflammation, excision is reserved for those rare cases where reposition is impossible
Lens	+++	–	Even a partially retained lens capsule can cause inflammation and contribute to destruction of the ciliary processes
Vitreous	+++	–	Vitreous removal should be complete and atraumatic
Retina	(+)	+++	Excision is permissible only in those very rare cases where reposition is physically impossible, but either way the retina must be carefully inspected ab interno, and any pathology properly addressed (see Chap. 2.14)

scleral and posterior, and there is subconjunctival hemorrhage. If presence of a non-self-sealing wound is confirmed at the slit lamp, there is no need to have a definite answer as to whether a tissue prolapse is also present; this should be determined intraoperatively.

2.4.3 Specific Conditions

2.4.3.1 Iris

The iris is the most mobile tissue after the vitreous; therefore, it is easily externalized along with the escaping aqueous. If the wound is corneal, the prolapsed iris is easy to visualize (Fig. 2.4.1); if the wound is scleral, the diagnosis may be more difficult since chemosis, blood, or an intact and congested conjunctiva can hide it. The irregular shape of the pupil ("peaking" toward the wound) should raise suspicion.

2.4.3.1.1 Management

Occasionally, a small prolapse through a small wound may be eliminated by using miotic drugs if the prolapse is peripheral and by mydriatic drugs if the prolapse is more central. It is usually safer, however, to deal with the problem surgically. The surgeon has two options: reposition or excision.

2.4.3.1.1.1 Reposition

This is the primary choice: unless the iris is contaminated and cannot be cleaned, the surgeon should try to save the iris so that it can continue to compartmentalize the eye and regulate the size of the pupil. The iris must first be cleaned of *organisms* that may cause infection, *foreign material*, especially if the injury was caused by explosion, and *epithelial cells*, which could possibly lead to epithelial downgrowth (see Chap. 2.18) [5].

Cleaning of a contaminated iris can be achieved via:

- Removing particles with a Wechsler sponge or forceps

- Directing a strong jet stream onto the iris from a 10-cc syringe, using an irrigation fluid that contains antibiotics.[4] A combination of the two techniques is often necessary.

The iris may also be *macerated*, especially if its prolapse is not fresh. It is a judgment call in such cases whether to reposit or excise it. An iris that is "barely hanging on" to its root is not worth repositing.

The *technique* of iris reposition is simple: if the prolapse is through the cornea or at the limbus, the surgeon should pull, rather than push, the tissue. This is not only more gentle but much more effective than pushing the iris back.[5] A paracentesis needs to be made at a convenient location (90–180° from the wound), and, using a properly long spatula, the iris is swept out of the wound. Once the iris is repositioned, viscoelastics or air can be injected to prevent a recurrence of the extrusion.[6] This is especially important if additional surgical maneuvers are planned.

Pearl

The closer the wound is to the limbus, the higher the risk of iris (re)prolapse and anterior synechia formation.

If the prolapse is through a scleral wound, reposition is done via gentle pushing. If the IOP is high, the prolapse may recur; the assistant should in such cases hold the iris back with a spatula while the surgeon introduces the sutures (see Chap. 2.3). Injecting a strong miotic agent into the anterior chamber (AC) can also help keeping the iris from reprolapsing.

Time was once considered essential in determining whether the iris should be reposited or excised ("excision if extruded for over 24 h"). We now consider the iris' condition (see above) the decisive factor.

---

4 The same concentration should be used as for intravitreal injections (see Chap. 2.17).

5 Pushing is recommended only if the prolapse is very small.

6 Viscoelastics are used to keep the iris from reprolapsing, *not* to push the iris back into the AC.

2.4.3.1.1.2 Excision

Excision is recommended if the iris is impossible to clean or if it is very necrotic, but the area of excision should be kept to the minimum, and reconstruction of the diaphragm should always be on the surgeon's mind (see Chap. 2.6). Diathermizing the iris before cutting is advisable if the iris is non-necrotic to prevent a major bleeding.

If a significant hemorrhage occurs during excision or reposition, it must be stopped using the endodiathermy probe to prevent blood accumulation in the AC or in the vitreous.

2.4.3.2 Ciliary Body and Choroid

Their prolapse is much less common than that of the iris. Recognition is straightforward once the scleral wound has been identified.

2.4.3.2.1 Management

A prolapsed *choroid* should be reposited since the risk of intraoperative hemorrhage and postoperative inflammation is significant if excision is performed. Gentle diathermy of the choroid makes it shrink, easing reposition.

If the *ciliary body* is extruded, its reposition is especially crucial. The goal is not only to avoid complications such as hemorrhage and inflammation, but to minimize the risk of phthisis (see Chap. 2.8). Special attention must be paid to avoid incarcerating the ciliary body in the wound. Ciliary body trauma is presumed to play a role in the development of sympathetic ophthalmia (see Chap. 1.8).

2.4.3.3 Lens

Both the *diagnosis* and *management* are straightforward: the extruded lens (or IOL), whether it is intact or fragmented, must be removed with forceps or a Wechsler sponge. Occasionally, parts of the capsule may remain attached to the zonules [1]. If the capsule is partially extruded in a young person, removal of the capsule must be very carefully done since the capsule is strongly adherent to the zonules; enzymatic zonulolysis[7] is advised first to

7 Alpha-chymotrypsin in a 1 to 5,000/10,000 dilution

avoid a major hemorrhage. Extreme caution in young people is also necessary because the posterior lens capsule is adhering to the anterior hyaloid as well. Use of the vitrectomy probe, rather than a forceps, allows prevention of vitreous-related complications.

2.4.3.4 Vitreous

Vitreous is the most mobile intraocular tissue.[8] Recognition of vitreous prolapse is also influenced by the condition of the tissue: a formed vitreous is easily visualized in the wound, while a less formed one may be difficult to visualize. TA is very helpful: its adherence to the vitreous fibrils is much stronger than to smooth tissues such as the sclera or choroid. If the wound is in the anterior sclera, and the AC and lens are clear, strands in the anterior vitreous are usually visible at the slit lamp visible as lines converging toward the wound (Fig. 2.4.1).

2.4.3.4.1 Management

All vitreous must be thoroughly excised. If the prolapse is through a corneal wound, the surgeon is advised to also remove the vitreous from the AC (see Chap. 2.5).

Cave

Although it is technically possible to thoroughly remove the prolapsed vitrectomy at the wound using Wechsler sponges[9] and scissors, this is not without risk. The vitreous first needs to adhere to the sponge and then be lifted from the eye before it is cut. The traction exerted on the extruded vitreous is unavoidably transmitted to the peripheral retina and may cause a break.

8 A healthy vitreous requires more force to extrude than one that has lost most of its gel properties.

9 The surgeon should avoid touching the corneal endothelium with the sponge.

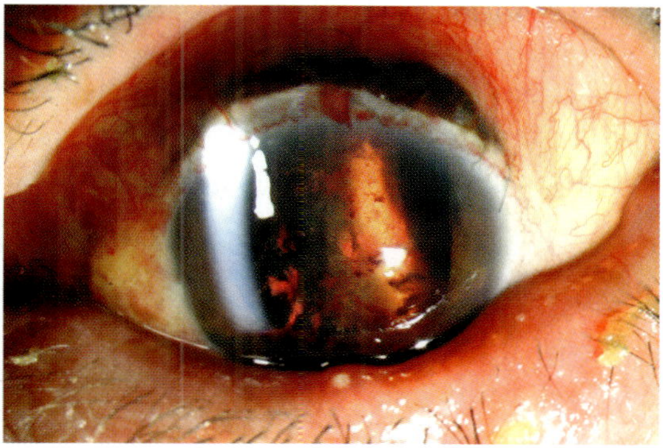

Fig. 2.4.1 Rupture of a cataract wound with iris prolapse and vitreous "streaks". The iris has prolapsed into the limbal wound and tamponaded it. The running suture has been severed. It is not possible to determine whether there is extraocular vitreous prolapse, but the vitreous has prolapsed into the AC and has a few dots of blood on its anterior surface. The vitreous configuration is such that it points the examiner toward the wound (Courtesy of V. Mester, Abu Dhabi, U.A.E.)

The vitrectomy probe is the preferred instrument for removing vitreous from the wound, irrespective of whether the wound is corneal[10] or scleral. It is possible that the higher incidence in the USEIR of retinal detachment associated with scleral compared with corneal wounds (23 vs 11%, respectively; see Tables 2.2.1, 2.3.1) is due not only to the injury itself but also to inappropriate management of vitreous prolapse. This assumption is supported by the finding that the retinal detachment rate is 78% if the scleral wound is at the ora serrata but only 16% the wound is posterior [4] as well as by the clinical experience that the breaks causing the retinal detachment are typically found either at the wound or a 180° away. Failure to fully excise the prolapsed vitreous greatly increases the risk of retinal detachment [2].

10 Unlike the sponge–scissors combination, the vitrectomy probe also allows removing the vitreous from the internal aspect of the wound (see Chap. 2.5).

If vitreous is found to have extruded through a wound posterior to the ora serrata, the retina must also have been injured,[11] and this must be taken into consideration when the management plan is designed. If the scleral wound is very posterior, it may be impossible to remove the vitreous prolapse completely, and management of the condition must be addressed ab interno (see Chap. 2.14).

2.4.3.5 Retina

If retina has prolapsed through the wound, this is easily recognized (Fig. 2.4.2), unless it is completely necrotic and/or blood covers it.

2.4.3.5.1 Management

As a general rule, the retina should not be excised but reposited. Even if it appears that the eye's condition is hopeless, successful retinal reposition may be accompanied by functional improvement.

- A *small* prolapse[12] is dealt with by first removing any vitreous from the retinal surface, then gently introducing the suture into one of the edges of the scleral wound, having the assistant hold/push the retina back with a spatula, putting the needle through the opposing edge of the wound, and tying the suture while the spatula is still underneath the suture, preventing a retinal reprolapse.
- If the prolapse is *large*, its underlying cause must be addressed first: the IOP is high, presumably due to a hemorrhage, which is pushing the retina forward. Patience is needed – waiting for tens of minutes if necessary. The intraocular bleeding must stop first,[13] and the IOP may have to be lowered.[14] Once the IOP is low, the material behind the

---

11 This statement is another example reflecting a proactive, rather than reactive, treatment philosophy (see Chap 1.8).

12 Small implies small area *and* small elevation.

13 The anesthesiologist should be asked to lower the patient's systemic blood pressure as much as possible.

14 This contradicts what is said about ECH in Chap. 2.8; however, a retinal prolapse requires special treatment. Usually, it is retinal prolapse that needs to be prevented if an intraocular hemorrhage occurs; once a retinal prolapse has occurred, the situation changes dramatically, and a different logic takes over.

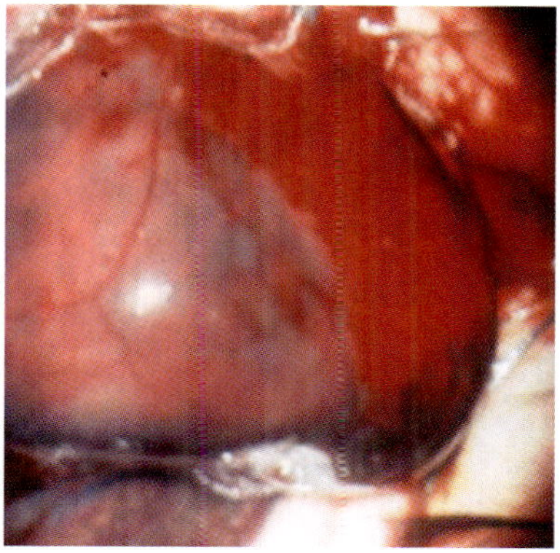

Fig. 2.4.2 Retinal prolapse in a ruptured eye. The retinal extrusion is caused by an ECH. Fresh blood is visible on the right side of the image. Although the prognosis is poor, the eye is not necessarily unsalvageable; primary enucleation is not justified (see the text for management details)

retina (may be vitreous or blood) can be slowly removed, through a retinotomy if necessary. The wound is then gradually closed, using the technique described above.

- If the retina cannot be completely pushed back, it should be cauterized in as small an area as possible, sacrificed, and the scleral wound closed, saving most of the retina.

Pearl

Incarcerating a prolapsed retina in the scleral wound is the lesser of "two evils." Retinal incarceration can be addressed in subsequent surgeries; only enucleation takes away the anatomical and functional hopes (see Chap. 1.8).

- The retina may be incarcerated despite the best efforts by surgeon and assistant [3]. The incarceration may be caused by the retina (a) being caught by the needle/suture, (b) prolapsing into the wound while the wound is being closed, and (c) subsequently being captured by the developing scar.

Regardless of the mechanism of incarceration, the choroid and retina must soon be liberated (i.e., excised) in this area (see Chap. 2.14).

DO:

- try to salvage as much of the uvea and retina as possible
- try to remove as much of the prolapsed vitreous as possible

DON'T:

- enucleate an eye just because there is retinal prolapse; in most cases, the retina can be reposited and the retinal incarceration dealt with later

Summary

Tissue prolapse is a common consequence of open globe injury. Knowledge of a few simple rules of how to deal with the prolapsed tissue greatly increases the eye's chances of anatomical and thus functional recovery.

References

[1] Blomquist PH (2003) Expulsion of an intraocular lens through a clear corneal wound. J Cataract Refract Surg 29: 592–594

[2] Cleary PE, Ryan SJ (1978) Posterior perforating eye injury. Experimental animal model. Trans Ophthalmol Soc U K 98: 34–37

[3] Han DP, Mieler WF, Abrams GW, Williams GA (1988) Vitrectomy for traumatic retinal incarceration. Arch Ophthalmol 106: 640–645

[4] Hsu HT, Ryan SJ (1986) Experimental retinal detachment in the rabbit. Penetrating ocular injury with retinal laceration. Retina 6: 66–69

[5] Nagra PK, Raber IM (2003) Epithelial ingrowth in a phakic corneal transplant patient after traumatic wound dehiscence. Cornea 22: 184–186

2.5 Anterior Chamber

Ferenc Kuhn

2.5.1 Introduction

The anterior chamber (AC) is an aqueous-filled compartment whose important bordering structures include the cornea, angle, iris, and the lens. Injuries to all neighboring tissues are discussed in their respective chapters; here we describe trauma-related pathologies involving the AC itself.

2.5.2 Evaluation

The ophthalmologist should evaluate the following variables in/of the AC:

- Depth
- Transparency (clarity)
- Presence of foreign material[1]
- Angle recession
- Abnormal tissue configuration (i.e., synechia)

The normal *depth* of the AC is 3 mm [6]; a significantly shallower or deeper AC is easily recognized by the reduced or increased distance between the cornea and the iris.

---

1 e.g., IOFBs (see Chap. 2.13), fibrin, lens particles; see below

Pearl

It is often easier to judge AC depth with the naked eye (rather than at the slit lamp) because this permits instant comparison with the normal fellow eye.

The AC depth may be uniformly or only partially abnormal. Lens dislocation is the most common cause, although other etiologies also occur.

Reduced clarity of the aqueous, presence of foreign material, or abnormal tissue configuration are also often recognizable with a penlight; nevertheless, the slit lamp remains the most effective diagnostic tool. The presence of white blood cells and flare are signs of anterior uveitis. Recognition of an angle recession requires a contact lens, although the UBM is an excellent alternative [7].

2.5.3 Specific Conditions

2.5.3.1 Depth

2.5.3.1.1 Shallowing of the AC

Possible causes of shallowing include:

- Leakage of the aqueous through a cornea/limbal wound[2]
- Dislocation of the lens into the AC
- Swelling of the lens
- Aqueous misdirection (malignant glaucoma; see Chap. 2.18)
- Severe intraocular hemorrhage (ECH). A combination of these etiologies is also possible

The *treatment* is determined by the underlying cause. Once aqueous loss through the wound is stopped (via spontaneous tissue tamponade or wound suturing), the AC rapidly reforms. Similarly, removal of the dislocated or swollen lens restores normal AC depth. In eyes with an ECH, treatment is

2 A scleral wound may also lead to shallowing of the AC, although this is much more rare.

much more complex (see Chap. 2.8). It is important to restore normal AC depth to prevent synechia formation.

2.5.3.1.2 Deepening of the AC

Possible causes of deepening include:

- Loss the lens (extrusion or posterior dislocation)
- Partial zonulolysis
- Presence of a posterior scleral wound [14]

Unlike a shallow AC, a deep one does not by itself represent a risk for additional complications. The AC always remains deeper in any eye if the lens has been removed.

2.5.3.1.3 Concomitant Shallowing and Deepening of the AC

The condition is caused by a complete posterior synechia, with the pupillary margin tightly adhering to the anterior lens capsule. Aqueous accumulates in the posterior chamber, pushing the iris forward in its mid-section (here the AC is shallow), and pushing the lens backward close to the iris periphery (here the AC deepens). Such an iris bombans can lead to secondary glaucoma (see Chap. 2.18).

2.5.3.2 Reduced Transparency

2.5.3.2.1 Blood (Hyphema)

This is the most commonly diagnosed pathology; the incidence varies with injury type. (Table 2.5.1). The blood usually clears spontaneously after a few days and mostly through the trabecular meshwork. The significance of hyphema lies in the secondary complications blood in the AC can cause (see below) as well as in the coexistent posterior segment injuries, which remain hidden from the examiner by the hemorrhage[3] (Table 2.5.2). In the USEIR, 53% of eyes with trauma-related hyphema showed some type of posterior pathology; in the HEIR, the rate reached 61%.

3 The ophthalmologist may not even suspect that any posterior segment pathology is present.

Table 2.5.1 The incidence of hyphema (%) in various types of trauma in the USEIR database

Type of trauma	Percentage of eyes with hyphema
Contusion	14
Rupture	21
Penetrating trauma	25
Perforating trauma	6
IOFB injury	4
Overall in open globe injuries	45

Based on injuries

Table 2.5.2 The incidence of various posterior segment pathologies (%) in eyes with hyphema in the USEIR database

Pathology	Incidence if hyphema caused by contusion	Incidence if hyphema is caused by open globe trauma
Vitreous hemorrhage	40	52
Retinal break[a]	6	6
Retinal detachment	8	19
Macular hole	1	0.002
Choroidal rupture	9	5
Total no. of cases	672	2196

Based on 2878 injuries

[a]Includes any type of peripheral break, e.g., dialysis, tear, hole

2.5.3.2.1.1 Consequences[4]

- Reduced visual acuity, which may drop to LP even if no other pathology is present [12].

4 See also section 2.5.3.2.1.4.

- Difficulty recognizing coexisting anterior segment abnormalities (e.g., cyclodialysis cleft, IOFB in the angle, angle recession).
- Difficulty recognizing coexisting posterior segment abnormalities (e.g., vitreous hemorrhage, retinal detachment).
- Elevated IOP, occurring in up to a quarter of eyes (see below and Chap. 2.18).
- Corneal blood staining, which can make visualization of intraocular pathologies even more difficult. It interferes with visual rehabilitation (see Fig. 2.2.14) and its effect can last for months. The risk is especially high if the hyphema is total, blood absorption is slow, and the IOP is high. If the endothelium is dysfunctional, blood staining can occur even if the IOP is normal [1]. The dark color of a total hyphema (see below) signals a lack of oxygen in the AC, which represents a risk factor for endothelial damage.
- Formation of posterior synechiae.

2.5.3.2.1.2 Evaluation

Taking a *systemic history* is especially important since hyphema is more common and potentially much more severe in patients with sickle cell disease. In addition, it needs to be known whether the patient suffers from bleeding disorders or is on anticoagulant therapy[5]. The *slit lamp* is the best tool to identify the presence and amount of blood[6] (Table 2.5.3). Ultrasonography, the UBM, and radiological tests may have to be performed to determine whether there is coexisting damage to anterior or posterior segment structures. Laboratory tests should also be ordered if sickle cell disease is suspected (sickle cell preparation, hemoglobin electrophoresis, bleeding tests) or if systemic antifibrinolytic therapy is planned (kidney and liver functions).

5 Although it has not been proven that such therapy increases the risk [5].

6 This is usually not possible if the patient is in bed and the blood cannot settle.

Table 2.5.3 Various methods to describe the size of hyphema

Method	Comment
Millimeters	The height of the pooled blood is given; however, a "12-mm" hyphema is described as total
Percentage	0 if there is no blood in the AC and 100 if a total hyphema is seen
Clock hour	The face of the clock is used to describe the height of the meniscus of the blood at the limbus
Grade	I: <1/3
	II: 1/3–1/2
	III: 1/2 to near total
	IV: Total[a]

[a] Often referred to as eight- or black-ball hyphema [9, 11]. The dark color is caused by deoxygenization of the hemoglobin

2.5.3.2.1.3 Management

Controversial

In eyes with *open globe trauma*, the blood can be evacuated at the time of primary repair. The benefits are that additional pathologies can be visualized early and that blood-related complications may be prevented; the disadvantages are that this increases inflammation and is an unnecessary procedure if the blood would rapidly absorb on its own.[7]

2.5.3.2.1.3.1 Medical Treatment

Medical treatment consists of:

- Cycloplegics/mydriatics to reduce pain and the risk of the posterior synechia formation
- Topical corticosteroids to reduce the inflammation

7 Which is impossible to prognosticate

- Topical and/or oral[8] aminocaproic acid to reduce the risk of rebleeding [10]
- TPA, an fibrinolytic agent (10 µg injected intracamerally)
- Oral antifibrinolytic therapy (tranexamic acid 25 mg/kg 3× daily for 6 days) [13]
- Antiglaucoma treatment as necessary

Controversial

It is not known whether aspirin therapy should be discontinued; the ophthalmologist should directly consult with the patient's treating physician.

2.5.3.2.1.3.2 Complementary Treatment[9]

- No bedrest necessary
- No hospitalization necessary
- No patching necessary

2.5.3.2.1.3.3 Surgical Treatment

Mechanical evacuation of the blood is indicated in either of these two scenarios:[10]

- Spontaenous blood absorption is too slow to allow treatment of a retinal pathology.
- The IOP cannot be medically controlled and corneal blood staining threatens. Surgery is 20 times more likely to be necessary if there is rebleeding [3]. Several surgical techniques are available. The selection is partially based on whether the blood has clotted and partially on surgeon preference.

8 Must not be used by persons having liver or renal disease; side effects are common and include diarrhea and postural hypotension.

9 These recommendations should be reversed if the patient is a noncompliant child or has sickle cell disease or a rebleeding.

10 The intervention is more pressing if the patient has sickle cell disease.

- The initial step is the preparation of a *paracentesis*. To be efficient, and reduce the risk of intra- and postoperative complications, the paracentesis must satisfy several criteria (Fig. 2.5.1a,b). The working paracentesis should be on the temporal side to increase convenience and minimize interference from the patient's nose.
- When the blood is *liquid*, simple irrigation is sufficient. The washout can be accomplished via a single paracentesis or via two.
  - If a *single* paracentesis is used, the irrigation cannula must be relatively small (23 g suffices) to fit the channel *and* to allow fluid[11] to egress (Fig. 2.5.1c). While the cannula is in the AC, it must be angled by the surgeon so as to minimize the risk to the endothelium and to the lens in a phakic eye. The surgeon can use both hands to hold the syringe (5 or 10 ml), and press the lower corneal wound lip down to gape the wound.
  - If *two* paracenteses are used, a larger cannula may be selected; the second paracentesis should be made on the opposite side of the eye where fewer manipulations are required. The surgeon uses a spatula to depress the wound lip here to gape it for easier fluid egress.
- When the blood is *clotted*, it must be evacuated using the vitrectomy probe or a fine forceps. Especially if the vitrectomy probe is used, an AC maintainer (Fig. 2.5.2) must be placed first to avoid collapse of the AC. Extreme caution is needed to prevent injuring the endothelium, lens, or the iris[12]; viscoelastics should *not* be used until the blood has been removed.
- A fairly thorough evacuation of the blood is recommended, but not all circulating red blood cells need to be removed.
- If a rebleeding is detected, it can be halted with viscoelastics and then the source cauterized if vitrectomy instrumentation is available.
- Whether air or viscoelastics needs to be left in the AC at the conclusion of surgery depends on the specifics of the case. The main goal is to

11 A mixture of blood and BSS, used for irrigation.

12 This can cause severe intraoperative bleeding.

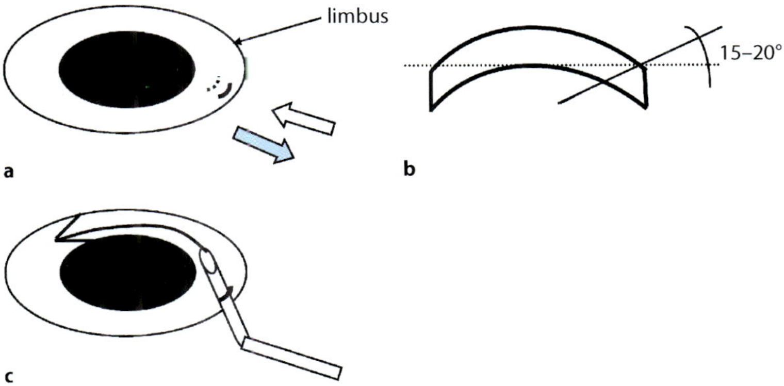

Fig. 2.5.1 The technique of paracentesis and AC irrigation. **a** The eye is held firmly with forceps (not shown here); ideally, the conjunctiva is grasped at a convenient location on the *same* side as the paracentesis: this allows the eye to be held against (*blue arrow*) the force of the MVR (*white arrow*). The MVR blade should be placed slightly central from the limbus to avoid pushing stem cells into the AC and to reduce the risk of synechia formation. The *solid line* shows the slice in the epithelium, the *dotted line* in the endothelium. The channel created by the blade is obviously a slit, yet it allows simultaneous fluid transport in both directions if the irrigation cannula is correctly used.[1] **b** The angle of blade direction is also important: too shallow a path leaves a large scar, limits maneuverability of the instruments introduced through the channel, and causes image distorsion[2] by compressing the cornea; too deep a path also limits instrument maneuverability and makes it less likely that the paracentesis will be self-sealing. An angle of 15–20° allows easy manipulations in the AC while alleviating the need for suturing. **c** The cannula must be kept parallel to the iris (reduce the injury risk both the endothelium the lens in the phakic eye), and its tip is kept over the iris at all times. The jet stream is not too forceful and is roughly parellel with the plane of the iris; the angle is irrigated with a gentle stream. As long as blood flows out from the AC freely, there is little need to modify the cannula's position. If the blood is sticky in certain places, this can usually be "uprooted" with a directly aimed jet stream

[1] i.e., the cannula is gently pushing down on the lower lip of the corneal wound to gape the wound, as described in the text and Fig. 2.5.2.

[2] This is also true for manipulating any instrument inside the AC whether the paracentesis was performed for blood washout or any other purpose.

have the AC reformatted and the IOP restored. If viscoelastics are left behind, the IOP may rise significantly, and prophylactic antiglaucoma treatment with close follow-up is necessary. Air takes longer to absorb from the AC than from the vitreous cavity.

Pearl

If viscoelastics must be left in the AC, use a cohesive, not a dispersive, one (see below). This tends to reduce the risk and length of IOP elevation.

2.5.3.2.1.4 Complications

Complications include:

- Recurrent bleeding. The incidence is between 3 and 26% [13]. The complication rate following a rebleeding is much higher than after the initial hemorrhage. Risk factors include sickle cell disease, being on systemic anticoagulant therapy, and larger initial bleeding.
- Corneal blood staining. This pathology is best recognized with the slit lamp, using high magnification and a narrow beam to find yellowish-brownish discoloration of the posterior cornea. Even though the condition has been reported at low IOP [1], the most important risk factor is a persistently elevated IOP. Patients with elevated IOP must be closely monitored, and surgical intervention should be early if signs of corneal staining appear. If staining has occurred and posterior segment surgery is indicated, TKP vitrectomy (see Chap. 2.15) or endoscopy (see Chap. 2.19) can be performed.
- Glaucoma. Since this is a rather common complication[13] (the incidence is up to 14% with the initial and 25–67% with recurring hemorrhage [13]), gonioscopy should be performed a few weeks after the hemorrhage has disappeared to lower the risk of rebleeding. Chapter 2.18 provides the details of treating eyes with elevated IOP in eyes with hyphema.

---

13 Elevated IOP in an eye with hyphema is not necessarily the consequence of the hemorrhage; the two may be independent pathologies caused by the same trauma.

2.5.3.2.2 Fibrin, Fibrinous Membranes, and Inflammatory Debris

While small amounts of *fibrin* do not require intervention, larger amounts or fully developed membranes should lead to the consideration of intervention. If surgery is not otherwise planned, 25 µg TPA may be injected intracamerally [4]. If surgery is performed,[14] surgical removal is another viable option.

The membrane is very elastic; it can usually easily be extracted with aspiration (through a paracentesis using a cannula or the vitrectomy probe; see above). If it is possible to completely occlude the cannula's port with the membrane, there is no need for an AC maintainer. To prevent AC collapse, however, it is safer to insert one first.

Alternatively, a fine intravitreal forceps is utilized. The membrane is grasped and gently pulled, then patiently held under traction until it detaches.

Pearl

Cohesion of a *fibrinous membrane* is stronger than its adhesion to the tissues it covers. Under the proper amount of tension, the membrane will break from the tissue, and allow the surgeon to remove it in a single piece.

A thorough irrigation of the AC is also needed to remove the *inflammatory debris* from the angle. Irrigation may have to be repeated throughout surgery, especially in children and in eyes with endophthalmitis.

2.5.3.2.3 Lens

Lens particles floating in the AC represent a serious secondary glaucoma risk as well as an obstacle to visualizing the deeper structures of the eye. Removal of the lens particles is rather urgent. The technique depends primarily on whether vitreous prolapse is present or threatens (see Chap. 2.18).

14 The presence of fibrin alone is almost never an indication by itself.

2.5.3.2.4 Vitreous

If vitreous is present in the AC, two factors determine whether removal is indicated:

- Presence of a corneal wound, which gives convenient access for the vitrectomy probe to be introduced to trim the vitreous. It is especially important not to leave vitreous fibrils to remain attached to the inside of the wound:[15] this is a source of traction and thus a risk factor for retinal detachment.
- The presence and type of secondary complications.
- A luxated lens requires surgery even in a contused eye.
- If the lens is subluxated but there is no corneal touch by the lens or vitreous, intervention is not necessary (see Chap. 2.7).

Recognition of the vitreous in the AC is not necessarily easy;[16] an indirect sign is a deformed pupil that cannot be explained by other reasons. Intraoperative diagnostic tools include air and TA (see below).

Regarding surgical technique:

- An infusion (typically, an AC maintainer) is almost always necessary. As always, the AC maintainer is placed in such a way that its tip it is unable to injure the lens (Fig. 2.5.2). The infusion is opened as the first and removed as the last of the maneuvers.
- A paracentesis is made on the *temporal* side, even if this does not coincide with the surgeon's better (dominant) hand. The vitrectomy probe must be held in the proper plane, and the nose of the patient must not interfere (see above).
- Vitreous that is clearly visible is removed.
- The vitrectomy probe should be held as deep in the AC as possible, and its port should be facing the surgeon to avoid injury to the lens or to the iris.

---

15 Irrespective of whether the incarceration occurred as the wound spontaneously closed or it is the result of the surgeon's actions.

16 Pigment dispersion on the vitreous surface is a giveaway.

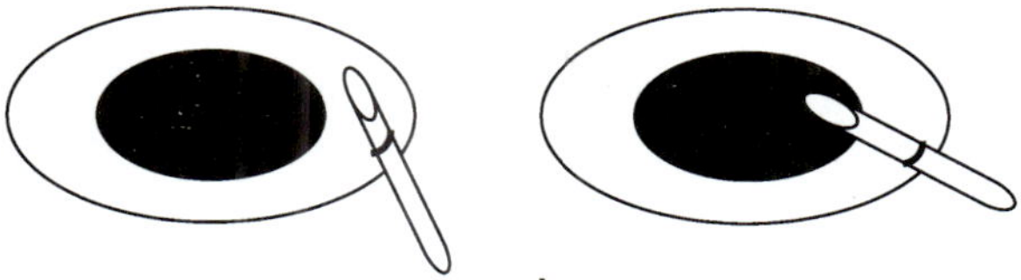

Fig. 2.5.2 The correct and incorrect placement of an AC maintainer in a phakic eye. **a** The correct placement of the cannula has its tip over the iris. Even if the cannula is pushed/pulled during surgery, its tip is unable to injure the lens. **b** The incorrectly placed cannula's tip is over the lens. Should any inadvertent force[1] be applied on the cannula,[2] the lens capsule can easily be breached

[1] e.g., the surgeon's hand, the assistant's instrument, the nurse's manipulation of the drape.

[2] The cannula does not have to be displaced to injure the lens: a downward push of its tip (i.e., elevation of its distal end around the fulcrum represented by the paracentesis wound) is sufficient.

- The cutting should be turned on continually to avoid traction of the peripheral retina via the pulling on the prolapsed vitreous.
- A small amount of TA is injected, which clearly shows any remaining vitreous. Injecting too much of the drug creates a "snowfall" phenomen and extends the surgical time.
- The iris is a great vehicle for demonstrating whether vitreous is still left. If the iris shows undulating movement as the vitrectomy probe is cutting at at area distant from the iris, it shows that vitreous remains adherent to the iris.

In a phakic eye, it is usually impossible to completely remove the vitreous; however, if only a thin layer is left, and it has lost its bridges to the cornea and is severed from the intravitreal vitreous, the risk of tractional retinal detachment is extremely low.

2.5.3.2.5 Air

Occasionally, air is introduced into the AC during the injury or injected during an intraocular injection. An air bubble actually forming inside the eye raises the possibility of infection by gas producing bacteria [2], a potentially leathal infection. Air is usually introduced by the surgeon to:

- Prevent the formation of anterior synechiae or iris prolapse into a wound (although an effective tool and devoid of the risk of IOP elevation, the air reabsorbs in only a few hours[17] or days)
- Determine the presence of certain foreign materials

Pearl

Air is the supreme tool to show the presence of vitreous or viscoelastics in the AC. Under normal circumstances, the air bubble takes on a regular dome shape. If vitreous or viscoelastic is present, the air bubble is deformed.

Removal of an air bubble is rarely necessary, but if deemed so, simple irrigation is sufficient. The eye (patient's head) should be turned so that the paracentesis is at the highest point of the eye. The BSS is injected when the tip of the cannula is *distal* from the wound so that the fluid can esaily push the air bubble outward. If multiple small air bubbles need to be removed, this is best done by injecting *more* air first so that the many small bubbles coalesce into a single large one, which is then easily irrigated out.

2.5.3.3 Viscoelastic Use

Viscoelastics have two distinct features: they can coat and maintain space. As an additional feature, they are also excellent in stopping a hemorrhage[18]:

- *Coating.* This attribute is utilized when the endothelium must be protected during manipulations of the lens or condensation of fluid on the IOL's or capsule's surface must be fought in an air-filled eye. In general,

17 The air bubble's presence is especially short-term if it was introduced during general anesthesia using nitrogen-dioxide.

18 Working as a tamponading agent.

viscoelastics of low viscosity (e.g., Viscoat[19]) are used for this purpose (dispersive viscoelastic).

- *Space tactics.* Viscoelastic materials are incompressible and hard to dislodge. If they are placed underneath a corneal wound, for instance, they tend to stay there and prevent the iris from adhering to the wound; they are also able to counter silicone oil prolapse into the AC irrespective of whether the eye is aphakic, pseudophakic, or phakic.[20] These cohesive or viscous viscoelastics (e.g., Healon[21]) have a much wider use in ocular traumatology, including pre- and even subretinal applications (see Chap. 2.9).
- When a cohesive viscoelastic is injected, it is especially crucial to use a low force[22] to avoid increased resistance ("backfiring") by the material.
- Before injection, a plan must be designed to make viscoelastic use efficient.
- Viscoelastics are not intended to push tissue back into the eye. The material is to be used after the prolapsed tissue has been repositioned (see Chap. 2.4). The viscoelastic should be injected through a paracentesis, not through the original wound.
- When a space is to be created/filled, injection should be started at the most distal point and advanced backwards (i.e., as the surgeon is slowly withdrawing the cannula).
- If the viscoelastic is used for breaking a synechia, it must be kept in mind that the material works indiscriminately: where the tissue breaks is not necessarily where the surgeon wanted it to break.

As mentioned above, viscoelastics are occasionally left in the AC to prevent silicone oil prolapse or synechia formation. The risk of IOP elevation is higher with *less* viscous materials, and they are also more difficult to re-

19 Alcon, Fort Worth, Texas.

20 Prophylactic filling of the AC with a cohesive viscoelastic should be considered in every eye undergoing silicone oil implantation.

21 Advanced Medical Optics, Santa Ana, Calif.

22 Think about a bulldozer instead of a hammer.

move during surgery. Just as when injecting the viscoelastic, the key during viscoelastic removal is to start distally and limit the force with which the BSS is applied.

2.5.3.4 Silicone Oil

- If silicone oil prolapses into the AC in an eye with an intact iris diaphragm, the prolapsed oil eventually breaks off from the large intravitreal bubble, and a single intracameral droplet is formed. This droplet cannot be forced back into the vitreous cavity.
- If the droplet is relative small, does not interfere with the patient's vision, and is mobile,[23] it can be left in situ.
- If the intracameral droplet does need to be removed, two paracenteses are prepared: one for the injection of a viscoelastic and one to drain the silicone oil. Injection of the viscoelastic requires a special technique (see above).
- The surgeon must make sure during the exchange that the silicone oil is in constant contact with the drainage paracentesis; otherwise, the droplet gets "lost," floating to the highest point of the AC. Reestablishing contact between the oil droplet and the paracentesis is not always easy. Inserting a spatula into the AC during drainage in such cases is very helpful. It can press the lower wound lip downwards but also reach into the inside of the silicone oil droplet. If this is achieved, the oil can be completely drained along the spatula even if the droplet itself is not in the immediate vicinity of the paracentesis. The viscoelastic must be left in the AC to prevent further silicone oil prolapse.
- If the silicone oil emulsifies (Fig. 2.5.3), removal becomes more difficult. If possible, the intravitreal oil must be removed first; otherwise, it provides an endless resupply of droplets. The technique of removal does not differ significantly from that described above, but it takes a lot

23 i.e., it does not press against the endothelium continually at the same site.

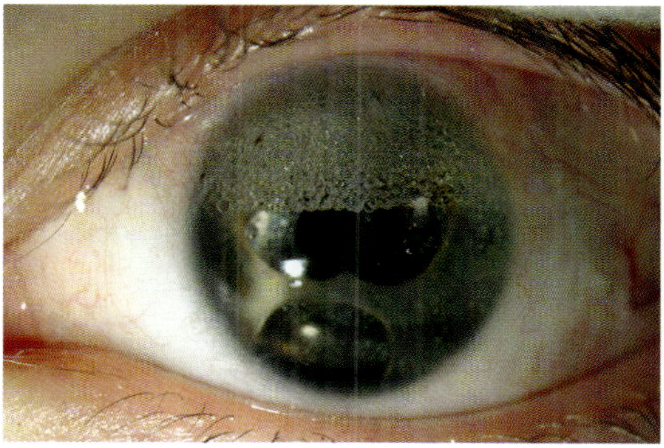

Fig. 2.5.3 Emulsified silicone oil in the AC. The inferior iridectomy is open; the eye is pseudophakic, yet the emulsified silicone oil fills at least 40% of the AC superiorly. Silicone oil bubbles are also seen through the iridectomy to adhere to the posterior capsule (See the text for more details.)

longer to "chase out" all the droplets.[24] The viscoelastic may be removed since no silicone oil resupply is possible.

2.5.3.5 Synechia

An *anterior* synechia is formed when the iris is caught in a corneal/limbal wound or adheres to an area with endothelial damage. A *posterior* synechia is diagnosed when the iris is attached to the lens. The condition is made worse when secondary scarring develops, which may grow into the angle and interfere with aqueous outflow.

Whether surgical intervention is indicated depends on the consequences of the condition; duration of the synechia is another factor to consider.

24 In fact, it is virtually impossible to leave the eye completely bubble-free. It takes many months for all the bubbles to clear through the trabecular meshwork; the IOP must be followed closely.

Cave

A blunt tool is best suited to break acute synechiae, but the blunt instrument can cause major tissue damage if used to deal with a chronic synechia.

Table 2.5.4 shows the recommended treatment modalities for synechiae of various types.

Table 2.5.4 Management of various types of synechiae

Synechia	Comment
Acute anterior	The iris should be freed from the wound before suturing the wound. Freeing is best done with a blunt spatula introduced into the AC through a paracentesis that is both at a distance[1] from the incarceration and at a convenient location. The spatula is used to gently sweep the iris away from wound, pulling it back into the AC. If there is a tendency of iris reprolapse, viscoelastic can be injected from the paracentesis site, leaving a viscoelastic "bolus" underneath the wound
Acute posterior	Dilating (constricting in the rare case of a wide pupil) the pupil with a drug such as intracameral synephrin usually suffices; surgical breaking of the synechia rarely becomes necessary. If mechanical breakage is needed, again the spatula is the optimal tool. Viscoelastic should *not* be used: since it would be injected under the iris, its effects would be blocked from the surgeon's view
Chronic anterior	Intervention solely for the purpose of breaking the synechia is necessary only if the IOP is elevated.[2] Synechiolysis often becomes part of a complex anterior segment reconstruction (Fig. 2.5.3). The tissue to be freed is usually vascularized and a strong scar present; blunt dissection is not an option any more because tissue tearing and severe bleeding threaten. Proper diathermization and prophylactic injection of viscoelastics are recommended first. The tissue is cut with a sharp instrument; there is no need to fully remove it from the cornea to avoid ripping off Descemet's membrane. Careful freeing of the angle is a more important, albeit difficult and somewhat dangerous, part of the procedure; it should be attempted only if the IOP is high and cannot be controlled medically

Table 2.5.4 *(continued)* Management of various types of synechiae

Synechia	Comment
Chronic posterior	Indicated only if the synechia prevents aqueous traffic between the two chambers[3] and laser iridectomy has not been effective. A spatula can be used to very carefully break the connection between the lens capsule and the iris. The risk of breaching the lens capsule is rather high, and this must be understood by the patient before the procedure is undertaken. If the spatula cannot be introduced for the lack of space between the two tissues at the pupillary margin, a peripheral iridectomy can be performed superiorly and the spatula introduced through the iridectomy. This has the additional advantage of being able to break the synechia 360° in a single sweep. Strong anti-inflammatory treatment must be used postoperatively to prevent synechia recurrence, and the pupil must be kept mobile[4]

[1] Typically at 90–180° from the wound if it is limbal; if the wound is more toward the central cornea, the primary factor in determining the paracentesis location is convenience for the surgeon.

[2] Cosmesis may be another indication if the synechia is large; the patient must understand the risks of the procedure before the surgeon consents to the patient's wish.

[3] i.e., an iris bombans is present

[4] i.e., short-acting dilatation is to be used, not atropin; a wide pupil may have to be constricted even though this risks increasing the inflammation

2.5.3.6 Comprehensive Anterior Segment Reconstruction

Several structures of the AC and adjacent tissues may be damaged during the injury, and posttraumatic scarring may make the condition worse. The scar tissue can destroy the cornea and the angle, elevate the IOP, and seriously impede vision (Fig. 2.5.4). Reconstruction of such eyes requires a surgeon skilled in both anterior and posterior segment techniques, ranging from PK to vitrectomy. Chapters 2.1–2.15 and 2.18–2.20 describe various elements of the intervention, which must also be carefully planned.[25]

25 The reconstruction is typically done as a late procedure, the details of which are beyond the scope of this book.

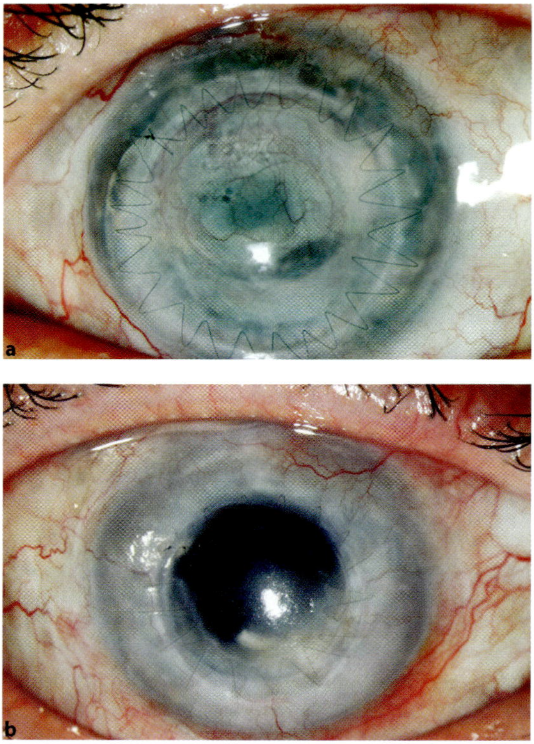

Fig. 2.5.4 Comprehensive anterior segment reconstruction. The patient had bilateral injuries several years ago; multiple surgeries (repeat PK, lens removal, IOL implantation, repeat vitrectomies) have been performed, but visual acuity is LP in both eyes and the IOP is under 8 mmHg. The two eyes look virtually identical. **a** Preoperative image of the right eye. The graft is clear but the peripheral cornea has multiple layers of new vessels. There is a large, vascularized retrocorneal membrane. The iris is barely visible; even its color is difficult to determine. **b** Postoperative image of the left eye. Most of the corneal vessels have been closed. The retrocorneal membrane has been removed. The angle has been freed. The IOL has been respositioned. The vitreous cavity has been lavaged. Visual acuity improved to 20/160, the IOP is 16 mmHg

2.5.3.7 Angle Recession

A condition that often leads to glaucoma, angle recession is discussed in Chap. 2.18.

DO:

- determine whether sickle cell disease has played a role in hyphema development
- prevent corneal blood staining by aggressively bringing the IOP down and by removing the intracameral blood early if staining threatens
- learn the basics of viscoelastic properties and use to maximize their benefits and reduce the risks of their use

DON'T:

- start hyphema removal before planning all aspects of surgery including timing, instrumentation, and wound preparation
- forget that damage to other intraocular structures are very common in eyes with hyphema
- leave vitreous incarcerated into a corneal wound

Summary

The AC has a wide variety of pathologies; in addition to knowing how to deal with each, the surgeon should also learn some basic rules such as space and tissue tactics. Of the major pathologies, hemorrhage has the greatest importance.

References

[1] Beyer TL, Hirst LW (1985) Corneal blood staining at low pressures. Arch Ophthalmol 103: 654–655

[2] Bhargava S, Chopdar A (1971) Gas gangrene panophthalmitis. Br J Ophthalmol 55: 136–138

[3] Edwards W, Layden W (1973) Traumatic hyphema. Am J Ophthalmol 75: 110–116

[4] Erol N, Ozer A, Topbas S, Yildirim N, Yurdakul S (2003) Treatment of intracameral fibrinous membranes with tissue plasminogen activator. Ophthalmic Surg Lasers Imaging 34: 451–456

[5] Katz J, Feldman MA, Bass EB, Lubomski LH, Tielsch JM, Petty BG, Fleisher LA, Schein OD (2003) Risks and benefits of anticoagulant and antiplatelet medication use before cataract surgery. Ophthalmology 110: 1784–1788

[6] Mandell MA, Pavlin CJ, Weisbrod DJ, Simpson ER (2003) Anterior chamber depth in plateau iris syndrome and pupillary block as measured by ultrasound biomicroscopy. Am J Ophthalmol 136: 900–903

[7] Ozdal MP, Mansour M, Deschenes J (2003) Ultrasound biomicroscopic evaluation of the traumatized eyes. Eye 17: 467–472

[8] Park S, Marcus D, Duker J, Pesavento R, Topping P, Frederick A, D'Amico D (1995) Posterior segment complications after vitrectomy for macular hole. Ophthalmology 102: 775–781

[9] Parrish R, Bernardino V Jr (1982) Iridectomy in the surgical management of eight-ball hyphema. Arch Ophthalmol 100: 435–437

[10] Pieramici DJ, Goldberg MF, Melia M, Fekrat S, Bradford CA, Faulkner A, Juzych M, Parker JS, McLeod SD, Rosen R, Santander SH (2003) A phase III, multicenter, randomized, placebo-controlled clinical trial of topical aminocaproic acid (Caprogel) in the management of traumatic hyphema. Ophthalmology 110: 2106–2112

[11] Sholiton DB, Solomon OD (1981) Surgical management of black ball hyphema with sodium hyaluronate. Ophthalmic Surg 12: 820–822

[12] Striph G, Halperin L, Stevens J, Chu F (1988) Afferent pupillary defect caused by hyphema. Am J Ophthalmol 106:

[13] Walton W, Hagen S von, Grigorian R, Zarbin M (2002) Management of traumatic hyphema. Surg Ophthalmol 47: 297–334

[14] Weissman JL, Beatty RL, Hirsch WL, Curtin HD (1995) Enlarged anterior chamber: CT finding of a ruptured globe. Am J Neuroradiol 16: 936–938

2.6 Iris and Pupil

Ferenc Kuhn

2.6.1 Introduction

The two most important attributes of the iris are its *regulatory* function, controlling the amount of light reaching the retina,[1] and its *barrier* function, separating the two main chambers of the eye.[2] In addition, the iris has a cosmetic function, whose significance should not be underestimated. Restoration of the injured iris to its normal anatomy is one of the most neglected aspects of ocular traumatology.

The presence of major iris damage is an indicator of ciliary body trauma: if traumatic aniridia is found, the risk of eventual phthisis increases.

2.6.2 Evaluation

Major abnormalities are easily seen with the naked eye, especially if the iris is light colored. A penlight is used to compare the injured iris' color with that of the fellow eye.[3]

1 Examination of the iris always includes examination of its aperture, the pupil.

2 Dividing the globe into anterior and chambers is especially important in an aphakic or pseudophakic eye filled with silicone oil.

3 Heterochromia is obviously impossible to diagnose without inspecting the fellow eye. Color difference is much more difficult to notice at the slit lamp since the two eyes cannot be viewed simultaneously.

The slit lamp remains the most important diagnostic tool. The iris must be inspected for the presence of wounds, membranes, and IOFBs, as well as for its shape (i.e., iridodialysis). Examination of the pupil is crucial (see Chap. 1.9 and Table 2.6.1), and includes evaluation both static (e.g., shape) and dynamic components (e.g., reaction to light). Inflammation, which always accompanies trauma, makes the pupil small[4] and may make it appear "muddy" due to swollen vessels and protein debris.

If an abnormality such as an irregular pupil size or iris discoloration is found, the ophthalmologist must ask the patient about preexisting conditions (previous injury, drug use) and diseases (uveitis). If necessary, an old photograph should be used for comparison to determine whether a heterochromia is congenital or a sign of siderosis. A greenish iris discoloration is often observed in (pre)phthisical eyes.

2.6.3 Specific Conditions

2.6.3.1 Mydriasis

Whether caused by central (third nerve palsy) or local (i.e., sphincter muscle damage, retroiridal scarring) pathology or other etiologies [6], the condition requires surgical correction if it results in photophobia that compromises vision. If mydriasis represents a major cosmetic problem for the patient, this is also an indication for corrective surgery.

Scarring usually occurs in the context of anterior PVR, and treatment of the mydriatic pupil should be addressed during vitrectomy. The goal is to remove the scar tissue that lines the pars plana, ciliary body, and the back surface of the iris. If the lens is present, it must be sacrificed. Endoscopy-assisted vitrectomy offers several advantages traditional viewing cannot match (see Chap. 2.20). Complete scar removal is not always possible, and even if it is, return of iris/pupil mobility is not guaranteed.

4 Unless the inflammation is being treated.

Table 2.6.1 Evaluation of the pupil in patients with eye injury

Variable	Comment
Size	Should be within normal range, depending on the power of the illumination, and not differ from the size of the uninjured fellow eye. In case of anisocoria, the pupil may be miotic or mydriatic. If miotic, the differential diagnosis includes synechia and Horner's syndrome; if mydriatic, consider: Preexistent condition (pharmacological, synechia, siderosis) Parasympathetic nerve damage (typically after a contusion) Adie's syndrome Third-nerve palsy
Position	Should be central; if dislocated, the cause can be iris or vitreous prolapse (see Chap. 2.4), or iridodialysis
Shape	Should be round; if not, the most likely cause is posterior synechia or iridodialysis
Color	Should be black;[1] a pupillary membrane causes color change, as does a cataract
Reaction to accommodation	The pupil should constrict
Reaction to direct light	The pupil should constrict – if lacking a reaction, it must be determined whether this is due to a problem with afferentation (no perception of light), efferentation (injury to the parasympathical system), or there is a local cause (injury to the sphincter muscle or the presence of posterior synechia)
Reaction to indirect light	Consensual (Fig. 1.9.1)

[1] Except, of course, if the illumination is coaxial (red reflex)

If a radial laceration causes the dysfunction of the sphincter muscle, a single transcameral suture [10] is usually sufficient to restore anatomy and function (Fig. 2.6.1).

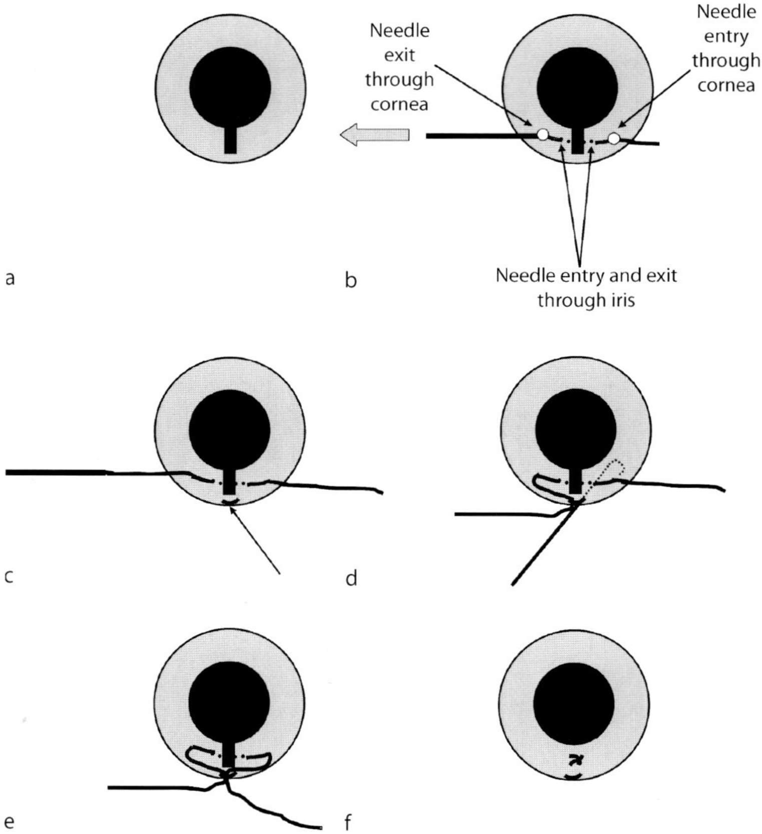
a
b
Needle exit through cornea
Needle entry through cornea
Needle entry and exit through iris
c
d
e
f

Fig. 2.6.1 Transcameral suture for damaged iris sphincter muscle.[1] The initial step is to assure that there is no synechia; if there is, this must be broken before suture introduction (see Chap. 2.5). **a** The iris lesion may involve the pupillary margin or may be more peripheral. **b** A long, straight or curved needle is used to enter the AC through the cornea at a convenient location but outside the visual axis. The needle enters the torn iris on both sides of the lesion, and exits the cornea on the opposite side (*thick arrow*). Do not enter/exit the AC in the limbus; it is easier to catch the suture later during the procedure if the suture is in an area with greater AC depth. Once the suture has been pulled through, the needle is cut off. **c** A paracentesis is made somewhere in the middle plane between the two needle entry/exit points, over the iris lesion (*arrow*). As described in Chap. 2.5, the angle of the paracentesis must allow easy maneuvering as well as watertightness without suture. The paracentesis should not be far away from where the knot will be (see below). **d** A hook fashioned at the tip of a hypodermic needle or a vitrectomy forceps is used to engage the two sutures above the iris and pull them out from the AC through the paracentesis. **e** The sutures are tightened. The iris must be sufficiently loose because it will be tented as the suture is tightened. This is the reason why the paracentesis must be strategically placed, and placed *after*, and not before, the sutures are introduced into the iris. If the iris is rigid or the lesion is wide, *intraocular suture tightening* may have to be performed or the lesion is treated only partially.[2] *Internal* tightening of the knot requires a paracentesis on both sides. The suture enters the AC via one paracentesis, picks up the iris as described above, and exits the AC through the other paracentesis. The suture is then partially withdrawn[3] and tied using the loop: the knot is formed inside the AC, without tenting the iris. The needle is then pulled back through both paracenteses and the entire procedure is repeated. An alternative is not to bring the iris edges in apposition but leaving a small gap between them. **f** The iris is left to slide back in place; the suture remains visible, but the gap in the iris should disappear or become very small. If need be, additional sutures may be introduced in the same way. The procedure can also be performed in a phakic eye, after first carefully injecting cohesive viscoelastics under the iris

[1] Viscoelastics are typically not necessary, although the surgeon should apply them if the AC gets shallow.

[2] A description of these two techniques are given here, but neither is shown.

[3] The needle remains outside the eye.

Transcameral needles are not easy to use (Fig. 2.6.2). The needle's path through the cornea acts as a fulcrum; the more forward the needle's position in the AC is, the smaller a movement with the needle holder is needed to cause in a large movement of the needle's tip. To make needle use easier, the surgeon should either bring the needle's entry point as close to its intracameral target as possible, or use another instrument (e.g., a vitrectomy forceps) to guide the needle inside the AC.

Cave

Any suture placed into the iris must provide a permanent lock: there is no iris healing. The suture material must be nonabsorbable [10/0 or 9/0 polypropylene on a straight (STC-6) or curved (CIF-4) needle][5] and the knot must be made very secure. The suture must not exert undue tension on the iris to avoid "cheesewiring."

If the sphincter muscle is completely nonfunctional, an iris cerclage (purse string) suture should be used (Fig. 2.6.3).

2.6.3.2 Laceration/Coloboma

Surgery should be considered if the lesion prevents proper pupillary function, visual disturbance[6], or causes a significant cosmetic problem. The surgical technique is identical to the one described above for sphincter muscle damage (Fig. 2.6.1).

2.6.3.3 Iridodialysis

The pathognomic sign of the condition – tearing of the peripheral portion of the iris root from the ciliary spur – appears as a black slit at the limbus.[7]

5 Ethicon/Johnson & Johnson, New Brunswick, N.J. Every suture mentioned in this chapter is one of the two types described above.

6 Monocular diplopia, photophobia.

7 It is usually visible to the naked eye, although the slit lamp is often needed to confirm the diagnosis. If the iridodialysis is large enough, a red reflex is apparent where it should not be (Fig. 2.7.2).

An iridodialysis also deforms the shape of the pupil. Angle recession and glaucoma are common associated pathologies.

Surgical reconstruction is recommended if the condition causes visual disturbance (monocular diplopia, glare, photophobia). The treatment concept is based on the McCannel suture [8]. A double-armed suture is used in either of the two techniques (Fig. 2.6.4).

2.6.3.4 Acute Traumatic Aniridia: "the Case of the Missing Iris"

It is not uncommon to find the iris completely extruded in severe ruptures. It is also possible that the iris is not actually lost, it is just rolled up and pulled posteriorly by fibrin initially and scar tissue subsequently ("pseudoaniridia"). The earlier such an iris retraction is discovered, the easier its unrolling is. If done before scar tissue develops, careful pulling on the iris at the pupillary margin with vitrectomy forceps introduced through a paracentesis is often able to reestablish the iris diaphragm. Pulling of the iris back to its normal position is not without risk.

- If scarring has already started, the iris can be torn from its root.
- If the pulling is too forceful, severe bleeding may occur.
- If the forceps holding the iris is squeezed too strongly, the pupillary margin can be seriously damaged.

Sutures may be necessary to maintain the recreated smaller pupil (see above).

Controversial

It is not always possible to explain how the iris can disappear after a severe rupture. Often there is no sign of iris extrusion, nor is the iris found during surgery. One must presume an acute dissolution of the tissue, although it is difficult to comprehend how this can occur so instantly.

For true traumatic aniridia, some type of correction is advised because of the associated photophobia and/or cosmesis. The options range from the simple to the complex (Fig. 2.6.5; Table 2.6.2), including prostheses that also have built-in refractory correction (IOL).

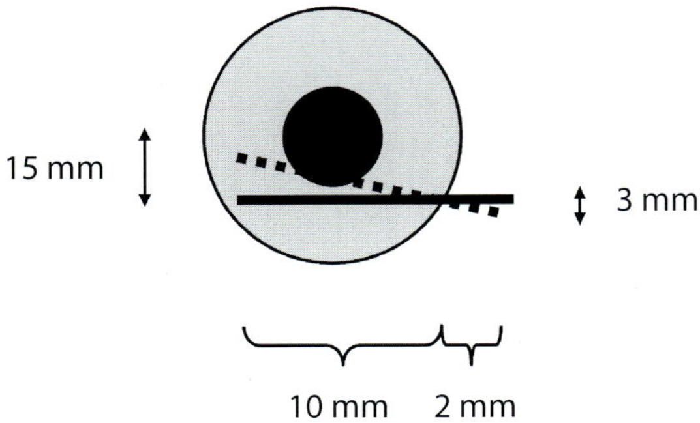

Fig. 2.6.2 The difficulties using a long transcameral needle. If the needle is 10 mm long inside and 2 mm outside the AC, a 3-mm movement at its external end with the needle holder results in a 15-mm movement of the needle's tip in the AC. Because in real life this is three-dimensional – not two-dimensional – the difficulty is even greater than what this schematic drawing suggests

Fig. 2.6.3 Purse string suture to constrict a wide, nonreactive pupil. **a** Three or four paracenteses are created. A long, straight needle is used to enter the AC through one paracentesis. The needle catches the iris at the pupillary margin several times before exiting at the next paracentesis. **b** The needle is then turned around and returned through the same paracentesis to catch the iris as described above. This is repeated until the needle arrives at the initial paracentesis. During entry, the needle must be wiggled inside each paracentesis tunnel so that corneal tissue does not get caught with the suture. **c** The suture is tied and the suture/iris released back into the AC. A 27-g needle inserted through the paracentesis toward which the straight needle is advancing helps guide the straight needle and makes the otherwise difficult procedure easier. **d** Preoperative picture. **e** Postoperative picture (Courtesy of B. Hamill, Houston, TX)

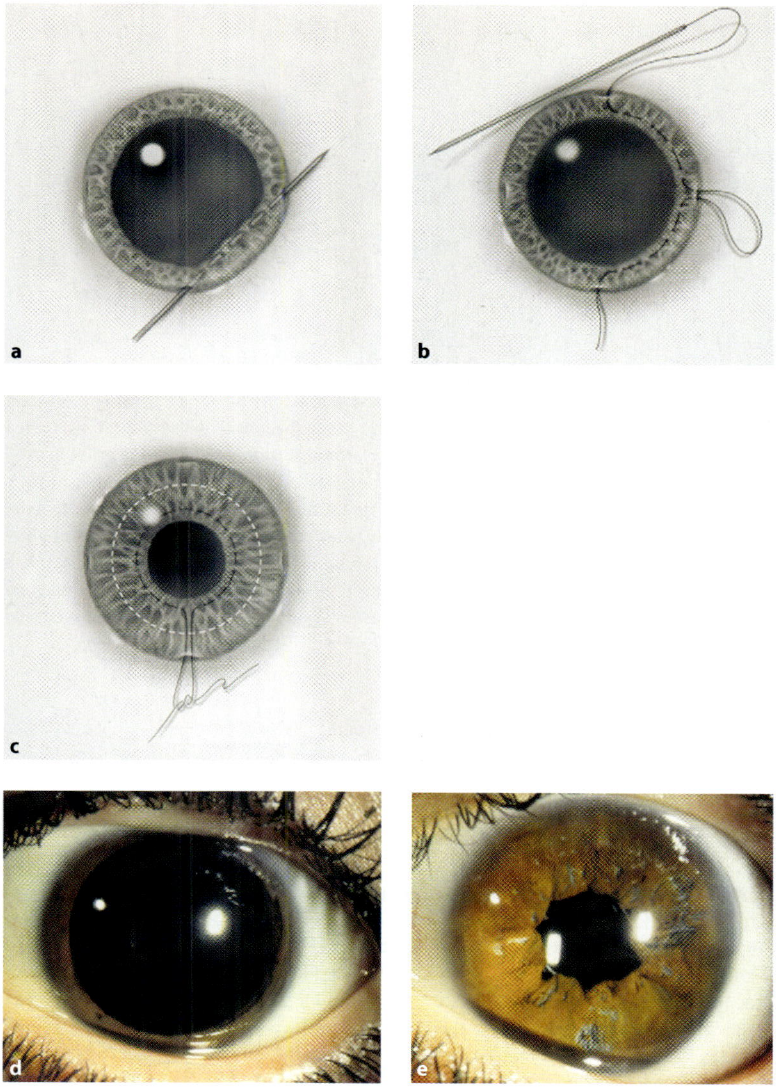
a
b
c
d
e

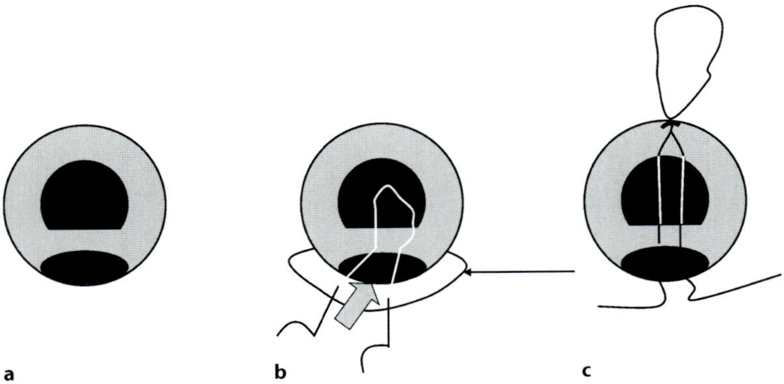

a b c

Fig. 2.6.4 Suturing of an iridodialysis.[1] **a** The iris root is torn and the pupil is deformed. **b** Direct suturing. A half-thickness scleral bed is prepared next to the iridodialysis area (*arrow*), then a limbal wound is created (*block arrow*). A double-armed suture with curved needles is used to first catch the iris root and to pass into the scleral bed.[2] The needles are cut, the suture is tightened, and the scleral bed closed. More than one suture may be necessary. **c** Transcameral suturing. A paracentesis is created at a convenient location (90–180° away). A straight double-armed suture is passed through the incision, carefully avoiding the capture of corneal tissue with the needle (see above). The needles are passed through the iris root then exit the sclera at 1 mm from the limbus, cut away, and the suture is tightened. The knot is compressed (see Chap. 2.2) and turned into the scleral channel

[1] The conjunctiva is not shown here.

[2] Both needles go through iris first and sclera second.

Fig. 2.6.5 Corrective options for traumatic aniridia.[1] **a** Aniridia ring to be placed in the capsular bag (it also serves as a capsular tension ring). Implantation and proper dialing of *two* devices reconstitute the iris. **b–d** Combined iris/IOL prostheses. **b** This implant can be placed in the bag or sutured into the bag; it has an inferior "iridectomy" in case silicone oil is also used. **c,d** The iris prosthesis is colored. **c** A prosthesis for scleral fixation. **d** This implant can be placed in the bag or sutured into the bag. **e** Preoperative image. This 38-year-old woman ruptured her eye 13 years after RK surgery, and lost both the lens and the iris. **f** Postoperative image 3 months after implantation of an Ophtec device (model 311 sutured into the sulcus) (Photographs E and F courtesy of M. Price, Indianapolis, IN)

[1] **a** and **b**: Morcher GmbH, Stuttgart, Germany; **c** and **d**: Ophtec, Groningen, Netherlands

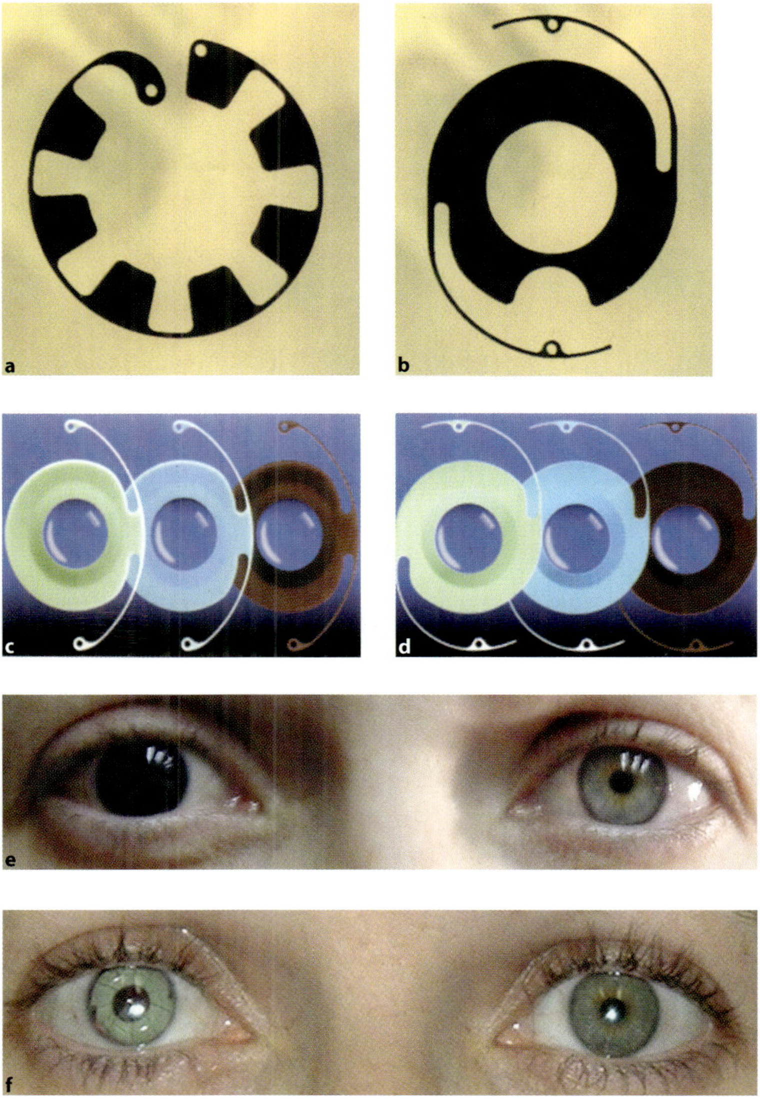
a
b
c
d
e
f

Table 2.6.2 Management options for traumatic aniridia

Option	Comment
Iris print contact lens [5]	Simple and easily reversible but has all the limitations associated with contact lens wear
Corneal tattooing [1, 4]	Simple and effective; permanent; epithelium healing over the tattooed region, however, may be slow. Various techniques have been described for the introduction of the pigments [6], and the color of the new "iris" can also be customized
Implants (iris prosthesis) [2, 3, 7, 9, 11]	Various devices are available; they may be used for partial or total loss of the iris, and certain types combine an IOL as well (Fig. 2.6.5). Various materials, including Gore-Tex paired with silicone[2], are available, and the color can also be customized. The major disadvantage is that a large incision is required for insertion

[2] HumanOptics AG, Erlangen, Germany

2.6.3.5 Prolapse

Regarding prolapse, see Chap. 2.4 for details.

2.6.3.6 Iritis

Inflammation of the iris is a consequence of virtually any eye injury. Its most important complication is synechia formation (see Chap. 2.5). The treatment of traumatic iritis is straightforward:

- Topical *corticosteroids*; use prednisolone acetate, hourly if the inflammation is severe, and do not taper it too early. The suspension needs to be shaken properly beforehand.
- If a very severe uveitis is present, the corticosteroid may be injected subconjunctivally.[8] If systemic administration is necessary,[9] start with a bolus (100 mg/day), taper quickly, then use 20 mg/day for 3 months.

8 The effect of this injection lasts longer than an intravitreal one.

9 In the exceptional, severe cases, which involve the posterior uvea as well.

- *Cycloplegics*; homatropin is usually sufficient, although scopolamide or even atropine may be necessary.

DO:

- reconstruct the iris if it cannot serve as a divider between the AC and the vitreous cavity or if the pupil lost functionality
- remember that sutures in the iris will not be supported by scar formation; the sutures must permanently hold the tissue on their own

DON'T:

- constrict the pupil to too small a size, especially if posterior segment surgery is expected
- give up too easily if iris is not found after the injury; it may be "hidden" underneath

Summary

The iris plays important functional and anatomical roles in the eye. Restoration of the diaphragm and of an operational pupil should be one of the goals of trauma management.

References

[1] Beekhuis WH, Drost BH, van der Velden–Samderubun EM (1998) A new treatment for photophobia in posttraumatic aniridia: a case report. Cornea 17: 338–341

[2] Beltrame G, Salvetat ML, Chizzolini M, Driussi GB, Busatto P, Giorgio G di, Barosco F, Scuderi B (2003) Implantation of a black diaphragm intraocular lens in ten cases of post-traumatic aniridia. Eur J Ophthalmol 13: 62–68

[3] Brown MJ, Hardten DR, Knish K (2005) Use of the artificial iris implant in patients with aniridia. Optometry 76: 157–164

[4] Burris TE, Holmes-Higgin DK, Silvestrini TA (1998) Lamellar intrastromal corneal tattoo for treating iris defects (artificial iris). Cornea 17: 169–173

[5] Grunauer-Kloevekorn C, Habermann A, Wilhelm F, Duncker GI, Hammer T (2004) Contact lens fitting as a possibility for visual rehabilitation in patients after open globe injuries. Klin Monatsbl Augenheilkd 221: 652–657 [in German]

[6] Kirchhof B (2002) Iris. In: Kuhn F, Pieramici D (eds) Ocular trauma: principles and practice. Thieme, New York, pp 146–156
[7] Marullo M, Scupola A, Pasqua R, Agostini N, Balestrazzi E (1997) Iris diaphragm implantation in post-traumatic aniridia and tractional retinal detachment. Eur J Ophthalmol 7: 171–173
[8] McCannel M (1976) A retrievable suture idea for anterior uveal problems. Ophthalmic Surg Las 7: 8–103
[9] Menezo JL, Martinez-Costa R, Cisneros A, Desco MC (2005) Implantation of iris devices in congenital and traumatic aniridias: surgery solutions and complications. Eur J Ophthalmol 15: 451–457
[10] Shin DH (1982) Repair of sector iris coloboma. Closed-chamber technique. Arch Ophthalmol 100: 460–461
[11] Thumann G, Kirchhof B, Bartz-Schmidt KU, Jonescu-Cuypers CP, Esser P, Konen W, Heimann K (1997) The artificial iris diaphragm for vitreoretinal silicone oil surgery. Retina 17: 330–337

2.7 Lens

Ferenc Kuhn and Viktória Mester

2.7.1 Introduction

Lens injury is much more common than one would presume from literature reports (Table 2.7.1). While the prognosis of the lens pathology itself is excellent, the outcome is generally much poorer because of the associated injuries (Table 2.7.2). Furthermore, several issues related to the management of eyes with lens injury remain controversial. Fig. 2.7.1 provides an overview of the trauma-related lens conditions. If the eye was pseudophakic at the time of injury, additional pathologies, such as IOL dislocation or haptic breakage, can occur.

2.7.2 Evaluation

The slit lamp is by far the most reliable method of diagnosing virtually all lens abnormalities.[1] The slit lamp is also crucial for the detection of important accompanying lesions such as vitreous prolapse into the AC in an eye with dislocated lens (see Chap. 2.5). Uneven depth of the AC may be the only sign of a slightly subluxed lens, although its edge may also be visible

1 Possible exceptions include a subconjunctivally extruded lens (see Fig. 2.12.2) or a deeper/shallower AC (see Chap. 2.5), which may be more readily recognizable by the naked eye.

Table 2.7.1 The incidence of lens injury in the USEIR database (%)

Injury type (*n*)	Cataract	All other types of lens trauma combined
Contusion (1497)	14	9
Rupture (2117)	17	20
Penetrating (4220)	34	10
IOFB (1235)	46	7
Perforating (464)	29	13
Total	2682	1139

Based on 14,523 injuries involving the globe

Table 2.7.2 The significance of lens trauma as related to posterior segment damage

Variable (source)	Lens damage present (%)	Lens intact (%)	Statistical significance
Endophthalmitis [23]	14	1	$p < 0.004$
Vitreous hemorrhage (USEIR)	42	23	$p < 0.0001$
Retinal detachment (USEIR)	12	7	$p < 0.0001$
Final vision of <20/40 [15]	72	34	$p < 0.0001$
Final vision of <5/200 [15]	30	11	$p < 0.0001$

Fig. 2.7.1 Trauma-related lens pathologies. The lesions can occur alone or in combination.

[a] This term is used in some literature reports to describe luxation, as opposed to subluxation, of the lens.

[b] May be accompanied by lens swelling. Intralenticular FBs are discussed in Chap. 2.13

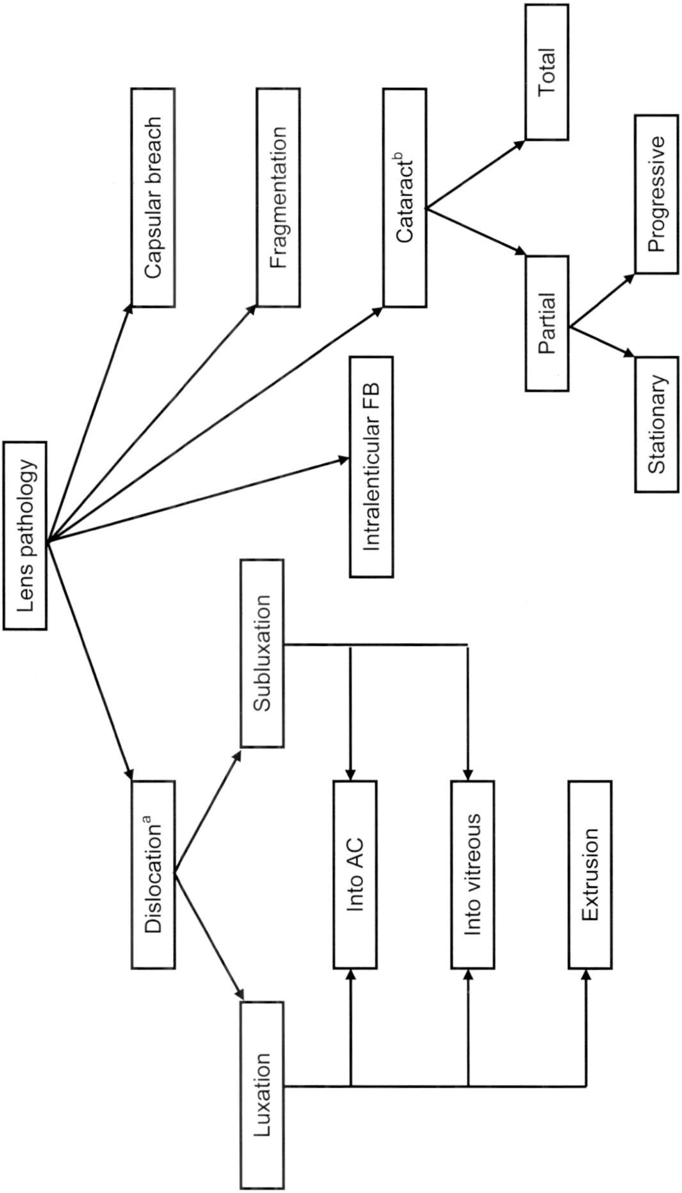
Lens pathology
Capsular breach
Fragmentation
Cataract[b]
Intralenticular FB
Total
Partial
Progressive
Stationary
Dislocation[a]
Subluxation
Luxation
Into AC
Into vitreous
Extrusion

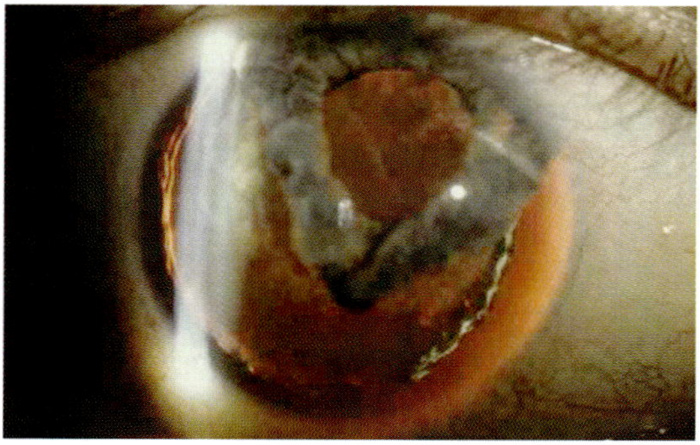

Fig. 2.7.2 Lens subluxation with iridodialysis. The lens is dislocated toward 10 o'clock; the iris is torn from its root between 2 and 11 o'clock. Red reflex is visible through the pupil as well as in the area of the iridodialysis. The edge of the lens is easily discernible

on retroillumination if the pupil is wide (Fig. 2.7.2). Typically, the lens and the iris show characteristic oscillatory movements when the eye or head moves (phacodonesis and iridodonesis, respectively). Depending on the site and area of zonular damage, the symptom may be present when the patient is in the erect but not in the supine position [10]. Vitreous prolapse is common: in the HEIR database, 34% of eyes with lens trauma showed vitreous prolapse into the AC.

The ophthalmoscope can supplant information if the lens is luxated into the vitreous. Ultrasonography may help to identify lens dislocation, posterior capsular rupture, or the presence of lens particles in the vitreous cavity. The CT is able to reveal lens damage even if the clinical examination is negative [4]. As always, injuries to any and all tissues of the eye must be suspected and sought.

It is important to realize that the preoperative and intraoperative findings may be quite different (Table 2.7.3); this has a major impact on surgical planning (see Chap. 1.8). As mentioned previously, intracamerally injected TA is able to show the presence and configuration of vitreous in the AC;

Table 2.7.3 Comparison of pre- and intraoperative findings (%) among 196 eyes undergoing extraction of a traumatic cataract

Capsule	Breach presence	Finding	
		Preoperative	Intraoperative
Anterior	Definite	69	71
	Questionable	3	0
Posterior	Definite	23	45
	Questionable	10	8

From the HEIR database

it reveals for the surgeon when the incarcerated vitreous has been severed (see Chap. 2.5).[2]

Table 2.7.4 provides a summary of questions that need to be answered during the examination.

2.7.3 Specific Conditions

2.7.3.1 Dislocation

The lens is either partially (subluxation) or completely (luxation) torn from the zonules; in the latter case, it may be still inside the eye or extruded[3]. Both subluxation and luxation can occur anteriorly (AC) or posteriorly (vitreous cavity), and both can happen in the context of open or closed globe trauma.

2 This is especially important in a phakic eye with corneal open globe trauma: traction on the peripheral retina must be prevented by severing the vitreous bridge reaching into the wound, but iatrogenic lens damage should also be avoided (see Chap. 2.5).

3 The lens may be under the conjunctiva (see Fig. 2.12.2) or completely lost.

Table 2.7.4 Diagnostic questions related to lens injury

Is the lens extruded?
Is the lens dislocated/luxated into the AC?
Are there lens particles in the AC?
Is the lens swelling?
Has vitreous prolapsed into the AC? If yes, is it also incarcerated into the wound?
Has the anterior capsule been breached?
What additional anterior segment pathologies are present? What is the IOP?
Is there an IOFB inside the lens?
Is there a cataract? If yes, is it partial or complete?
Has the posterior capsule been breached? If yes, has the vitreous prolapsed into the lens?
Is the lens subluxated/luxated into the vitreous cavity? If luxated, is the lens fragmented?
What posterior segment pathologies are present?

If the eye has an open globe injury, many of these questions will be answered during, rather than before, surgery

Whether, when, and what type of intervention is necessary are primarily determined by the type of injury[4], the visual acuity, the position of the lens, and the severity of secondary complications including vitreous prolapse, cataract, and glaucoma. Obviously, the range of independently coexisting pathologies is endless.[5]

4 Open vs closed globe (see Chaps. 2.10, 2.11)

5 Indications for, and types of, intervention for pathologies other than the lens are discussed in the appropriate chapters; this chapter focuses on the implications of the lens trauma itself.

2.7.3.1.1 Subluxation

If the visual acuity is normal and there is no vitreous incarceration into the wound, no treatment is necessary. If the lens needs to be removed, the type of intervention should be determined by a careful consideration of all variables.

- *Phacoemulsification* or *ECCE* is acceptable if there is no vitreous prolapse into the AC or into the lens – this is why it is crucial to preoperatively determine whether the posterior capsule is intact.
- If there is a small vitreous prolapse into the AC and it can first be removed with the vitrectomy probe, or if only a small posterior capsular lesion is present and viscoelastics[6] can effectively keep the vitreous from prolapsing, careful phacoemulsification may be attempted. The surgeon must keep in mind that the viscoelastic plug covering the capsular breach may be dislodged and the vitreous prolapse may recur; TA should periodically be used to check for vitreous reprolapse.
- A capsular tension ring can be inserted if the area of zonular rupture is verifiably small. A Cionni ring may be used if the zonular damage extends for a few clock hours.[7] Since the ring, and thus the capsule, is suture-fixed to the sclera, the capsular bag is given extra stability [1, 5].

6 A small amount of cohesive viscoelastic injected behind the lens capsule. Such use of viscoelastics, however, is a double-edged sword. It may be able to keep the vitreous behind the posterior capsule, but it also makes recognition of vitreous reprolapse even more difficult.

7 The damaged zonular area must not exceed 12 clock hours.

Cave

If the surgeon cannot be absolutely certain that vitreous has not prolapsed into the lens, phacoemulsification or ECCE must not be the method of choice to remove a subluxated or cataractous lens. Lensectomy using vitrectomy instrumentation is recommended to avoid exerting traction on the peripheral retina via aspirating vitreous. It must also be emphasized again that once lens removal has started, recognition of vitreous presence becomes difficult, and when it is recognized, it is often too late.[8]

- *Intracapsular cataract extraction* is recommended if most or all of the zonules are torn; again, the surgeon must make sure that there is no vitreous present before the cryoapplicator is applied.
- *Lensectomy* is the preferred method if vitreous is confirmed or suspected to have prolapsed into the lens.[9] Lensectomy is very safe and can be combined with IOL implantation [7].
  - If the *limbal* route is used, the posterior capsule can usually be preserved.
  - If the *pars plana* approach is chosen, the anterior capsule is preserved.[10] The pars plana route has distinct advantages: increased maneuverability and access to potential posterior segment abnormalities.[11]

---

8 The editor recently operated on an eye whose injury (*corneal penetrating trauma with an intravitreally located FB causing a visible anterior capsule lesion and cataract; Fig. 2.7.3*) made it obvious that the posterior capsule had also been breached. Lensectomy was therefore the selected lens removal method, but the probe malfunctioned: aspiration was applied without cutting (i.e., as if phacoemulsification or ECCE had been done). This was soon realized and the probe was replaced; nevertheless, during vitrectomy (performed in the same surgical setting), a large inferior retinal dialysis was found: an iatrogenic complication, not one caused by the original injury.

9 Prolapse of vitreous into the AC is easier to deal with (see above).

10 A three-piece IOL can be implanted into the sulcus on top of the retained capsule(s).

11 In the HEIR, 48% of eyes undergoing removal of a traumatic cataract had coexisting posterior segment injury, and 79% of these eyes had to undergo vitrectomy.

- Infusion is always needed: an AC maintainer is suitable in all cases. If a pars plana infusion is used, this should not be turned on unless the cannula's position can be verified (see Chap. 2.9). If the surgeon is experienced in bimanual surgery, a good alternative solution is to keep inside the capsular bag a needle attached to the infusion line: this method assures that the vitreous is not unnecessarily violated, the eye remains pressurized, and the lens gets hydrated, making removal easier.

Pearl

The usual vitrectomy settings need to be modified for the lensectomy procedure.[12] The aspiration should be somewhat higher (200 mmHg), as should the infusion pressure be (40 mmHg), and the cut rate is significantly reduced (200 cpm). The low cut rate prevents the escape of lens particles from the aspiration port and the collapse of the globe[13], should the port become unoccluded.

2.7.3.1.2 Luxation

A *subconjunctivally* extruded lens [21] is easily removed with forceps or a cryoapplicator. *Anterior* luxation of the lens is rare; this, however, requires rather urgent intervention to prevent endothelial damage. *Posterior* luxation, even if the lens capsules are intact, triggers an inflammatory response; removal is not an emergency but should not be deferred indefinitely. The removal technique depends on the hardness of the nucleus (mostly determined by the age of the patient) and on the surgeon's personal preference.

- *Phacofragmentation.*[14]
  - The energy of the ultrasound should be set at no more than 20%.
  - The infusion pressure must be set at no less than 40 mmHg.

---

12 As in virtually every trauma case, 20-g systems are recommended (see Chap. 2.9).
13 A preferred alternative is a flow-based system (peristaltic pump; see Chap. 2.9).
14 An ultrasonographic handpiece designed for intravitreal use.

- The aspiration must be linear; if the port is not occluded, instantaneous globe collapse occurs.
- The lens should be lifted into the midvitreous cavity using minimal aspiration and then the ultrasound is turned on. A second instrument,[15] inserted into the lens, is very helpful in keeping the lens from falling back onto the retina – even then, smaller lens particles will be falling down and need to be picked up repeatedly. The ultrasound must always be off when the probe is close to the retina. The lens often resembles Emmental ("Swiss") cheese before removal is completed.
- If phacofragmentation is performed for complications[16] of cataract surgery, the postoperative retinal detachment rate is around 5% [17]; in trauma-related cases the rate is probably significantly higher.

Pitfall

To reduce the risk of retinal detachment, a complete vitrectomy must be done *before* the onset of phacofragmentation. If a retinal dialysis or horseshoe tear and then detachment develop shortly after phacofragmentation, the surgeon may conveniently blame the complication on the original injury. Such retinal complications, however, may well have been caused by improper surgical techniques.[17] As a general rule, the shorter the time between injury/cataract removal[18] and the development of retinal detachment, the more suspect the technique of lens extraction is.

- *Lensectomy.* The vitrectomy probe can also be used to remove the lens, even if the nucleus is hard (e.g., in patients in their sixties). The nucleus is crushed into small pieces between the vitrectomy probe and another

15 e.g., pick light probe
16 i.e., "dropped nucleus" (see below)
17 e.g., the selection of an inappropriate method of lens removal (e.g., phacoemulsification instead of lensectomy)
18 Using phacoemulsification or ECCE

instrument (even the light pipe suffices), and the small pieces are removed one by one. The process is lengthy[19] but reduces the risks associated with intravitreal ultrasound use.

- Removal *in toto*. The lens can be extracted using an intraocular cryoprobe or with a vectis after floating it up with PFCL [14]. In the latter case, a complete PFCL fill is necessary, and the initial injection of the PFCL must be carefully done so that it gets underneath, not on top of, the lens. During fill-up, the lens may temporarily disappear from view: the initial shape of the enlarging PFCL bubble is more of a sphere, making the lens slide sideways. For *in toto* lens removal, a large limbal incision is necessary. Obviously, the eye must be aphakic.[20]

2.7.3.2 Capsular Breach

A breach in the *anterior* capsule is usually easy to see at the slit lamp, although good dilatation is needed if the lesion is peripheral. A posterior capsular breach is much more difficult to visualize, although it is often detectable on ultrasonography [12] or even at the slit lamp if posterior cortical material has "sunk" into the vitreous: an empty space is seen in the anterior cortex of the cataract. It is important to remember that a posterior capsular rupture can occur in isolation, i.e., without any other lens or even ocular pathology [16].

Common sense must be used: in the presence of an anterior capsular lesion and a posterior segment IOFB, it is very unlikely that the posterior capsule is intact (Fig. 2.7.3). The surgeon must be prepared for intraoperative surprises regarding capsular injury (Table 2.7.3).

Regarding management, no treatment is necessary for the breach itself, and its presence does not imply that subsequent cataract formation is inescapable since the break may spontaneously seal.

---

19 Especially because the vitrectomy probe may get clogged and needs flushing repeatedly.

20 This is why in case of a "dropped nucleus" IOL implantation may be ill-advised before the lens is removed (see below).

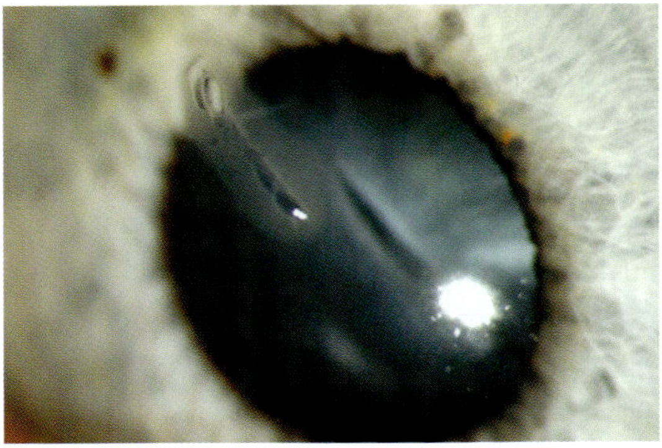

Fig. 2.7.3 Injury to the anterior lens capsule. The FB caused a corneal penetrating wound, an anterior capsule lesion, and a cataract. The corneal and capsular injuries provide trajectory information: a straight line drawn from the corneal wound and through the two capsular lesions should indicate the location of the potential impact site in the retina

2.7.3.3 Fragmentation

If the lens is in pieces, this always causes major inflammation and IOP elevation (see Chap. 2.18). Intervention is urgent.

Regarding management, all lens particles must be removed; the method depends on the location of the particles, the coexisting pathologies, the hardness of the nucleus, and the surgeon's personal preference (see above). Intense anti-inflammatory treatment must accompany the surgical intervention. An admixture of lens particles, vitreous, and blood is a uniquely potent inciter for PVR development.

2.7.3.4 Cataract

This is the most common type of lens injury and the one with the most significant visual consequence.[21] It can occur as a result of mechanical as

21 It must be noted that it is not always easy to definitely establish that a cataract is present; even experienced surgeons can err on either side: diagnosing a traumatic cataract when the lens is clear or declaring the lens to be clear when in fact there is cataract.

well as nonmechanical[22] trauma. The cataract can be partial (localized, focal) or total; the former may be stationary or progressive. The progression from minor to total lens opacity may take only hours (especially short in children; see Chap. 2.16) or may take years. Swelling with consequent IOP elevation is another factor to consider when the management options (i.e., removal or observation) are contemplated. The decision whether and when to intervene should also be influenced by the presence of, or potential for, posterior segment pathologies (Table 2.7.2).

Regarding management, the various techniques of lens removal have been described previously.

Pitfall

The different implications of removing an age-related (elective) cataract vs a traumatic cataract must clearly be understood by the surgeon. In an elective case, preservation of the capsular bag is important; for the trauma surgeon, avoiding iatrogenic damage to the retina is the main goal. It is not whether the IOL is in the bag[23] that determines the visual outcome but the integrity of the retina.

If vitrectomy is performed in an injured eye that has a risk high of, or already developed, PVR, and the lens needs to be sacrificed, both capsules must also be removed to reduce the surface ("scaffold") available for the proliferative cells. Preserving the capsule further increases the risk of anterior PVR as well as of phthisis (see Chaps. 2.9, 2.19).

- The lens is removed using a technique required by the eye's condition (see above) or the surgeon's preference. Depending on the surgical technique employed, one of capsules is left intact.
- A complete vitrectomy is performed.
- A capsulectomy is made with the vitrectomy probe or the MVR blade.

22 e.g., electricity/lightning; laser, microwave, thermal, and UV energy
23 As opposed to being in the AC, iris-fixated, or in the sulcus

- Utilizing the capsulectomy, the capsule is grabbed with a forceps, slowly rolled up ("spaghetti technique"[24]), and carefully removed. If the zonules are especially strong,[25] alpha-chymotrypsin[26] should first be injected under the iris, then removed by thorough irrigation. If the capsule tears, the other sclerotomy can be used to regrasp it.
- Scleral indentation is performed to assure that all of the capsule has been removed and the ciliary processes have been freed of all tissues.

The *timing* of lens removal must be carefully considered. If the injury is a contusion, and the IOP elevation and inflammation can be controlled medically, the decision is easily deferred. If, however, a wound is present and requires acute surgery, the surgeon must weigh the benefits and risks of primary vs secondary lens removal (Table 2.7.5; the flowchart in Fig. 2.7.4 explains the surgical strategy).

If lensectomy is performed and the anterior capsule is retained, it must be polished with the vitrectomy probe at low vacuum (flow)[27] and without cutting. The best method to visualize the efficiency of the polishing is to switch off the microscope light, hold the endoilluminator at the limbus, and aim its light at the capsule.[28] Preserving the anterior capsule means that the risk of iris damage and constriction of the pupil is reduced during the procedure, and, at least theoretically, the incidence of postoperative synechia formation is also decreased.

2.7.3.5 Iatrogenic Lens Damage

Although the discussion of surgeon-induced trauma is beyond the scope of this book, two important issues deserve to be mentioned briefly here:

24 A term coined by C. Forlini, Ravenna, Italy

25 Such as in young patients

26 See Chap. 2.4

27 If such a vacuuming is carried out, the surgeon must continually keep the probe moving on the back surface of the anterior capsule to avoid aspirating it into the port.

28 i.e., the endoilluminator is outside the eye, and its light enters the eye through the peripheral cornea

Table 2.7.5 Arguments for and against primary removal of a cataractous lens

For	Against
Single surgery: convenience and cost	Diagnosis may be false
Posterior segment immediately visible and surgery can planned according to the injuries found	Optimal surgical conditions not always available: proper equipment, experienced surgeon
Prevention of secondary complications (e.g., IOP elevation)	Increased inflammation
Immediate visual rehabilitation possible	Difficulty to determine optimal IOL power
Postoperative synechia formation will make secondary IOL implantation more difficult	Increased risk of secondary complications such as inflammation (especially if primary IOL implantation is also performed)

- A *dropped nucleus* during phacoemulsification should not be appreciated as a dreaded complication; inappropriate management of the complication should. Ideally, when lens is lost into the vitreous, the cataract surgeon instantly becomes an ocular traumatologist – or immediately calls for such a colleague's help.
  - The only acceptable management is vitrectomy, as described previously; never should "fishing" for the lens particles be performed [2].
  - If vitrectomy in the same session cannot be performed, the eye should be closed, anti-inflammatory therapy instigated, and vitreoretinal consultation sought.
  - The cataract surgeon may implant an IOL[29], but its disadvantages must be understood: it limits the removal options of the lost lens particle(s) (see above), and may make it more difficult to thoroughly clean the capsular bag.

29 Since it was the original goal of surgery, there is a strong desire on the surgeon's and the patient's part to have an IOL implanted at the termination of a cataract surgery.

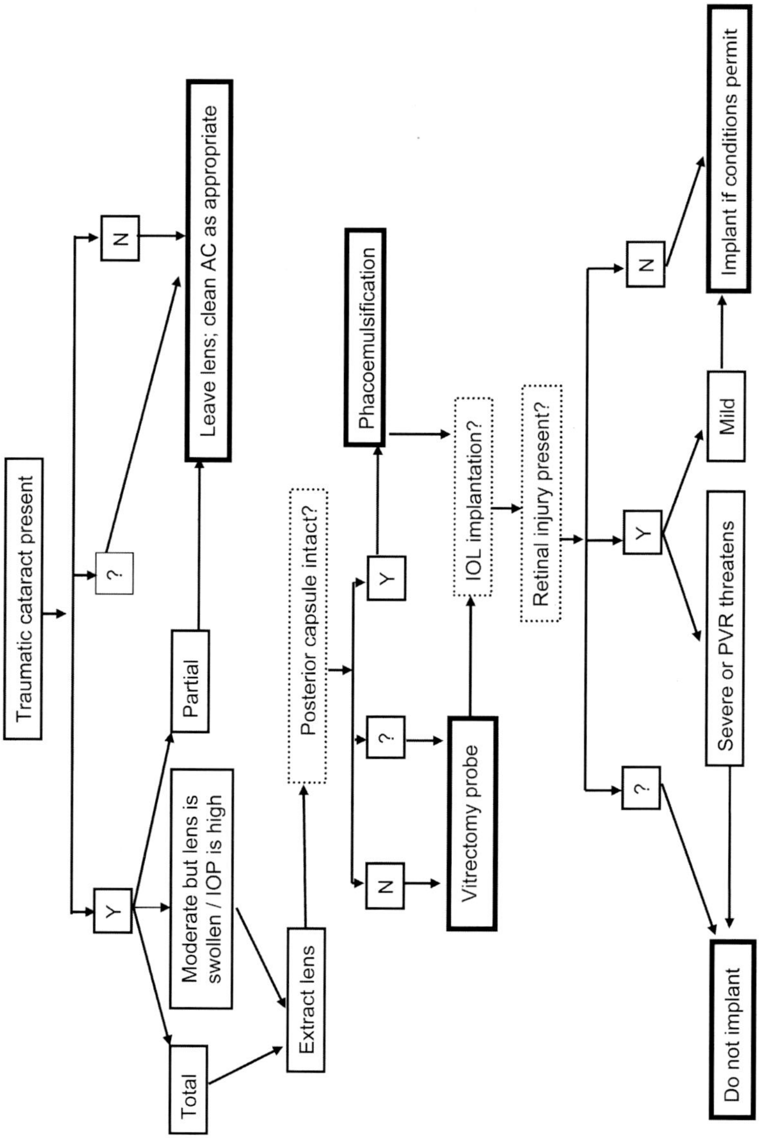
Traumatic cataract present
Y
?
N
Total
Moderate but lens is swollen / IOP is high
Partial
Leave lens; clean AC as appropriate
Extract lens
Posterior capsule intact?
N
?
Y
Vitrectomy probe
Phacoemulsification
IOL implantation?
Retinal injury present?
?
Y
N
Severe or PVR threatens
Mild
Do not implant
Implant if conditions permit

Fig. 2.7.4 The management flowchart for eyes with traumatic cataract. *Y* yes, *N* no

Lens touch during vitrectomy is a rare complication. The risk is higher if anterior PVR or retinal detachment is the indication because a judicious anterior vitrectomy is one of the goals of surgery. Paradoxically, wide-angle viewing systems have increased the risk since they make it more difficult to visualize the posterior capsule.

Pearl

Injecting a small air bubble into the anterior vitreous helps identify the plane of the posterior capsule and reduce the risk of lens touch.

If lens touch has occurred, the surgeon should not panic: unless the capsule is actually broken, cataract formation is not inevitable. If, however, major lens opacity does develop intraoperatively and interferes with visualization, cataract extraction must be performed to allow completion of the vitrectomy and unhindered postoperative viewing of the retina.

Lens "feathering" is described in Chap. 2.9.

2.7.3.6 IOL

2.7.3.6.1 Implantation

There are several methods to restore the eye's lost refractive power after cataract extraction.[30] Of these methods, the IOL is the one that is most convenient for the patient, although it has its own disadvantages.[31] Details of

30 Prescription glasses, contact lens, epikeratophakia

31 e.g., the optimal power is difficult to determine in children whose eye is still growing (see Chap. 2.16), and implantation represents additional trauma to the eye, especially if the IOL needs to be sutured into the sulcus

IOL implantation are beyond the scope of this book; only a few important issues are discussed briefly here:

- *Timing.* Whether primary [11, 13] or secondary [6] implantation should be performed remains a controversial issue. Primary implantation is important for a child in the amblyopic age, or if the patient is unable to afford a second procedure or return for one. Primary implantation causes increased postoperative inflammation and may interfere with subsequent retinal procedures due to visibility issues.[32] A careful individual decision must be made, but as a general rule, secondary implantation is recommended.

Cave

Primary IOL implantation should not be performed if the eye has a serious retinal injury or if the risk of PVR is high (see Chap. 2.9).

- *Type of implant.* Ideally, the IOL is placed in the bag; however, if this is not possible for the lack of adequate capsular support, the lens can be placed in the AC [20], fixated to the iris [22], or sutured into the sulcus.
- *Material of the implant.* Silicone IOLs should to be avoided, especially if posterior segment surgery with silicone oil use is expected; the oil may adhere to the IOL surface, making its removal very difficult [19].
  - One method to deal with silicone oil that is coating the IOL's surface is to grab a small piece of cotton[33] with a vitrectomy forceps, and wipe the IOL's surface with it. The oil cannot be removed completely, but it can be pushed toward the IOL's periphery to reduce its interference with the patient's vision.
  - If the zonules are weakened, use of a *capsular tension ring* may be considered; however, in a trauma case there are several unknowns,

32 The IOL's edge can be disturbing; opacification of the capsule is another issue to consider.

33 e.g., torn from a cotton-tipped applicator

and late, "unexplained" luxation of the IOL or even of the capsular tension ring itself may occur [9] if the zonules are weaker than expected.

2.7.3.6.2 Trauma to the IOL Already in Situ

Subluxation is usually treatable by simple repositioning; often it is only the haptic that is partially dislodged. If one of the scleral-fixated IOL's haptics is loose because its suture is broken, the intravitreally hanging haptic can be resutured using a simple technique.

- Prepare a scleral bed in the area where the IOL haptic needs to be fixated.
- Introduce a long, straight intracameral needle (see Chap. 2.6) 1 mm from the limbus through the scleral bed; the needle must be passed *behind* the haptic and *in front of* the optic of the IOL, and then partially[34] out of the AC on the other side.
- A 27-g hypodermic needle is passed into the AC 1 mm from the limbus through the scleral bed at some distance from the suture. This needle is passed *in front of* the haptic *and* optic of the IOL.
- The straight needle is pushed back into the barrel of the 27-g needle. The polypropylene suture is now looped around the free-hanging haptic.
- The 27-g needle is withdrawn from the eye, bringing the suture with it: the suture can now be tied, trimmed, and the scleral flap reattached.

Luxation into the vitreous may involve only the IOL or the IOL may still be inside the capsule (Fig. 2.7.5). The IOL luxation does not itself represent a major complication: erosion of the retina is unlikely, but vision is compromised because of the lost IOL power and because of the presence of a large floating object inside the vitreous cavity.

---

34 The suture end of the needle remains in the AC, only about a half of the needle is externalized.

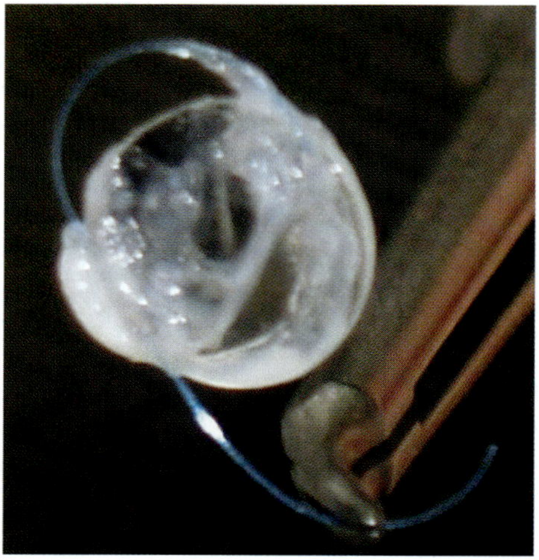

Fig. 2.7.5 Luxation of an IOL and its capsular bag. This IOL was removed from the vitreous cavity after a contusion injury; the IOL is still in the bag (Courtesy of Z. Slezak)

- If the capsular bag is sufficiently strongly held by the zonules and there is a large enough capsule left, the IOL can be replaced into or onto the bag. The following is a simple and effective technique:
  - Use an independent light source[35] so that a second instrument can be utilized if necessary.
  - Complete the vitreous removal, including that of the posterior hyaloid face.
  - Coat the endothelium with a dispersive viscoelastic.
  - Grab the *distant* haptic of the IOL with forceps: the forceps is in front of the optic of the IOL.[36]

35 e.g., Torpedo (Insight Instruments Inc., Stuart, Fla.).

36 Carefully avoid injuring the retina with the forceps as the haptic is grasped and not dragging the IOL over the retina.

- Rotate the IOL 180° so that the forceps is now *underneath* the optic of the IOL.[37]
- Place the proximal (superior) haptic into the capsular bag.[38]
- Bring the distant (inferior) haptic into the bag and release it.[39]
- The IOL can be removed through the pars plana [20] or the limbus [24]. If the lens is a foldable one, it can be re-folded or transected so that a smaller removal incision is needed.

Controversial

It remains to be determined whether intracameral manipulations to reduce IOL size (cutting or folding) so that a smaller incision is needed for extraction or the creation of a larger limbal wound is more traumatic to the eye long term.

- The IOL can also be sutured into the sulcus ("lasso" technique [8]) or fixed to the iris with a suture [3]. An excellent alternative[40] to suturing the IOL in a vitrectomized eye is to prepare two sclerotomies with a 24 g needle 1.5 to 2 mm from the limbus at 180° apart. The needles are also used to prepare two limbus-parallel sceral tunnels next to these sclerotomies. The haptics of the IOL are first externalized through the sclerotomies with a 25 g intravitreal forceps, and then buried into the tunnels, followed by final positioning of the IOL. This technique allows for great IOL stability without the need for keeping the eye open for extended periods of time during manipulations such as those necessary for sulcus-fixation. Instead of a pars plana approach, this technique can

37 The Revolution handle from Alcon (Fort Worth, Texas) or the "Syntrifugal" handle from Synergetics (Synergetics, East Windsor Hill, Conn,) offers easy rotation after grabbing.
38 Into the AC if the IOL must be removed.
39 The IOL can also be removed if both of its haptics are brought into the AC: a limbal wound is prepared and the IOL extracted. A replacement IOL can be inserted through the same wound.
40 The "sutureless intrascleral PCIOL fixation" technique was developed by Gaber B. Scharioth, Recklinghausen, Germany.

also be performed via corneal side port incisions and with the help of an AC maintainer.

The endoscope is of great help when dealing with a displaced IOL [18].

DO:

- carefully evaluate the lens to determine the nature of its injury so that the most optimal type of treatment can be selected
- be careful during cataract removal not to aspirate vitreous, presuming that vitreous prolapse is not present

DON'T:

- rush to remove the lens: what appears as cataract at the slit lamp may be fibrin only
- try to preserve at all cost the posterior capsule for in-the-bag IOL implantation; the eye may have a much better prognosis if the capsule is removed
- rush to implant an IOL primarily; secondary IOL implantation has distinct advantages

Summary

The vast majority of ophthalmic surgeons are knowledgeable about the elective removal of an age-related cataract. Treating an eye with a lens pathology caused by trauma, however, is different: the surgeon must not force his own favored extraction method on the eye but select an option that is optimal for the eye's specific condition, even if this means referral of the patient to a colleague more experienced in ocular traumatology.

References

[1] Ahmed, II, Crandall AS (2001) Ab externo scleral fixation of the Cionni modified capsular tension ring. J Cataract Refract Surg 27: 977–981

[2] Arbisser LB (2004) Managing intraoperative complications in cataract surgery. Curr Opin Ophthalmol 15: 33–39

[3] Aurich H, Korte P, Wirbelauer C, Haberle H, Pham DT (2007) Iris sutures for refixation of decentered intraocular lenses. Klin Monatsbl Augenheilkd 224: 28–31 [in German]

[4] Boorstein JM Titelbaum DS, Patel Y, Wong K, Grossman R (1995) CT diagnosis of unsuspected traumatic cataracts in patients with complicated eye injuries: significance of attenuation value of the lens. Am J Roentgenol 164: 181–184

[5] Cionni RJ, Osher RH (1995) Endocapsular ring approach to the subluxed cataractous lens. J Cataract Refract Surg 21: 245–249

[6] DeVaro JM, Buckley EG, Awner S, Seaber J (1997) Secondary posterior chamber intraocular lens implantation in pediatric patients. Am J Ophthalmol 123: 24–30

[7] Kazemi S, Wirostko WJ, Sinha S, Mieler WF, Koenig SB, Sheth BP (2000) Combined pars plana lensectomy-vitrectomy with open-loop flexible anterior chamber intraocular lens (AC IOL) implantation for subluxated lenses. Trans Am Ophthalmol Soc 98: 247–251

[8] Lawrence FC 2nd, Hubbard WA (1994) "Lens lasso" repositioning of dislocated posterior chamber intraocular lenses. Retina 14: 47–50

[9] Levy J, Klemperer I, Lifshitz T (2005) Posteriorly dislocated capsular tension ring. Ophthalmic Surg Lasers Imaging 36: 416–418

[10] Loo AV, Lai JS, Tham CC, Lam DS (2002) Traumatic subluxation causing variable position of the crystalline lens. J Cataract Refract Surg 28: 1077–1079

[11] Moisseiev J, Segev F, Harizman N, Arazi T, Rotenstreich Y, Assia EI (2001) Primary cataract extraction and intraocular lens implantation in penetrating ocular trauma. Ophthalmology 108: 1099–1103

[12] Nguyen TN, Mansour M, Deschenes J, Lindley S (2003) Visualization of posterior lens capsule integrity by 20-MHz ultrasound probe in ocular trauma. Am J Ophthalmol 136: 754–755

[13] Pavlovic S (1999) Primary intraocular lens implantation during pars plana vitrectomy and intraretinal foreign body removal. Retina 19: 430–436

[14] Peyman GA, Schulman JA, Sullivan B (1995) Perfluorocarbon liquids in ophthalmology. Surv Ophthalmol 39: 375–395

[15] Pieramici DJ MacCumber MW, Humayun MU, Marsh MJ, de Juan E Jr (1996) Open-globe injury. Update on types of injuries and visual results. Ophthalmology 103: 1798–1803

[16] Rao SK, Parikh S, Padhmanabhan P (1998) Isolated posterior capsule rupture in blunt trauma: pathogenesis and management. Ophthalmic Surg Lasers 29: 338–342

[17] Ruiz-Moreno JM (1998) Repositioning dislocated posterior chamber intraocular lenses. Retina 18: 330–334

[18] Sasahara M, Kiryu J, Yoshimura N (2005) Endoscope-assisted transscleral suture fixation to reduce the incidence of intraocular lens dislocation. J Cataract Refract Surg 31: 1777–1780

[19] Sharma Y, Sudan R, Gaur A (2003) Droplets on posterior surface of intraocular lens in silicone oil filled eye. Indian J Ophthalmol 51: 178–180

[20] Steinmetz RL, Brooks HL Jr, Newell CK (2004) Management of posteriorly dislocated posterior chamber intraocular lenses by vitrectomy and pars plana removal. Retina 24: 556–559

[21] Stoller GL, Barone R, Fisher YL (1997) Traumatic dislocation of the lens into posterior Tenon's space. Retina 17: 557–558

[22] Tahzib NG, Eggink FA, Odenthal MT, Nuijts RM (2007) Artisan iris-fixated toric phakic and aphakic intraocular lens implantation for the correction of astigmatic refractive error after radial keratotomy. J Cataract Refract Surg 33: 531–535

[23] Thompson W, Rubsamen P, Flynn H, Schiffman J, Cousins S (1995) Endophthalmitis after penetrating trauma. Risk factors and visual acuity outcomes. Ophthalmology 102: 1696–1701

[24] Wong KL, Grabow HB (2001) Simplified technique to remove posteriorly dislocated lens implants. Arch Ophthalmol 119: 273–274

2.8 Ciliary Body and Choroid

Ferenc Kuhn

2.8.1 Introduction

By secreting aqueous, the ciliary body plays a crucial role in the structural and functional integrity[1] of the eye: even if all other tissues, including the retina, are healthy, loss of aqueous production eventually results in a phthisical, blind eye. The choroid is an elastic tissue that supplies blood for the external retinal layers and the entire anterior segment.

2.8.2 Evaluation

The ciliary body is located in a "blind spot" for the examiner, making direct preoperative inspection impossible. Certain pathologies are detectable: gonioscopy may help identifying cyclodialysis, but a more reliable noninvasive method[2] is with the ultrasound biomicroscope (UBM) [8]. Intraoperatively, the ciliary body can be examined with deep scleral indentation[3] or with the endoscope; the latter has several advantages: it gives an image of high resolution and magnification, and without distortion caused by the

1 Keeping the eye pressurized ("inflated"), nourishing the cornea, accommodation.
2 Gonioscopy is less likely to reveal presence of a cyclodialysis cleft because of interference from commonly coexisting pathologies such as corneal edema and hyphema.
3 Aniridia greatly enhances inspection of the ciliary body.

indentation (see Chap. 2.20). The surgeon needs to determine whether the ciliary body is detached and the ciliary processes are healthy.

Monitoring the IOP is the best method to judge the functional viability of the ciliary body, although other factors can also cause hypotony.

Preoperatively, the choroid is best examined with the ophthalmoscope or on ultrasonography.

2.8.3 Specific Conditions

2.8.3.1 Ciliary Body[4]

2.8.3.1.1 Cyclodialysis

Detachment of the meridional ciliary muscle fibers from the scleral spur (Fig. 2.8.1) allows direct communication between the AC and the suprachoroidal space; even if aqueous production remains unaffected by the trauma[5], hypotony ensues because of the increased uveoscleral outflow. The size of the cleft has not been proven to correlate with the degree of hypotony.

Regarding *treatment*, if the cleft does not close spontaneously, it should be treated, especially if secondary complications, such as hypotony maculopathy, develop [17]. In addition to the UBM and pre- or intraoperative examination using a gonioscopy lens, transillumination during surgery helps determine the exact location of the cyclodialysis. Several options are available to achieve ciliary body reattachment:

- Conservative. Topical atropine to deepen the AC and prevent synechia formation. Anti-inflammatory drugs, such as corticosteroids, are ineffective.

4 Several of the ciliary body pathologies (e.g., angle recession, ciliochoroidal detachment, phthisis) are discussed in Chaps. 2.18 and 2.19.

5 Most commonly: contusion.

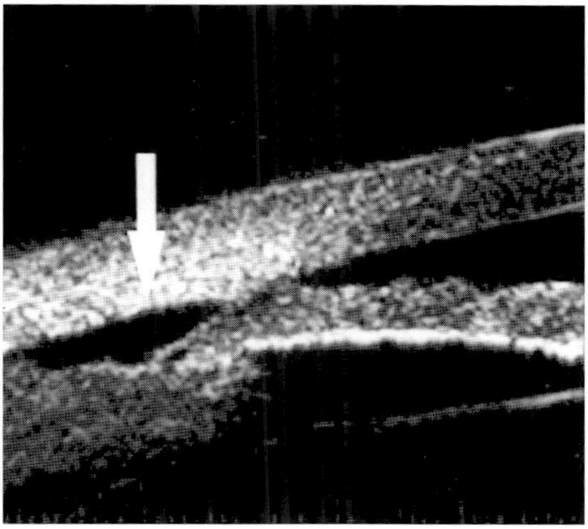

Fig. 2.8.1 Cyclodialysis cleft imaged on UBM. Expansion of the suprachoroidal space due to detachment of the ciliary body (*arrow*) (Courtesy of M. Modesti, Rome, Italy)

- Argon laser applied continually over the margins and inside the clefts [1][6] to block aqueous outflow via choroidal swelling and inflammation (iridocyclitis) [4].
- Transscleral YAG[7] [5] or diode[8] laser [2].
- Cryopexy with deep indentation applied directly over the sclera in the area of the cyclodialysis in a continuous row [3].

- Surgical.
  - Diathermy, incorporating both the sclera and the ciliary body [14].
  - Suturing, using any of the methods described for iridodialysis (see Chap. 2.16).

6 "91 burns, 0.45 mW power, 300-μm spot size, 100 μm, 1-s duration"

7 "20 applications in two rows of ten applications, 2–3 mm behind the limbus, at a power setting of 6 J, with a defocus setting of 9"

8 "Two rows of 14 applications in a post-traumatic at a power setting of 2500 mW and duration of 2000 ms"

- Anterior scleral buckling to close the gap between sclera and ciliary body by indenting the sclera [13].
- Vitrectomy with gas tamponade [17].

Cave

Once the ciliary body is successfully reattached, a surge in the IOP should be expected [10]; prophylactic antiglaucoma treatment is crucial (see Chap. 2.18). Monitoring for, and immediate treatment of, the IOP elevation are a must. Miotics must be avoided [16] to prevent ciliary body redetachment.

2.8.3.1.2 Ciliary Body Scarring (Anterior PVR)

Proliferative cells, blood, fibrin, and eventually PVR membranes may grow over the ciliary body, destroying the ciliary processes and shutting down aqueous production.[9]

Prevention is far more effective than treatment. Complete vitreous and blood removal is necessary in the periphery (see Chap. 2.9, 2.20), and sacrificing the lens is often advised. If the lens is removed, neither capsule should be preserved since it is expected to schrink and exert traction on the ciliary processes with their eventual destruction (see Chaps. 2.7, 2.9, 2.19).

Treatment is thorough vitrectomy, which should be performed early to prevent irreversible damage to the ciliary epithelium. In aphakic or pseudophakic eyes judicious scleral depression can greatly aid the surgeon, even if traditional viewing is used. Endoscopy-assisted vitrectomy offers the best option for cleansing the ciliary body surface (see Chap. 2.20).

9 Not uncommonly, this is the reason why vision is gradually lost in eyes with an otherwise functioning retina.

2.8.3.2 Choroid

2.8.3.2.1 ECH

No fewer than 19 terms have been used in the literature to describe this condition [11], which is the most devastating complication of open globe surgery. Its incidence in the context of trauma is much less investigated and its importance is certainly underappreciated. In the editor's own survey of the pathological specimens of 30 eyes enucleated after severe trauma, all had large amounts of suprachoroidal blood, but none of the clinical charts mentioned this complication (see Chap. 1.10).

2.8.3.2.1.1 Prevention

The surgeon can reduce the bleeding risk via the follwing:

- The ECH potential must always be kept in mind if an eye sustained serious trauma, whether open or closed globe. Even if suprachoroidal bleeding is not apparent through the pupil and no wound is visible, an ECH may have started but could have been stopped early by the increasing IOP (self-tamponade). Careless examination or reopening of the wound may cause the bleeding to recur or even be its primary cause.
- Avoid putting pressure on the eye during examination (see Chap. 1.9).
- Use caution when reopening the wound for toilette and suture closure. Remember the ECH potential when the timing of intervention is considered: delay of surgery reduces the risk (see Chap. 1.8).
- Topical corticosteroid use reduces vascular engorgement and thus the ECH risk. The drug should be used *hourly* in the first couple of days.

2.8.3.2.1.2 Recognition

The characteristics for recognition are:

- Pain
- Hardening of the eye
- Dark crescent appearing deep inside the eye, disappearing red reflex
- Intraocular tissues pushed forward with eventual extraocular extrusion (Fig. 2.8.2; also see Fig. 2.4.2)

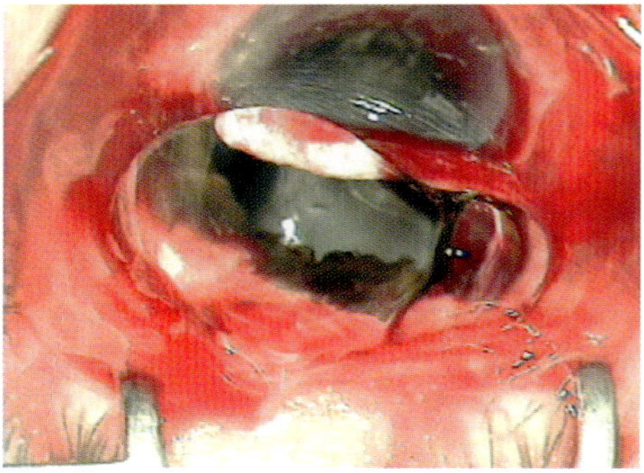

Fig. 2.8.2 Intraoperative photograph of an impending ECH. During reconstruction of a ruptured eye, a large prolapse of formed vitreous is visible in the limbal wound. The eye is collapsed, and the ciliary body is in direct view

- Fresh blood streaming from inside the eye.[10]

2.8.3.2.1.3 *Treatment*

If a true ECH is occurring, the only chance the surgeon has to save vision is to immediately close the eye. The wound can be held together with forceps or even with a finger pushing the wound lips together; actual suturing should wait until the built-up IOP stops the bleeding. Even if tissues get incarcerated as the wound is sutured, this represents a small late risk compared with losing all intraocular contents acutely if the wound is kept open. Secondary wound toilette can be performed a few days later, after intense topical corticosteroid therapy has reduced the vascular engorgement.

Pearl

Immediate apposition of the wound lips, regardless of the method utilized to achieve it, is the only option the surgeon has to save the eye if an ECH is occurring.

10 Remember, the bleeding is arterial, not venous.

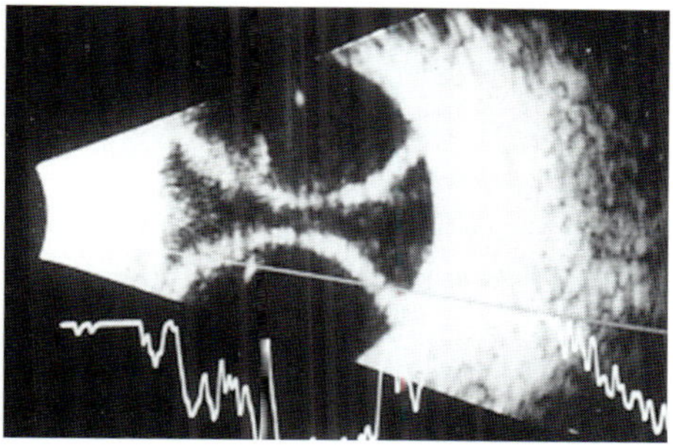

Fig. 2.8.3 "Kissing choroidals" caused by an ECH. The large amounts of suprachoroidal blood push the choroid and retina centrally, until the retinal surfaces are "bridged"

An entirely different situation arises if a *retinal prolapse* is present. The goal is to preserve as much of the retina as possible by reducing the IOP, repositing the retina without retinectomy if possible, suturing the wound, and addressing the retinal incarceration during a subsequent vitrectomy (see Chap. 2.4).

Drainage is rarely necessary in the acute phase. If there is persistent hypotony or retinal complications, such as retino-retinal bridging ("kissing choroidals"; Fig. 2.8.3), careful reconstruction by a posterior segment surgeon is needed. Timing is important: if the blood is still clotted, it is very difficult to remove, requiring "thrombectomy" [12] with the vitrectomy probe. It takes an average of 10 days for the blood to liquify. Ultrasonography is used to determine when the solid mass turns to fluid.

The procedure is as follows:

- Place an infusion in the AC or through the pars plana if the cannula's position is possible to verify; a long cannula should be used. The infusion is opened at a pressure of ~35 mmHg. Air or PFCL [7] can be used instead of BSS.
- Identify the highest point of choroidal elevation.[11]

11 The ophthalmoscope or ultrasonography is used to identify the best location for the sclerotomy.

- Carefully open the sclera. The incision should be perpendicular to the limbus and approximately 2 mm long.[12] The blood usually drains spontaneously once the sclera is fully opened. The color of the blood characteristically resembles dark, liquid chocolate.
- Gentle pressure is occasionally necessary to apply over the sclera in the vicinity of the incision: a cotton-tipped applicator is rolled toward the incision to push the blood toward the sclerotomy.
- The same procedure may be repeated elsewhere if high elevation of the ciliary body and choroid after the initial drainage still exists.
- Vitrectomy is performed as required by the intraocular pathologies.[13]

In most cases, the hemorrhage absorbs spontaneously. If vitreoretinal surgery is necessary for other reasons, drainage may be considered, especially if the suprachoroidal blood is located anteriorly and would interfere with scleral buckling.

2.8.3.2.2 Choroidal Rupture

Choroidal ruptures are breaks in the choroid, Bruch's membrane, and the RPE. Contusion is the most common cause. In the HEIR database, the incidence is 8% among eyes with contusion but only 1% in ruptures[14]. Choroidal rupture can occur at the site of impact (direct) or, more frequently, in the back of the eye as the shockwaves are traveling along the eye wall coalesce (contra coup mechanism; indirect). Direct choroidal ruptures are usually parallel to the limbus, whereas indirect ones are concentric to the disc or run in a straight, radial, or vertical line. Multiple ruptures may be present in up to

---

12 If necessary, the incision can also be longer or "L"-shaped.

13 Internal drainage of the suprachoroidal blood has also been advocated. This obviously requires a retinotomy, which represents a PVR risk factor and thus significant disadvantage. The advantages are that it is easy to identify the ideal site for the drainage, and that the blood evacuation can be complete even if the hemorrhage is posterior.

14 When the eye ruptures, this appears to act as a pressure valve, reducing the risk of choroidal rupture.

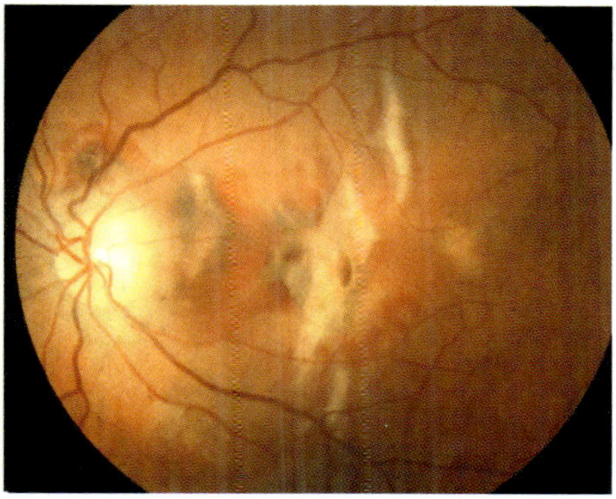

Fig. 2.8.4 Multiple choroidal ruptures with subretinal hemorrhage. Contusion-related multiple, indirect choroidal ruptures; subretinal hemorrhage is also visible in the maculopapillary bundle. An unusually wide, vertical choroidal rupture is located juxtafoveally. Visual acuity may remain surprisingly good unless reactive RPE changes subsequently reach into the fovea or CNV develops

a quarter of eyes. The presence of a choroidal rupture makes it three to seven times more likely that other serious pathologies have also occurred [18]. Unless the lesion runs directly through the macula, the prognosis is good [6].

2.8.3.2.2.1 Recognition

The fundus findings differ with time:

- In an *acute* injury, subretinal hemorrhage, which commonly occurs as the choroid ruptures, can block view of the rupture; consequently, a choroidal rupture should be suspected in every contused eye with subretinal hemorrhage.
- In *chronic* cases, the linear or crescent-shaped hypo- or hyperpigmented streak running subretinally is easy to recognize.

2.8.3.2.2.2 Management

The rupture itself is untreatable, but the visual acuity can remain excellent [15] even if the rupture runs very close to the fovea (Fig. 2.8.4). If a choroidal neovascularization develops[15] and causes late deterioration of vision, laser photocoagulation, photodynamic therapy [6], intraocular anti-VEGF injections[16], or surgical removal [9] may help.

DO:

- try to remove blood, membranes, fibrin from the ciliary body surface to prevent scarring
- reattach the ciliary body if a cyclodialysis is present and the IOP is low
- keep in mind that an ECH is always a threat in eyes with open globe injury; the bleeding may have occurred at the time of the injury or can occur during wound toilette and closure, even be caused by a careless examination

DON'T:

- forget that the IOP may dramatically rise after closure of the cyclodialysis cleft
- keep the wound open if an ECH occurs; immediate closure, by whatever means, is the key to saving the eye: the wound can properly be reconstructed in a secondary procedure
- give up on an eye whose vision deteriorates late after sustaining a choroidal rupture: it is often possible to treat the neovascularization that is most likely to be responsible

Summary

The ciliary body produces aqueous, without which an eye is unable to function, even if all other tissues, including the retina, have recovered from the injury. Early recognition and treatment of the ciliary body pathology therefore remain crucial for the ocular traumatologist. Injury to the choroid is relatively rare; the gravest acute danger of losing an eye, however, is an arterial bleeding originating in the choroid.

15 Expected in up to a third of cases and may appear years after the injury.

16 e.g., bevacizumab

References

[1] Alward WL, Hodapp EA, Parel JM, Anderson DR (1988) Argon laser endophotocoagulator closure of cyclodialysis clefts. Am J Ophthalmol 106: 748–749

[2] Amini H, Razeghinejad MR (2005) Transscleral diode laser therapy for cyclodialysis cleft induced hypotony. Clin Experiment Ophthalmol 33: 348–350

[3] Barasch K, Galin MA, Baras I (1969) Postcyclodialysis hypotony. Am J Ophthalmol 68: 644–645

[4] Bauer B (1995) Argon laser photocoagulation of cyclodialysis clefts after cataract surgery. Acta Ophthalmol Scand 73: 283–284

[5] Brooks AM, Troski M, Gillies WE (1996) Noninvasive closure of a persistent cyclodialysis cleft. Ophthalmology 103: 1943–1945

[6] Conrath J, Forzano O, Ricings B (2004) Photodynamic therapy for subfoveal CNV complicating traumatic choroidal rupture. Eye 18: 946–947

[7] Desai U, Peyman G, Chen C, Nelson NJ, Alturki W, Blinder K, Paris C (1992) Use of perfluoroperhydrophenanthrene in the management of suprachoroidal hemorrhages. Ophthalmology 99: 1542–1547

[8] Gentile R C, Pavlin C J, Liebmann J M, Easterbrook M, Tello C, Foster FS, Ritch R (1996) Diagnosis of traumatic cyclodialysis by ultrasound biomicroscopy. Ophthalmic Surg Lasers 27: 97–105

[9] Gross JG, King LP, de Juan E Jr, Powers T (1996) Subfoveal neovascular membrane removal in patients with traumatic choroidal rupture. Ophthalmology 103: 579–585

[10] Kronfeld PC (1954) The fluid exchange in the successfully cyclodialyzed eye. Trans Am Ophthalmol Soc 52: 249–263

[11] Kuhn F, Mester V (1998) Anterior globe injuries with vitreous prolapse and/or incarceration. In: Stirpe M (eds) Anterior and posterior segment surgery: mutual problems and common interests. Ophthalmic Communications Society, New York, pp 252–257

[12] Kuhn F, Morris R, Mester V, Witherspoon C (1998) Management of intraoperative expulsive choroidal hemorrhage during anterior segment surgery. In: Stirpe M (eds) Anterior and posterior segment surgery: mutual problems and common interests. Ophthalmic Communications Society, New York, pp 191–203

[13] Mandava N, Kahook MY, Mackenzie DL, Olson JL (2006) Anterior scleral buckling procedure for cyclodialysis cleft with chronic hypotony. Ophthalmic Surg Lasers Imaging 37: 151–153

[14] Kutschera E (1973) A simplified procedure in the treatment of the hypotony-syndrome. Klin Monatsbl Augenheilkd 166: 834–835 [in German]

[15] Raman SV, Desai UR, Anderson S, Samuel MA (2004) Visual prognosis in patients with traumatic choroidal rupture. Can J Ophthalmol 39: 260–266

[16] Shaffer RN, Weiss DI (1962) Concerning cyclodialysis and hypotony. Arch Ophthalmol 68: 25–31

[17] Takaya K, Suzuki Y, Nakazawa M (2006) Four cases of hypotony maculopathy caused by traumatic cyclodialysis and treated by vitrectomy, cryotherapy, and gas tamponade. Graefe's Arch Clin Exp Ophthalmol 244: 855–858

[18] Viestenz A (2004) Rupture of the choroid after eyeball contusion: an analysis based on the Erlangen Ocular Contusion Registry (EOCR). Klin Monatsbl Augenheilkd 221: 713–719 [in German]

2.9 Vitreous and Retina

Ferenc Kuhn

2.9.1 Introduction

In most cases the condition of the retina[1] determines the outcome of an injury. In all cases of ocular (or systemic; see Chap. 3.3) trauma when posterior segment involvement can be suspected, vitreoretinal consultation should be sought. The earlier such consultation takes place the better. Many vitreoretinal surgeons also prefer if they are the one who sutures the corneal/scleral wound so that optimal conditions are established for vitrectomy, which may have be to performed in a very short period of time[2] if this is deemed necessary to prevent secondary complications.

This chapter provides a summary of selected pathologies[3] of the vitreous and retina,[4] including management and certain prophylactic measures.[5]

---

1 More precisely, the viability the macula.

2 e.g., the corneal wound must remain watertight even if the IOP is raised during surgery, corneal edema must be minimized via the use of full-thickness sutures (see Chap. 2.2), and retinal incarceration into the scleral wound must be avoided.

3 Some of these conditions have a less obvious or direct relationship to trauma than others (e.g., vitreous opacities). Such conditions are discussed here because they may be a late, albeit rare, consequence of trauma.

4 The vitreous and retina are covered in a single chapter because many of their pathologies are interrelated.

5 Space limitations do not allow a complete description of all surgical techniques; for these the reader is referred to vitreoretinal textbooks.

2.9.2 Evaluation

If direct visualization of the vitreous and retina with the ophthalmoscope or at the slit lamp is not possible because of media opacity, several diagnostic tests are available that can provide important indirect information. These tests include determining the visual acuity (e.g., presence of LP and projection), ultrasonography, CT, MRI, UBM, and electrophysiology. Optical coherence tomography is an increasingly utilized test, although it requires clear media and its usefulness is mostly restricted for the chronic cases (Fig. 2.9.1). If concerns or doubts persist, surgical exploration (endoscopy or vitrectomy) must be considered (see Chap. 1.9).

2.9.3 Specific Conditions

2.9.3.1 Vitreous Penetration

Objects entering the vitreous cavity do not appear to cause adverse consequences if they are not contaminated, not retained, and do not cause concomitant damage[6]. In such cases the eye with vitreous penetration can simply be followed after wound closure[7], and any intervention be deferred until a complication does occur. If the object was contaminated, is retained, or complications resulted, intraocular surgery is needed accordingly (see below and Chaps. 2.10, 2.13).

2.9.3.2 Vitreous Base Avulsion

Although the incidence after contusion reached 26% in one study [21], this is a rarely diagnosed condition. Even if neurofibromatosis [25] is one of the possible etiologies, vitreous base avulsion is pathognomonic of trauma[8] [87].

---

6 e.g., significant vitreous hemorrhage or a retinal break
7 Wound closure is not always necessary (see Chaps. 2.2 and 2.3).
8 More precisely, contusion.

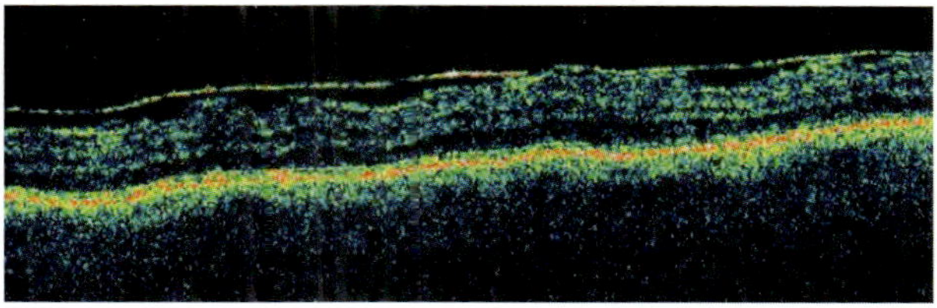

Fig. 2.9.1 Optical coherence tomography of an eye with traumatic macular pucker. The epiretinal membrane is clearly visible on the macular surface, causing full-thickness retinal folds

As a result of the blunt force applied to the eye, the vitreous base separates from the underlying retina and pars plana, which is recognized by a whitish line hanging from the periphery ("bucket handle sign"). No treatment is necessary unless secondary complications, such as retinal dialysis or tear, are also present. A careful retinal examination is therefore recommended.

2.9.3.3 Posterior Vitreous Detachment

This is perhaps the most commonly misinterpreted condition of all trauma-related posterior segment pathologies. By definition, this term should characterize a *complete* separation (Fig. 2.9.2a) of the postequatorial retina from the cortical vitreous, as opposed to a complete vitreous attachment (Fig. 2.9.2b). Posterior vitreous detachment (PVD) is often reported to occur in eyes with posttraumatic vitreous hemorrhage [16]. The vitreous may also be partially detached: there is strong vitreoretinal adhesion in an area surrounded by vitreoretinal detachment (Fig. 2.9.2c). Often, however, what is described after biomicroscopic, ultrasonographic, or OCT examination as a PVD is in reality a vitreoschisis (Fig. 2.9.2d). Such splitting of the vitreous can be present even if a Weiss ring is visible: separation of the vitreous from the retina at the optic disc does not necessarily imply that it has also detached at the macula [45].

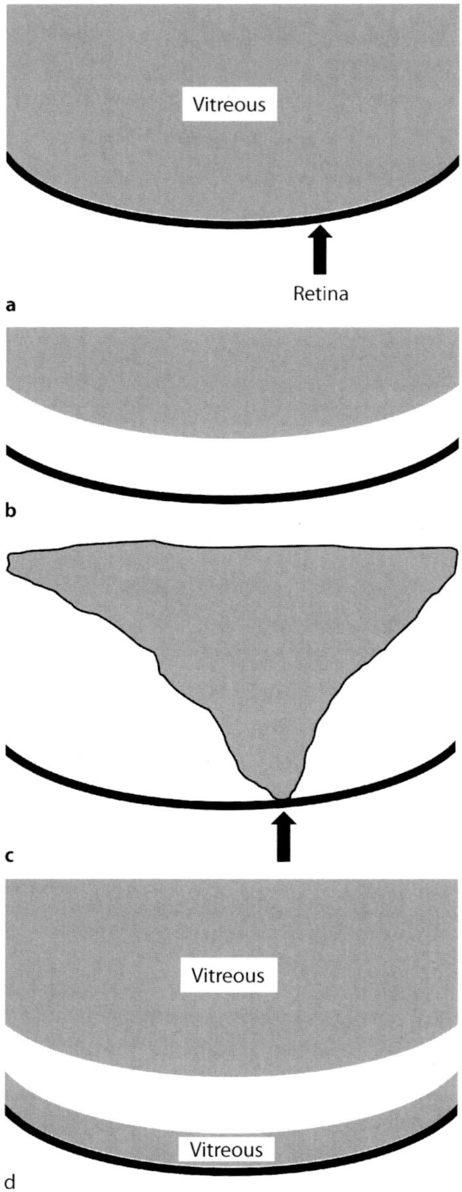
Vitreous
Retina
a
b
c
Vitreous
Vitreous
d

Fig. 2.9.2 Vitreoretinal configuration and the risk of retinal detachment. **a** The vitreous is completely attached. Even if there are areas with abnormally strong vitreoretinal adhesion, there is no risk of retinal break and subsequent detachment development formation since the vitreous gel is stable: it is unable to shift position[1] even with major and abrupt eye or head movement. **b** The vitreous is completely detached (true PVD). Although there is now room for the vitreous to shift with eye or head movement, it represents no risk for retinal break development lacking vitreoretinal adhesion.[2] **c** Partial PVD, the only condition carrying a significant risk of retinal break formation. With eye or head movement, vitreous movement follows, exerting traction at the point of adhesion (*arrow*). In principle, there are two therapeutic approaches: to surround the area of adhesion with *(laser)* scars to overcome the traction force or to perform vitrectomy to eliminate the traction.[3] **d** Vitreoschisis. Although the intravitreal presence of a hyaloidal face on examination suggests that a vitreous detachment has occurred, the vitreous in reality has split, and a layer is still adherent to the retina. There is fluid inside the vitreous pocket (syneresis)

[1] i.e., cause dynamic traction.

[2] Obviously, this is true only in the retinal area shown here: the risk may be substantial in other areas.

[3] Presence of such an adhesion by itself is not an indication for vitrectomy, but if vitrectomy is performed for any other indication, the surgeon must make sure that the vitreous removal is complete and there is no residual traction.

Cave

Based on current technology, it is impossible to preoperatively determine with absolute certainty that a true PVD has occurred. Even intraoperatively, only intravitreally injected TA can provide indisputable evidence whether or not a layer of cortical vitreous still coats the retinal surface.

The vitreous is much less commonly detached after trauma than generally presumed. A recent study found that in eyes undergoing vitrectomy for a posterior segment IOFB a median 9 days (range 5–18 days) after the injury, only 19% of eyes had a PVD [88].

2.9.3.3.1 Management Pearls Regarding the Vitreoretinal Interface Posteriorly

Issues regarding management are as follows:

- Vitreous abnormalities, such as PVD, syneresis, and vitreoschisis, commonly occur with age or in certain conditions, e.g., myopia. Trauma can accelerate the development of these abnormalities, but true PVD within the first few weeks after an injury is much less common than suggested.

Pearl

Since true PVD rarely develops in the first few weeks post-injury, this should not be a significant factor in determining the timing of vitrectomy (see Chap. 1.8). It is not recommended to delay vitreous surgery for the sake of PVD development, and it is best to assume during surgery that the vitreous is still attached.

- Posterior vitreous abnormalities do not require treatment unless they lead to secondary complications such as the development of an EMP or retinal tear.
- Very rarely, a posterior retinal break occurs as the vitreous with abnormally strong retinal adhesion detaches.[9] Mobility of the vitreous (i.e., detachment in at least the adjacent area) is an obvious precondition.
- In eyes with *complete* vitreous attachment or detachment the risk of retinal break formation is virtually nonexistent (Fig. 2.9.2A,B).
- If the PVD progresses and involves the retina anterior to the equator, the risk of the development of a (peripheral) retinal break and subsequent detachment dramatically increases.
- A central retinal break, which is itself rarely a complication of PVD, virtually never causes retinal detachment. The only exception is an eye with high myopia.

9 The dynamic traction exerted by the vitreous overcomes the strength of retinal cohesion and adhesion.

- The risk of retinal detachment is even higher if the PVD is symptomatic. Recent complaints of flashes/floaters, however, do not necessarily indicate that a retinal break has occurred or even that it is imminent.
- If an area of abnormal vitreoretinal adhesion or a true retinal break is found in an eye with a history of trauma, prophylactic laser treatment is indicated. If prophylactic treatment is performed in the periphery, endolaser cerclage is more effective than focal laser [63] since the retinal detachment often originates in an area that appeared normal during the examination.
- If no treatment is employed, educating the patient about the symptoms of PVD and retinal detachment is just as important as performing periodic follow-up examinations using the slit lamp and a contact lens[10].

2.9.3.3.2 Surgical PVD

The procedure should be part of every vitrectomy performed for trauma:

- If the retina and the vitreoretinal interface are visible and no significant traction is noted, the editor uses the postero-anterior technique [47], in which detachment of the posterior cortical vitreous takes precedence.
  - Minimal vitrectomy is initially performed in front of the disc and macula.
  - A tiny amount[11] of TA is injected to visualize the posterior vitreous.
  - If the cortical vitreous is still adherent, it is either elevated using the vitrectomy probe at the disc margin and then in an increasingly larger circle, or it is incised and lifted with a slightly barbed MVR blade.[12]

10 Traditionally, such examinations are advised at 3- or 6-month intervals. These intervals are arbitrarily chosen; there is no evidence why one interval would be preferable over any other.

11 Not exceeding 0.1 ml; if more is used, the clearing of the "intraocular snowfall" takes substantial time without contributing to the efficacy of the "staining."

12 To complete the vitrectomy, the entire vitreous is then removed while holding the vitrectomy probe in the midvitreous cavity. The last area to address is the periphery and the retrolental space.

- If there is significant vitreous opacity or vitreoretinal traction, the usual antero-posterior approach should not be used; the PVD *follows* the core vitrectomy. Areas of exceptionally strong vitreoretinal adhesion or of retinal necrosis require very careful decision-making and manipulations to avoid tearing and detaching the retina. If the risk is deemed high or the vitreous does not separate easily, it is safer to circumcise the vitreous (Fig. 2.9.3) with the vitrectomy probe, or, if the vitreous shows true sheets at the site, with scissors.
- One useful trick involves switching to air from BSS. The air will help keep the retina attached and the residual cortical vitreous somewhat compressed, providing decent visualization for the surgeon and allowing shaving of the inseparable vitreous.

Controversial

Pharmacological vitreoretinal separation and vitreolysis, using enzymes[13] [74, 81, 83], is a management option that holds promise for many conditions; it is probably most important in eyes with very strong vitreoretinal adhesion such as in young patients. Its efficacy in trauma remains to be determined.

2.9.3.4 Vitreous Opacities

Opacities may be present in the vitreous as a result several conditions such as inadequate absorption of a vitreous hemorrhage, infection, inflammation, or because of metallosis [73]. The only proven cure is vitrectomy; the patient's individual needs, rather than relying on an arbitrarily determined cut-off visual acuity level, should be the decisive factor in whether surgery is performed (see Chap. 1.4).[14]

13 e.g., plasmin, streptokinase, recombinant microplasmin, hyaloronidase, collagenase

14 Even if vision is 20/20, the floaters may cause major, unacceptable disturbance to some people. If the person understands and accepts the risks of surgery, this should not be denied by the ophthalmologist; if he feels strongly against the operation, the patient should be referred for second opinion.

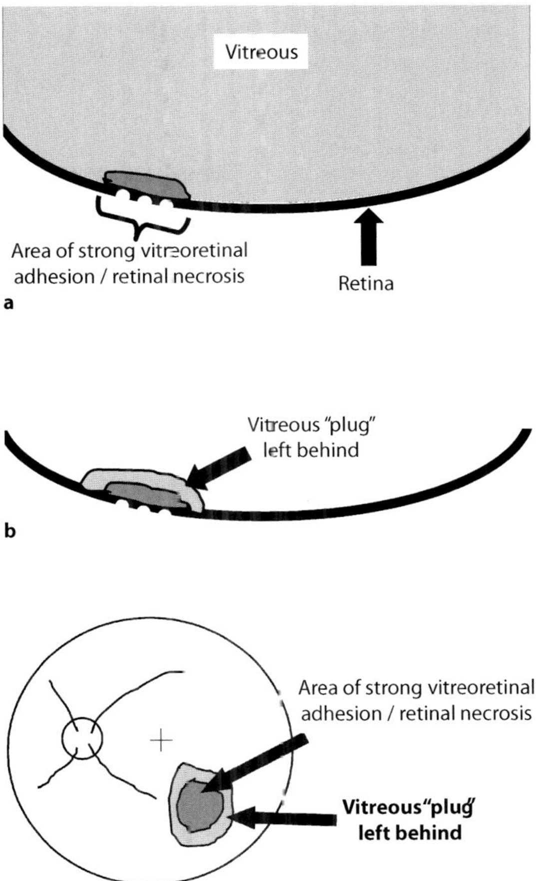

Fig. 2.9.3 The "circumcision" option during vitrectomy in eyes with strong vitreoretinal adhesion or retinal necrosis. If the vitreous cannot be safely separated from the retina, it should be left in situ but truncated: severed from all connections from the rest of the vitreous, which must then be removed. Only a vitreous "plug" is thus left behind, but this represents no threat since it cannot exert traction on the retina. **a** Preoperative view. **b** Postoperative, cross-sectional view. **c** Postoperative, anterior view

2.9.3.5 Vitreous Hemorrhage[15]

This is the most common injury-related vitreous pathology (Table 2.9.1); one-third of eyes with serious trauma have vitreous hemorrhage (USEIR datum). The source of the blood may be any tissue from the iris anteriorly to the optic nerve head posteriorly.

2.9.3.5.1 Significance

- Vitreous hemorrhage interferes with the patient's visual acuity and field.
- It makes it difficult or impossible for the ophthalmologist to inspect the retina.
- It can cause secondary complications such as glaucoma,[16] hemosiderosis [14], cataract, retinal gliosis and EMP, retinal detachment, PVR, myopia, and amblyopia [15, 30, 42, 50, 61, 78, 93].
- If the hemorrhage does not absorb spontaneously, it may be seeded with proliferative cells and undergo organization. The first sign of organization, a precursor to tractional retinal detachment and PVR, is decreased vitreous motility. Serial ultrasonography is often employed with the hope of detecting this complication early.

2.9.3.5.2 Treatment

Although there have been reports of successful nonsurgical treatment for trauma-related vitreous hemorrhage (recombinant activated factor VII [2], intravitreal hyaluronidase [52]), vitrectomy remains the mainstay of therapy. Vitrectomy achieves instantaneous clearing and allows instant treatment of any coexisting other intraocular pathology. The timing of vitrectomy remains a controversial issue; it is discussed in Chaps 2.10–2.14.

15 The blood may be located in the gel proper or in syneresis cavities; subhyaloidal bleeding is discussed separately.

16 Various types (see Chap. 2.18)

Table 2.9.1 The incidence of various vitreoretinal pathologies in different types of ocular trauma in the USEIR database (%)

Pathology	Contusion (1497)	Rupture (2117)	Penetrating (4220)	IOFB (1235)	Perforating (464)
Vitreous penetration	0	9	14	21	23
Vitreous hemorrhage	35	41	31	43	56
Retinal break[a]	8	8	10	18	14
Macular hole	2	0.2	0.1	0.2	1
Retinal hemorrhage	18	11	9	15	18
Retinal detachment	10	19	12	19	26

Based on 14,523 injuries

[a]Includes all peripheral lesions (tear, necrotic hole, dialysis). All numbers are rounded

Controversial

Not all eyes with contusion-related traumatic vitreous hemorrhage require vitrectomy, which has its own complications; however, surgery is much easier, less risky, and more effective if secondary retinal complications are not yet present; early vitrectomy can also *prevent* retinal complications. It therefore remains an individual decision how early a surgeon decides to remove the vitreous hemorrhage.

2.9.3.5.2.1 *Management Pearls for Vitrectomy for Trauma-induced Vitreous Hemorrhage*

The surgeon should keep in mind the following:

- The difficulties and risks associated with the procedure are proportional to the severity of the hemorrhage.
- A severe hemorrhage makes it hard to determine what lays immediately behind the vitrectomy probe surrounded by nontransparent vitreous.

Even if the retina has been confirmed to be attached preoperatively[17] and easy detachment of the posterior vitreous has been achieved in a large area, strong vitreoretinal adhesion may be present elsewhere. Careless vitreous removal can quickly lead to the development of a retinal break and detachment.

- Removal of the vitreous should be complete and compatible with safety.
- It may be difficult and dangerous to separate the vitreous in very young children; a judicious core vitrectomy is the compromise, leaving as thin a layer of cortical vitreous on the retina as possible (see Chap. 2.16).
- It is not always possible to completely remove the vitreous in the periphery; a thorough shaving is necessary in such cases.

Pearl

Vitreous-related complications in a seriously injured eye originate from vitreous left behind, not from vitreous removed: vitrectomy should be as complete as possible.

- If fresh, red blood is encountered in increasing amounts during vitrectomy, this may be caused by acute intraoperative bleeding.[18] It is also possible, however, that blood, previously trapped between vitreous layers or subhyaloidally, is now being freed.
- In vitreous containing older, yellow blood,[19] streaks of red blood may also be present. The tissue resembles, and can be very difficult to distinguish from, a necrotic, detached retina. (See Chap. 2.12 for a special surgical technique to deal with the problem.)
- The posterior vitreous may not spontaneously detach, even if the hemorrhage has persisted for several months: in a recent study only a quarter of eyes showed spontaneous PVD after an average 38 days with IOFB injury [22]. The posterior cortical vitreous may be delineated by

17 Which may not be a reliable information (Fig. 1.9.5).

18 May be a sign of ECH (see Chap. 2.8).

19 May persist for months or years, especially inferiorly.

the blood, though, making recognition and thus surgical detachment easier.

- The source of the hemorrhage is rarely found. Additional pathologies, however, are very common and must be meticulously sought.
- In the presence of a wound[20] [17] or a disrupted lens [86], the risk of PVR is significantly higher (see below). It therefore appears reasonable to indicate vitrectomy early, especially if the injury was a rupture.
- The gravest danger in an eye with severe vitreous hemorrhage is the development of a retinal detachment.

Cave

In eyes with severe vitreous hemorrhage the B scan is often unable to reliably distinguish a PVD from a retinal detachment (see Fig. 1.9.5).

2.9.3.6 Subhyaloidal Hemorrhage[21]

Occasionally, blood is not dispersed in the gel itself but remains trapped between the retina and vitreous. Even though the media are clear, the patient registers severe visual loss if the blood is in front of the macula. The bleeding may occur as a result of direct trauma to the eye [66] or indirectly (e.g., Valsalva mechanism [37]; see Chap. 3.3).[22]

Regarding treatment, spontaneous dispersion of the blood can improve vision and help prevent PVR and retinal detachment; however, these complications can occur as early as within 5 weeks [68]. Treatment should therefore be considered early, especially if the hemorrhage is large and/or thick. The following options are available:

- *SF_6* alone [69] or in combination with *TPA* [19].
- *YAG laser* [29]
- *TPA* and *C_3F_8* [46].

20 Especially if the wound was caused by rupture, rather than a laceration.

21 Technically, this is also a vitreous hemorrhage since the blood is in the vitreous cavity; however, because it does not enter the vitreous gel itself and has different implications, it is discussed separately.

22 Obviously, the differential diagnosis list includes nontraumatic causes as well.

- *Vitrectomy* is the definite treatment, indicated primarily if additional pathologies are present or the other modalities, listed above, have failed.

2.9.3.7 Contusion Retinopathy[23]

Areas of the retina may become opaque after a contusion. This condition is not caused by edema, as previously presumed, but by photoreceptor death [76], a finding recently confirmed on OCT [43].

- *Acutely*, a cloudy retina is noted, accompanied on occasion by hemorrhages. As in all contused eyes, choroidal rupture may also occur and full-thickness retinal necrosis may also develop [40]. Occasionally a retinal detachment follows [59]. If the macula is involved (contusion maculopathy), a full-thickness hole can form. The vision in the affected area is moderately to severely decreased.
- *Subsequently*, minor to major RPE disturbance is seen (Fig. 2.9.4). The vision may improve or remain unchanged.

There is no treatment for traumatic retinopathy; specific complications, as described above, require appropriate intervention. The surgeon must remain conservative regarding surgery if necrosis is present: the risk of postoperative retinal detachment is not negligible because retinal breaks can develop at the border of the contused area (see Chap. 2.10). Creating a protective barrier around the area with laser may be considered [79].

2.9.3.8 Chorioretinitis Sclopetaria

The name refers to a somewhat vaguely understood condition in which the eye sustains indirect damage from an object that penetrates the orbit with great momentum; the typical agent is a pellet or bullet. Other etiologies have also been described, including air-bag-related trauma, in which orbital penetration is unlikely [6]. The eye wall remains intact but various types of intraocular damage occur: tissue rupture; hemorrhage; and retinal

---

23 Also called commotio retinae or Berlin's edema.

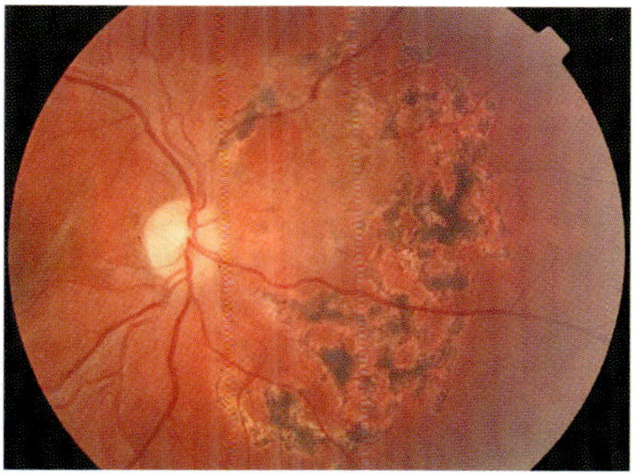

Fig. 2.9.4 Contusion retinopathy. Small to large islands of hyperpigmentation, often bordered by hypopigmentation, was the result of a large-object impact in this eye. The injury occurred via a contra-coup mechanism

necrosis. Retinal detachment is rare because of the developing chorioretinal scar [71].[24]

Intervention is necessary for findings such as a retinal tear or a nonresolving vitreous hemorrhage. Detaching the posterior vitreous in areas of retinal necrosis requires extreme caution (Fig. 2.9.3).

2.9.3.9 Retinal Break

A retinal break is defined here as a full-thickness discontinuity in the retinal tissue. Table 2.9.2 shows the various types of breaks and the recommended management. (For further details, see Chap. 2.10.)

24 It not clear why such scars do not evolve into PVR.

Table 2.9.2 Various types of retinal breaks

Type of break	Comment	Treatment
Laceration/ impact site	Direct retinal injury caused by an object penetrating the eye wall. The object impacts the retina either directly[1] or secondarily (transvitreally). The lesion develops instantly	It is advisable to surround the lesion with laser [88], although deep lacerations probably require prophylactic chorioretinectomy [49] (see above and Chap. 2.14)
Hole	Caused by slow disintegration of the retina; traction does not play a role in the pathogenesis. The lesion develops months/years after the injury	Treatment is rarely necessary; surrounding the hole with laser is probably more important for the ophthalmologist's peace of mind than for the prevention of retinal detachment
Necrotic hole	The retina is dissolved at the impact site; the choroid may also be involved. The necrosis can be evident immediately or manifest shortly after the contusion	It is advisable to surround the lesion with laser
Macular hole (see the text for more details)	The pathomechanism of the development of traumatic macular holes is unknown; traction probably contributes. The vast majority of cases are caused by contusion. The lesion develops within hours or up to a few weeks after the injury; its shape is often oval, not round	Traumatic macular holes have a stronger tendency to spontaneously close [92] than do idiopathic holes; conversely, surgery (vitrectomy, ILM peeling, and gas tamponade) is highly successful, even if other macular pathologies are present [51]
Dialysis	The retina is torn at the ora serrata; the condition is most common in the inferotemporal quadrant and pathognomonic of contusion. The vitreous remains attached to the torn retina. The dialysis presents very early but its progression to retinal detachment is slow [44]	It is advisable to wall-off the lesion with laser. A dialysis-related retinal detachment is the one most amenable to be treated with a scleral buckle, rather than with vitrectomy

Table 2.9.2 *(continued)* Various types of retinal breaks

Type of break	Comment	Treatment
Tear	The typical horseshoe appearance is a telling sign of strong vitreoretinal traction as the responsible factor. The vitreous is attached to the peripheral lip of the tear in the form of a strand; this is why symptoms[2] are common and the risk of retinal detachment development is high. Vitreous often remains adherent to the retina posterior to the tear	It is advisable to surround the lesion with laser
Giant tear	Tears exceeding 90° are discussed separately because they do not show the characteristic horseshoe shape and, more importantly, because they lead to retinal detachment much faster, with a significantly elevated risk of PVR	It is advisable to surround the lesion with laser; because of the large size and prominent traction, prophylactic scleral buckling should also be considered. Conversely, should a retinal detachment develop, it is best treated with vitrectomy *without* a scleral buckle to prevent slippage

[1] i.e., injuring the RPE first

[2] Floaters, photopsia

Pearl

Surrounding a retinal break with laser scars makes clinical sense if vitreoretinal traction is present or expected to develop, or the vitreous cannot be completely removed in the vicinity[25]. If, however, true PVR with strong traction evolves, adhesion provided by the laser (cryo) scars rarely have the strength to prevent retinal detachment.

If a break is treated, laser is the preferred option since cryopexy has a much greater tendency to incite inflammation, which is a known precursor to PVR [9]. If cryopexy is used,[26] its power must be kept to the minimum necessary[27] and placement must be carefully controlled (Fig. 2.9.5).

2.9.3.10 Macular Hole

Although macular holes caused by injury may close spontaneously, delaying surgery is not without risks. Even if serious additional damage in the macular area is present (e.g., contusion maculopathy, choroidal rupture), surgery may improve vision [51]. The OCT allows following the patient with a posttraumatic macular hole in more detail than what biomicroscopy can provide.

Regarding treatment, complete vitrectomy should be performed. Removal of the ILM is strongly advised. Staining of ILM makes the surgery less traumatic to the retina and less frustrating to the surgeon. Table 2.9.3 shows the various methods of ILM staining; Table 2.9.4 provides an overview of ILM removal techniques and instrumentation.

25 i.e., in the periphery: here the vitreous is shaved rather than removed. Conversely, full-thickness retinal lesions can be left without "pexy" in the posterior retina where a complete PVD has been accomplished.

26 e.g., because media opacity interferes with laser delivery or there is a substantial amount of subretinal fluid present.

27 Stop the cryo application as soon as the retina starts turning white. If the retinal detachment is high, never try to freeze the fluid over and wait for the retina to turn white; watch the RPE closely instead and stop the cryopexy as soon as the RPE becomes pink.

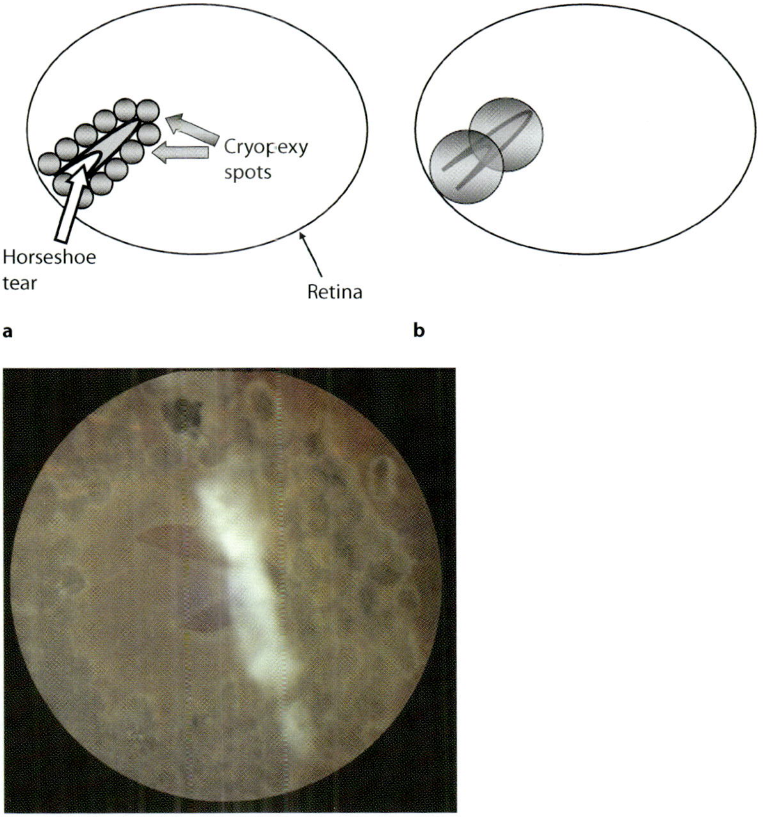

Fig. 2.9.5 Cryopexy or laser treatment of a retinal break. **a** The properly placed cryopexy spots are confluent and are in normal retina. The base ("RPE floor") of the break is spared of any cryopexy. Although ideally the entire lesion is to be surrounded, the most important areas to be treated are inferiorly and centrally from it. **b** It is technically easier and faster to apply a few large (and thus strong) spots. This, however, is dangerous and contraindicated. It leads to intraoperatively visible dispersion of RPE cells and dramatically increases the postoperative PVR risk.[1] **c** Laser scars surround this horseshoe-spaded break, the shape of which reveals that there is residual traction, which at the moment is weaker than the strength of the laser-induced scars. The light reflex is an artifact

[1] It is not uncommon to read a note in the patient's chart, stating that: "PVR developed *despite* the good cryopexy scars." The note should read instead: "PVR developed *due to* the too good cryopexy scars."

Table 2.9.3 Methods of intraoperative staining of the ILM in eyes with a traumatic macular hole[1]

Dye (reference)	Technique and comment	Advantage	Disadvantage
None [65]	It is highly advisable to incise the ILM first; the safest tool is a slightly barbed[2] MVR blade; a vertically acting forceps (see Table 2.9.4) is used to find the ILM's edge. If the edge is lost because the ILM tore, it must carefully be searched for; changing the direction of the intraocular light helps if reflex from the ILM is noted[3]	Dye toxicity is avoided	It is potentially very traumatic for the retina if the surgeon has to search for the ILM's edge; the instrument is dragged over areas already denuded of the ILM's protection. It is much more common than with staining to be deeper with the instrument than intended, resulting in hemorrhages and possibly nerve fiber damage
TA[4] [34]	This is not truly staining; the crystals simply settle on the surface. In areas of ILM removal, the TA is also removed, which helps identify the approximate location of the ILM's edge	Simple and inexpensive	Does not help in the initial phase when ILM peeling is started; it is not determined whether toxicity is a risk if the crystals are left inside the hole
ICG [8, 31]	The drug is dissolved, diluted, injected, and left for a few seconds over the posterior pole. The hole can be protected by plugging it with a viscoelastic, or the dye itself can be mixed with viscoelastic	Excellent staining; the cost is greatly reduced if multiple doses are prepared from the same original bottle	Toxicity remains an issue

[1] Other dyes, such as sodium fluorescein, Chicago blue, Patent blue, etc., are also under investigation; staining the tissue during surgery is becoming more prevalent, increasingly effective, and even has its own name: "chromovitrectomy."

Table 2.9.3 *(continued)* Methods of intraoperative staining of the ILM in eyes with a traumatic macular hole

Dye (reference)	Technique and comment	Advantage	Disadvantage
Infracyanine [84]	Same as with ICG	Same as with ICG	None reported so far
Trypan blue [55]	The drug is now available in a package ready to use	Toxicity does not appear to be an issue if the dye is properly used	Staining is much weaker than with the two green dyes, which requires a longer staining duration; the posterior lens capsule should be protected

[2] The barb is made by pressing, not hitting, the tip of the MVR blade against a metallic object. The barb should be small and its angle is ideally around 45°.

[3] Performing surgery using illumination from a slit lamp attached to the microscope is of great help.

[4] The drug must be filtered through a Millipore filter (0.45 µm) and then diluted to its original concentration with BSS.

Table 2.9.4 Internal limiting membrane removal techniques and instrumentation: an overview

Tool/technique	Comment
Tano membrane scraper	If the ILM has been properly stained, the instrument is able both to initially tear and then separate the ILM from the retina;[5] however, the maneuver is dangerous and *not recommended.* If the ILM has not been stained, the risk of damaging the nerve fibers is especially high and use of the Tano membrane scraper is contraindicated [48]
MVR blade	Incision of the ILM prior to forceps use is useful especially if the peeling is done without staining and if the surgeon is less experienced: the blade gives greater depth control than the forceps. In principle, an ILM-rhexis, similar to a capsulorhexis, can also be executed with the barbed MVR blade, but this maneuver requires exceptional dexterity, has not benefit, and is risky

Table 2.9.4 *(continued)* Internal limiting membrane removal techniques and instrumentation: an overview

Tool/technique	Comment
Forceps: vertical action	These forceps[6] have platforms that are horizontal; the lower blade can slide under the ILM, grasp is accomplished by the upper blade being lowered onto the ILM/lower blade platform. These forceps are most useful when the ILM is not very adherent; they should not be employed, however, if the retina is not healthy (e.g., CME is present)
Forceps: horizontal action	These forceps have vertically positioned platforms, which grab the tissue simultaneously from two sides. By definition they must be pressed down during the initial grab[7] and even later if the ILM tears so that the remaining edge is still adherent to the retina. There are two basic designs: one with a large platform,[8] which allows relatively easy initial grasp because the ILM tends to "rise up" in front of the forceps that pushes the retina down; the grasp remains firm throughout the peeling and the ILM's tendency to tear is reduced because its contact area with the forceps is large. The disadvantage of these forceps is the loss of visual control of maneuvers performed on the retinal surface. The second design[9] has the great advantage of coming down to the retina at an angle and its shafts are hollowed, which allow continual observation of all maneuvers: the shaft or the platforms never block the surgeon's view. The disadvantages of these forceps are the relatively small size of the platform (i.e., tearing of the ILM is more common) and the vulnerability of the instrument
Spatula	Rarely used today; it was originally conceived as a device that bluntly dissects and separates the ILM from the retina
FILMS	This is the most physiological and least traumatic method [62]: the ILM is separated by viscoelastic fluid gently injected underneath from a specially designed cannula. It is the only method where the retina is not elevated but actually gets pushed down while the separation occurs. Once the ILM is lifted, it is removed with any type of forceps. The FILMS technique *should not* be employed in eyes with unhealthy macula (e.g., CME)

[5] Similarly to a cataract surgeon using a sharp, pointed instrument to perform capsulorhexis. The ILM must also be flipped as it is being dialed around.

[6] e.g., Storz #E 1964 (Bausch and Lomb, St. Louis, Mo.)

[7] Ideally, the two actions: pressing down onto the retina and grabbing the ILM are separated in time, not done simultaneously.

[8] e.g., DORC #1286 (Zuidland, The Netherlands)

[9] e.g., Alcon #641.21 (Fort Worth, Texas)

Controversial

The use of ICG in eyes with a macular hole has been found by some authors to cause toxic damage to the RPE; Table 2.9.3 presents some alternatives and technical advice.

- After the ILM has been peeled, gas tamponade should be used and the patient should be informed about the importance of positioning.

2.9.3.11 Retinal Hemorrhage[28]

The condition in itself rarely justifies treatment; if the bleeding is under the ILM in the macula (submembranous hemorrhagic macular cyst [64]), however, surgical evacuation is advised. YAG laser may also be used to puncture the ILM and drain the cyst if other pathologies do not interfere [4].

2.9.3.12 Subretinal Hemorrhage

The photoreceptors may start dying as early as within 24 h [36], and early photoreceptor death ensues if the blood is not evacuated [57]. Late subretinal scarring is another threat that should force the ophthalmologist to consider fairly acute intervention if the blood is thick *and* submacular.

28 The term refers to bleeding into the retinal layers. Blood that originates in the retinal vasculature but accumulates elsewhere (e.g., subhyaloidal, intravitreal) is discussed elsewhere in this chapter.

Controversial

Being able to preoperatively determine whether the blood is under or in front of the RPE would be very helpful to the ophthalmologist. If the hemorrhage is sub-RPE, evacuation is probably not necessary; if it is under the neuroretina, removal is indicated. The OCT may be helpful in some cases, but the exact location of the blood is more difficult to determine in the context of large traumatic hemorrhage than in a small one caused by age-related macular degeneration.

The following options are available:[29]

- Intravitreal gas injection (e.g., 0.3 ml pure SF_6) and positioning.
- Laser (argon) retinotomy and positioning. Once the retina is perforated and the patient is upright, a nonclotted hemorrhage may "ooze" out [24].
- TPA. A subretinal injection of 0.1–0.2 ml of (12.5 µg/0.1 ml) of (recombinant) TPA subretinally helps liquefy the clotted blood, which can be displaced by positioning or surgery [13]. One of the disadvantages of the procedure is a long waiting period[30] while the drug takes effect, although a preoperative intravitreal injection (100 µg) may alleviate this problem.
- Surgical evacuation.
  - If the blood is still *fluidic*, one[31] small retinotomy is made at a convenient location and the subretinal space is irrigated with BSS. The flow must be kept low. Since the blood is drained into the vitreous, it obscures the surgeon's view and requires removal as well as repeated entries into the subretinal space. The desire to do a complete irrigation must be balanced with the need to minimize trauma to the photoreceptors and RPE cells.

---

29 The treatment modalities listed here may also be combined with each other.

30 Up to 45 min

31 There is no real advantage to creating two retinotomies (one for BSS entry, the other for the exit of BSS and blood): as soon as the view is lost due to the intravitreally "leaked" blood, the subretinal cannula must be withdrawn, the vitreous cavity irrigated, and then the entire procedure can be repeated.

- If the blood is still *clotted*, either TPA is injected and then irrigation performed as described above, or a slightly larger retinotomy is created and the blood clot is removed with forceps. The retina is very elastic, as is the clot: surprisingly, a large clot can be removed through small a retinotomy. Forceps use for removal of subretinal hemorrhage is not without risk; complications include unintentional grabbing of the retina or RPE, injury to the choroid, and extraction of large areas of RPE.

Pearl

It is mandatory to remove all vitreous from the retinal surface before a retinotomy is performed; if so, there is no need to surround the site with laser. The retinotomy is virtually impossible to detect the following day.

If the retina is detached over a large area because of the blood, this must be considered a hemorrhagic retinal detachment (see below).

2.9.3.13 Retinal Detachment

Traumatic retinal detachment is a prime example showing how proper (and timely) surgery can improve the prognosis after an injury: in one study ambulatory vision was achieved in 75% of eyes undergoing vitrectomy for retinal detachment after open globe injury, as opposed to only 37% of eyes without vitrectomy [56]. There are several types of posttraumatic retinal detachment; these may present alone or in combination. During the preoperative evaluation, it is insufficient to focus on break localization; if possible, the type of traction should also be investigated.

One of the consequences of retinal detachment is increased uveal aqueous outflow. Removal of the retina is a last resort in lowering the IOP (see Chap. 2.18).

2.9.3.13.1 Rhegmatogenous

A retinal break (see above) is present, which may have been caused by the injury or by the surgeon (see Chap. 2.7). The time from injury to retinal detachment development varies from hours to years, depending on the type, location, and size of the break as well as whether vitreous hemorrhage is also present.

Regarding treatment, even in the presence of a retinal break, the most important factor in the development of a retinal detachment is traction. Unless the vitreoretinal traction is addressed, therapy is likely to fail.

In terms of countering traction, vitrectomy and scleral buckling are the two main weapons:

- A *buckle* achieves its goal by shortening the distance between the endpoints of the traction force.[32] Since the traction forces may also act at different locations on the peripheral retina, a circumferential, rather than a segmental, buckle is preferred in the context of trauma. The buckle must carefully calibrated: if too broad and too high, anterior segment ischemia may follow.[33] The buckle is much more efficient in eyes with stationary[34] traction; less so if the traction is dynamic[35].
- *Vitrectomy* achieves its goal by eliminating the traction. It has the added benefit of allowing the treatment of the additional intraocular pathologies that may have occurred. Vitrectomy is able to address both stationary and dynamic tractions.

Cave

Vitrectomy for retinal detachment should always be complete; if vitreous (i.e., traction) is left behind, there is now more room for intraocular fluid movement (currents) and for vitreous movement (dynamic traction). The fluid can then easily enter through the retinal break, which is held open by the residual traction force.

- *Creating a chorioretinal adhesion around the break*: the retinopexy is delivered by laser or cryo (see above).

---

32 Thereby lessening or eliminating the power of the pulling force exerted on the retina.

33 It is not possible to analyze in great detail the advantages and disadvantages of each procedure. The reader is referred to appropriate textbooks specifically dedicated to these topics.

34 The traction is present continually and is not influenced by eye or head movement.

35 With sudden eye or head movement, the mobile vitreous, due to inertia, also moves. This movement is transmitted to the retina at the site of vitreoretinal adhesion and presents as a powerful traction force. Without head or eye movement, the traction disappears or at least greatly subsides.

2.9.3.13.2 Tractional

The cause is vitreoretinal traction but in the absence of a retinal break. The progression from injury to retinal detachment is usually slow.

Regarding treatment, the traction must be addressed. Although in principle a buckle is also an option, vitrectomy is preferred because it is able to deal with not only the anterior (peripheral) but also with the posterior and subretinal traction.

2.9.3.13.3 Hemorrhagic

The retina is lying on a dome-shaped accumulation of blood, which may be truly subretinal[36] or located between the RPE and the neuroretina (see above). This is a commonly underdiagnosed complication in ocular traumatology.

Regarding treatment, if the blood is under the macula and thick, it should be evacuated (see above). If the hemorrhage is very large, a retinotomy may have to be performed to allow direct access to the blood. The risk of PVR is significant.

2.9.3.14 PVR

Scar formation is the most common cause of vision loss after successful retinal detachment surgery, and it has been reported to occur in up to 40% of eyes after serious trauma [11]. With current techniques and technology, the initial surgery aimed at reattaching the retina after an injury is almost always successful; operations for PVR have a dramatically lower anatomical and functional success rate. The surgeon must understand the risk factors (see Table 2.14.1), prophylaxis possibilities, and treatment of PVR.

The timing of PVR occurrence depends on the type of injury: it presents earliest after perforating injuries (1.3 months), followed by ruptures (2.1 months) and IOFBs injuries (3.1 months) [11].

2.9.3.14.1 Risk Factors

The following variables have been found to increase the PVR rate:

36 i.e., sub-RPE

- Rupture [11, 49].
- Perforating injury [11, 49].
- IOFB injury (the incidence is as high as 21% [88]), especially if a deep impact has occurred [49].
- Vitreous hemorrhage [11].[37]
- Choroidal detachment [28].[38]
- Size of the retinal break [35].
- Extent of retinal detachment [35].
- Severe inflammation [35].
- Cryopexy [20].
- Incomplete PVD [10].
- Too early removal of silicone oil [77]: even if a longer tamponade does not reduce the PVR risk, it does improve the functional outcome[39] [38].

2.9.3.14.2 Prophylaxis

Since treatment of an established PVR has a poor prognosis, prevention remains the surgeon's best hope. The following list shows certain surgeon-controlled variables that may help reduce the PVR risk.

- Timing of surgery. Early vitrectomy in high risk eyes [18, 49] appears to reduce the PVR risk, probably by removing the inflammation-inciting elements from the eye.
- Foregoing cryopexy (see above) [9].
- Atraumatic surgery. Avoiding intraoperative complications such as hemorrhage or retinal damage (see above) eliminates certain PVR-inciting factors.
- Complete surgery. Removal of all vitreous, i.e., posteriorly (PVD), anteriorly (vitreous base and retrolental area), and all proliferative membranes [1], reduces the medium/scaffold on which cells can proliferate.
- Destruction of RPE cells in certain high-risk injuries. Since these cells are the primary culprit in PVR development, their elimination in the

37 Whether intra- or postoperative.
38 Whether intra- or postoperative.
39 By keeping the macula attached.

Table 2.9.5 Pharmaceutical options in preventing/treating PVR

	Drug (reference)
Experimentally	Protein kinase-C inhibitor, melatonin [32]
	All-trans retinoic acid [27]
	Cholcicine [54]
	Taxol [85]
	Daunorubicin encapsulated in liposome [75]
	(Radiation[11] [53])
Clinically	Intravitreal corticosteroids [58, 67]
	Daunorubicin [89]
	Low molecular weight heparin, fluorouracil [3, 5]
	Low molecular weight heparin and intravitreal corticosteroids [90]

[11] Mentioned only for completeness; this is obviously not a drug.

affected areas appears crucial ("prophylactic chorioretinectomy"; see Chap. 2.13).

- Silicone oil use. It appears that complete filling (see below) reduces the PVR risk [94] by taking away the space in which cells could multiply, especially if heavy silicone oil[40] is used [91].
- The true value of heavy silicone oil use is yet to be determined. The rationale is that it does not allow the accumulation of proliferative cells inferiorly, where PVR traditionally starts [82]. The early results of the efficacy of heavy silicone oil use are mixed [72, 82].
- Removal of the ILM during vitrectomy in eyes with high PVR risk may prevent the development of proliferative membranes in the macula, even keep the macula attached in eyes with otherwise total, PVR-related retinal detachment.
- Pharmaceutical approach (Table 2.9.5).

40 e.g., Densiron (Geuder GmbH, Heidelberg, Germany), Oxane (Bausch and Lomb, Rochester, N.Y.)

Pitfall

It appears that a long list of drugs is effective against PVR experimentally, but their efficacy in clinical use is limited at best [12].

2.9.3.14.3 Treatment

For a discussion of treatment, see Sect. 2.9.5.

2.9.3.15 Macular Pucker[41]

Seeding of the retinal surface in the macula by proliferative cells[42] leads to wrinkling of the ILM. Collagen production by these cells then results in focal traction with partial- or full-thickness folds, and (cystoid) macular edema. Traumatic EMP usually occurs after contusion, and it is more common after vitreous hemorrhage, retinal detachment, or incomplete vitrectomy (i.e., if PVD was not achieved). Inflammation is another contributing factor. The risk of EMP is lower in patients over 50 years of age. The condition may take years to develop.

2.9.3.15.1 Symptoms

- Decreased visual acuity
- Metamorphopsia, which is best followed by M-charts [60][43]
- Aniseikonia (micropsia or macropsia)
- Diplopia (monocular or binocular) due to foveal dragging [23]

The most important diagnostic tools are slit lamp biomicroscopy[44] and OCT (Fig. 2.9.1).

41 EMP is discussed here because, although a much less serious condition, it is reasonably perceived as a "mini PVR".

42 Mostly fibrous astrocytes, RPE cells, fibrocytes, myofibroblasts, and macrophages; the same as in PVR.

43 Serial Amsler grid testings are inappropriate to determine progression.

44 Use of a contact lens is necessary to detect early cases.

2.9.3.15.2 Treatment

The definite solution is vitrectomy; spontaneous EMP separation [26] is extremely rare. The indication (i.e., when to intervene rather than to observe) should primarily rest with the patient (see Chap. 1.4). The recommended surgical steps are shown on Fig. 2.9.6.

Pearl

Intentional removal of the ILM in EMP surgery reduces the recurrence rate from at least 5% to virtually zero.

2.9.4 Visibility and Vitreoretinal Surgery

Detailed discussion of this topic is beyond the scope of this book; only a few helpful suggestions are made here:

- Use a wide-angle viewing system. Conditions[45] that would otherwise make surgery much more difficult if not impossible lose at least some of their importance if a panoramic viewing system is used.
- Corneal edema is very common after corneal trauma and can be exacerbated by scleral indentation. The edema may be epithelial or stromal.
  - Scraping of the epithelium can dramatically improve visibility; however, it increases the postoperative edema and infection risk, and healing may be protracted and painful, especially in diabetics.
  - Alternatives to scraping include topical glucose (40%) and glycerin (50–95%). The solutions are applied by soaking a small piece of cotton, which is the placed on the cornea for a few minutes.
  - If Descemet's membrane is folded, the AC can be pressurized with viscoelastics. Filling the AC with viscoelastic is also helpful if BSS-fluid exchange or silicone oil implantation is performed in an eye that is pseudophakic or has weak zonules.

45 i.e., corneal edema, small pupil, lens opacity

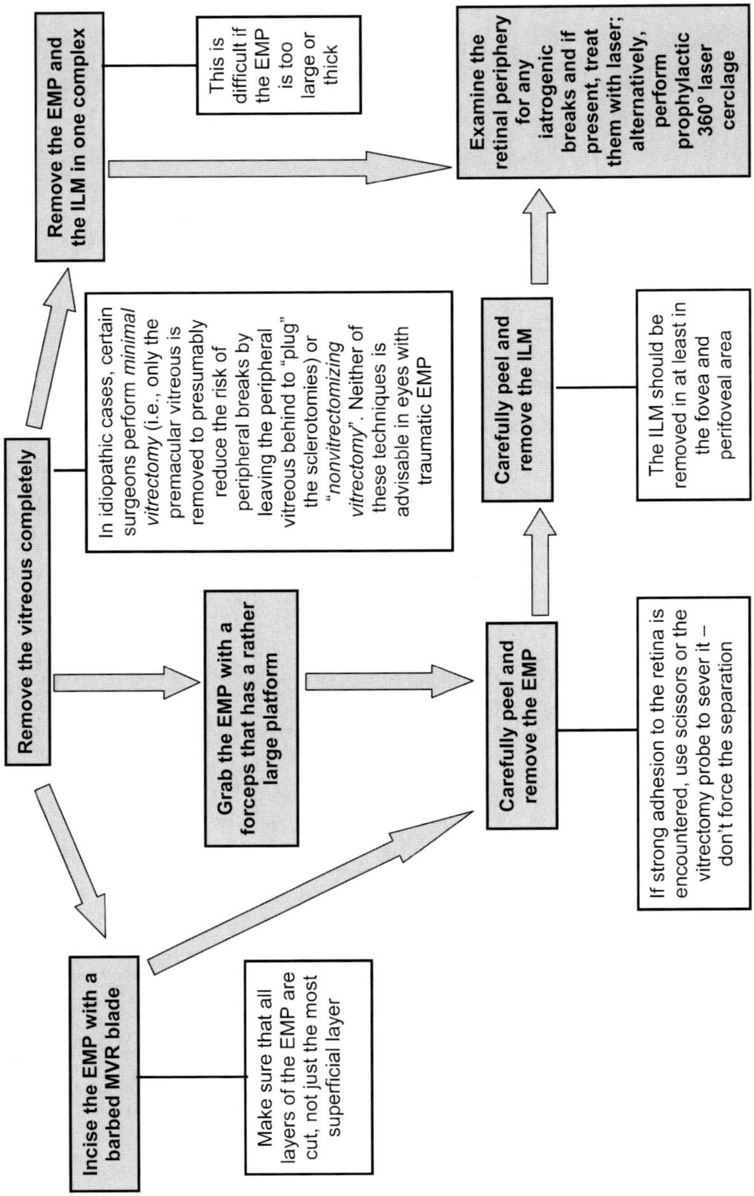
Remove the vitreous completely
In idiopathic cases, certain surgeons perform *minimal vitrectomy* (i.e., only the premacular vitreous is removed to presumably reduce the risk of peripheral breaks by leaving the peripheral vitreous behind to "plug" the sclerotomies) or "*nonvitrectomizing vitrectomy*". Neither of these techniques is advisable in eyes with traumatic EMP
Remove the EMP and the ILM in one complex
This is difficult if the EMP is too large or thick
Grab the EMP with a forceps that has a rather large platform
Incise the EMP with a barbed MVR blade
Make sure that all layers of the EMP are cut, not just the most superficial layer
Carefully peel and remove the EMP
If strong adhesion to the retina is encountered, use scissors or the vitrectomy probe to sever it – don't force the separation
Carefully peel and remove the ILM
The ILM should be removed in at least in the fovea and perifoveal area
Examine the retinal periphery for any iatrogenic breaks and if present, treat them with laser; alternatively, perform prophylactic 360° laser cerclage

Fig. 2.9.6 Flowchart: surgical tactics for EMPs

- If the surface of the IOL is dirty because of the settling of inflammatory debris on it, the surface can be cleaned by the Tano membrane scraper.[46]
- If there is fluid condensation on the back surface of an IOL[47] during BSS-air exchange, dispersive viscoelastic should be injected onto the IOL to coat it and wipe off the condensed fluid.
- Even though the wide angle system is helpful to overcome the visualization difficulties caused by a small pupil, good *mydriasis* dramatically increases surgical ease. If intracameral adrenaline does not help, iris retractors need to be used.[48]
- The use of strong illumination is particularly useful if the media are hazy and/or small gauge vitrectomy is performed.[49] The dangers of such a powerful light source must always be kept in mind (see Chap. 3.2).

46 Synergetics, East Windsor Hill, Conn

47 The eye already underwent a posterior capsulectomy.

48 Most iris retractors are made of plastic, not metal. It is not possible to bend them intracamerally. It is therefore crucial to aim well with the paracentesis (using a 27-g needle). The needle should be directed so that it is somewhere between where the pupillary margin is and where it needs to be. Too deep a path makes it very difficult to catch the iris; too shallow a path makes the iris tent. The parallaxis phenomenon must be taken into account when the angle of the needle path is made: objects appear closer to the cornea than they are in reality.

49 e.g., such as provided by the Photon (Synergetics, East Windsor Hill, Conn.)

2.9.5 Surgery for Eyes with PVR-related Retinal Detachment: Technical Issues

2.9.5.1 Timing

Selecting the optimal time for vitrectomy is not straightforward. Several factors need to be considered:

- PVR cycle. It appears that the proliferation takes a certain amount of time[50] before it spontaneously stops. This cycle is independent of whether surgery is performed during the cycle.

Controversial

If vitrectomy is performed before the PVR cycle is complete, retinal redetachment is virtually assured.[51] Conversely, early surgery with silicone oil implantation is usually able to keep at least the macula attached and prevent, in most cases, the development of a closed funnel.

- Presence of silicone oil tamponade. Silicone oil slows down the progression of the retinal detachment and makes reoperation less urgent.
- Condition of the macula. If the macula is on (and especially if there is silicone oil in the eye), the intervention can be deferred virtually indefinitely[52]. If the macula is off or the retinal detachment is rapidly threatening it, surgery should not be delayed.

2.9.5.2 The Goals of Surgery

All traction exerted on the retina should be eliminated, whether caused by pre-, intra-, or subretinal forces. The risk of traction recurrence should also be reduced. In addition to the factors already mentioned,[53] the surgeon should follow certain principles:

50 Usually several weeks.

51 Surgery is also much easier if the PVR membranes are established since they are visible.

52 i.e., depending on the complications caused by the silicone oil

53 See under PVR prophylaxis.

- Remove all vitreous, both posteriorly and anteriorly. In the periphery, scleral indentation must be used to assure that no residual vitreous is present. If the surgeon feels that the lens prevents completion of this task, the lens must be sacrificed (see below).
- The injection of trypan blue[54] is very useful to demonstrate the presence of membranes that are immature or difficult to notice.
- If the retina is shortened because of intrinsic traction, either a scleral buckle should be used[55] or a retinotomy be performed.
- When considering retinotomy,[56] the surgeon must be aware that if the retina is cut from its peripheral insertion, it can quickly "roll up like a rug" if traction persists/recurs centrally. Retinotomy should therefore be performed only if the PVR recurrence risk is low.
- The retinotomy may be carried out with scissors or the vitrectomy probe, but either should be preceded by sufficient diathermy to prevent bleeding.
- The peripheral retina should be removed with the vitrectomy probe (retinectomy).

Pearl

If retinotomy is performed, the surgeon should err on the side of "too much," not "too little." A common cause for failure is residual traction at the edges of the retinotomy if retinal shortening is present.

2.9.5.3 Lens-related Issues

Lens-related issues are as follows:

- If the *lens* interferes with the completeness of vitrectomy, it must be removed; however, "feathering" of the lens may also occur, especially

54 i.e., VisionBlue, DORC, Zuidland, The Netherlands

55 Encircling band (with a tire if necessary). Care must be taken not to make the band too tight so as to avoid anterior segment ischemia (see above).

56 This is circumferential retinotomy, followed by retinectomy, i.e., removal of the peripheral retina. Relaxing retinotomy, a radial cut, must also be considered; this is usually not followed by retinectomy.

if the eye is filled with air (gas). This is a temporary phenomenon, and sacrificing a lens in a patient who still has accommodation is an unnecessary price to pay.

- If the lens is removed, its posterior capsule should also be taken (see Chap. 2.7).
- If the eye is pseudophakic, the IOL is usually preserved.
- A posterior capsulectomy is often necessary since the capsule tends opacify faster in these eyes, especially if silicone oil tamponade is used.
- If the IOL is made of silicone and silicone oil is used, this makes subsequent silicone oil removal very difficult: the oil droplets tend to adhere to the IOL very strongly. Either the IOL must be removed or at the conclusion of silicone oil removal, an intraocular forceps holding a piece of cotton can be employed as a "window wiper" to collect the droplets or at least push them toward the periphery of the IOL (see Chap. 2.7).

2.9.5.4 Selected Retina-related Issues

Some retina-related issues are as follows:

- If a giant tear has caused the retinal detachment, implanting a scleral buckle does not improve the success rate, but it does increase the slippage risk (Table 2.9.2). Conversely, if PVR develops later, a scleral buckle should be considered during reoperation.
- Subretinal strands are often found in eyes with PVR.
  - If they are encountered in an eye without a prior retinal break, which would allow convenient access to the strands, it must first be determined whether the strands interfere with retinal reattachment, because not all strands do. A fluid–gas exchange must be performed to observe how the retina behaves; if reattachment easily occurs and the retinal contour is smoothly concave, the strands are best left behind.[57]

57 Both retinotomy and retinectomy increase the risk of PVR; they should be avoided unless their benefit exceeds the risk they pose.

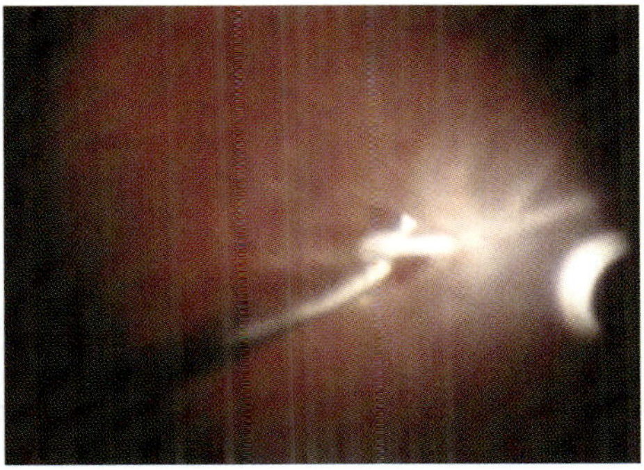

Fig. 2.9.7 Removal of a subretinal strand in an eye with PVR. In this intraoperative photograph, a subretinal strand that is too thick and elastic to allow retinal reattachment is being removed with forceps. The retinotomy has been created right on top of the strand

- If the strands do not permit retinal reattachment and no retinal break exists, a careful site selection for the retinotomy[58] is needed.
- Issues to consider include: dexterity of the surgeon;[59] proximity of the strand to the macula and major blood vessels;[60] and the likely choice of tamponade[61].
- It must also be decided whether the retinotomy should be right on top of the strand (Fig. 2.9.7) or at some distance from it; the latter has the advantage of allowing more room for manipulations, but it may be more difficult to firmly grasp the strand.
- The gravest danger during subretinal manipulations is choroidal injury and hemorrhage. All maneuvers must be performed with great caution.

58 More than one retinotomy may be required.

59 The dominant hand's side is preferred.

60 The retinotomy should be as far away from the macula and from major blood vessels as possible.

61 A site superior to the horizontal plane is recommended, especially if gas, rather than silicone oil, is to be used as postoperative tamponade.

  - If the subretinal strand is firmly attached to the retina or the RPE/choroid, forceful removal can result in the rupture of either. The retina can even be folded under and pulled through the retinotomy. In such cases the strand should be simply *severed*: this achieves sufficient traction relief.
- A closed funnel is no justification to abandon the eye.
  - All traction from the posterior retinal surface must be removed. Bimanual vitrectomy is especially important in these cases. Even if 360° retinotomy will be needed, the posterior retinal surface must be freed before the retina is completely cut. If the retinotomy is performed first, the remaining "retinal calyx" is very mobile and makes the removal of subretinal strands or membranes very difficult.
  - To open the funnel, a cohesive viscoelastic, not PFCL, needs to be used. This will not tip the retina over[62] even if the closed funnel developed in an eye with 360° retinotomy. The viscoelastic must be injected slowly to avoid tearing the retina if membranes/strands are exerting traction inside the funnel.

2.9.5.5 Selected Issues Related to Surgical Technique

2.9.5.5.1 Bimanual Surgery

Working with two hands makes manipulations technically easier and increases the chance of success. Several types of hands-free illumination devices are available from several manufacturers. The microscope can also be used for relatively reflex-free illumination of the fundus so that the surgeon can use both of his hands for intraocular manipulations (e.g., slit lamp, OFFISS[63] [41].

2.9.5.5.2 PFCL Use

A "third hand" is also available for the surgeon. The PFCL can stabilize the retina during surgery, keeping the posterior retina in position while the

---

62 As PFCL would
63 Topcon, Tokyo, Japan

surgeon works elsewhere, and is extremely useful when posterior subretinal fluid should be evacuated through a peripheral retinal break or a giant retinal tear must be flipped back.

The PFCL should not be used in eyes with a posterior break in the presence of residual traction or in an eye with a closed funnel (see above).

2.9.5.5.3 Tamponade

In almost all cases of vitreoretinal surgery for a serious injury, a tamponade is left in the eye. The tamponade helps keep the retina attached by resisting traction and by blocking the subretinal access of intravitreal fluid trough a retinal break.[64]

Pearl

For eyes with serious posterior segment trauma, silicone oil, not long-acting gas, is the preferred tamponade.

With regard to silicone oil tamponade:

- If it is possible to know before surgery that silicone oil will be used, it makes sense to determine the eye's axial length. The measurement is much less reliable in a silicone oil-filled eye. The reading comes handy when the silicone oil is removed; simultaneous IOL implantation can be performed should the lens become cataractous and be extracted at the time of silicone oil removal.
- Implant the silicone oil after a fluid–air exchange to achieve a complete fill.[65]
- There is BSS lining the retinal surface; it takes time for this fluid to collect at the disc during fluid–air exchange (Table 2.9.6). It takes much longer for this BSS to "trickle down" to the bottom of the eye if there

64 Detailed discussion of the indications for, and selection of, different tamponade options is beyond the scope of this book. Table 2.9.6 shows selected suggestions regarding intravitreal exchanges.

65 100% is not feasible, but the fill should be as close to it as possible.

Table 2.9.6 Exchanges in the vitreous cavity

Exchange from	Exchange to	Yes (+) or no (–)	Comment
BSS	Air/gas	+	It is easy to see the meniscus and thus do a complete job. There is always residual fluid on the retinal surface[12], which takes time to collect at the posterior pole; this is not a major issue if gas tamponade[13] is used, but becomes one if silicone oil is needed since it prevents the fill from reaching the desired 100%. If subretinal fluid is drained, the retinal break must be marked with diathermy prior to the exchange so that even when visibility is poor initially, the flute needle can be kept over the break and a complete drain can be achieved
BSS	Silicone oil	–	Too slow and the meniscus is difficult to discern. If silicone oil is needed, the BSS must be exchanged for air first, then the air is exchanged for oil
Silicone oil	BSS	+	The BSS simply forces (most of) the oil out
BSS	PFCL	+	The PFCL is easy to see; even if many small bubbles form initially, they quickly coalesce spontaneously or can be "mixed" into one with a little shaking. Unless the sclerotomy is very tight, there is no need to periodically withdraw the PFCL cannula because the excess BSS is able to escape. If the IOP does get elevated, this is easily seen at the disc, which turns white as the blood circulation stops – the disc therefore should continually be monitored by the surgeon
PFCL	Silicone oil	+	The meniscus is easy to see, but BSS remains trapped between the PFCL and the oil in virtually all cases.[14] This fluid must also be collected once the PFCL "sphere" is removed. The flute needle should be kept inside the PFCL bubble throughout the exchange to avoid leaving PFCL behind

12 Similar to a coffee mug: after all the coffee is thought to have been swallowed, it quickly accumulates at the bottom once the mug is replaced on the table.

13 Gas tamponade must not be used if the patient lives at high altitude or is expected to fly on airplanes while the gas is in the eye (see Chap. 3.3).

14 The rare exception is when the eye was *completely* filled with PFCL first.

is silicone oil, rather than air, in the vitreous cavity. In addition, visualizing the BSS/silicone oil meniscus is much more difficult than the BSS/air meniscus.

- Prophylactic removal of the lens[66] should be considered if the silicone oil is to be kept in the eye for extended periods of time. Serial ophthalmoscopic examinations (i.e., direct retinal inspection) are crucial in eyes with silicone oil and a cloudy lens is as aggravating for the surgeon as it is for the patient.
- If the lens is removed before silicone oil implantation, extracting the lens *in toto* should be considered (see Chap. 2.7). The posterior capsule is likely to become at least somewhat cloudy, and silicone oil may find its way around the zonules and prolapse into the AC.[67] If this complication occurs, the only option the surgeon has is to inject cohesive viscoelastic into the AC[68] and simultaneously evacuate the silicone oil.[69] The viscoelastic must be left in the AC: it will be absorbed within a few days.[70] The IOP must closely be monitored and prophylactic antiglaucoma medications should be used for a few days.

---

66 Especially in older patients whose eye has already lost accommodation capability

67 High myops are especially at risk.

68 Filling the AC with a cohesive viscoelastic before silicone oil implantation should always be considered (see Chap. 2.5).

69 A small silicone oil can be left behind in the AC. As long as it has enough room to be mobile, the threat to the endothelium is minimal.

70 Silicone oil prolapse will or will not recur.

- A peripheral inferior iridectomy must be created with the vitrectomy probe before oil implantation, preferably after diathermy to prevent bleeding. The iridectomy must be sufficiently large;[71] its subsequent scarring and thus closure of the iridectomy is a common cause of secondary glaucoma.
- For most cases, 1000 centistokes silicone oil will suffice. If the tamponade is felt to be necessary for several years, 5000 centistokes silicone oil is preferred. A more viscous silicone oil is more difficult to inject and remove.
- The aim is a 100% silicone oil fill (see above). The surgeon should check the IOP before removal of the infusion cannula[72] and the optic disc for circulation patency.
- If PVR recurs under silicone oil but the macula remains attached (see above), there is no urgency to reoperate unless the detaching retina pushes the oil into the AC or the retina suffers a tractional break[73] and silicone oil is found subretinally[74]. If any of these complications occur, a reoperation is necessary to remove the proliferative tissue and reattach the retina. It is the surgeon's preference whether the reoperation is performed under oil or after a silicone oil–fluid exchange. The latter has the advantage of "oil change," which starts the "emulsification cycle" anew. Removal of the subretinal silicone oil is difficult and does require removal of the intravitreal oil first; PFCL is not helpful in removing subretinal oil, which can be achieved only by active aspiration (e.g., using the flute needle or the vitrectomy probe).

---

71 A judicious posterior capsulectomy must also be performed in the area of the iridectomy.

72 Mild IOP elevation is actually preferred over a normal or low value to compensate for temporary space-filling factors such as tissue edema and residual intravitreal fluid.

73 This is recognized by its characteristically oval shape and typically very large size.

74 As the detaching, rigid retina pushes against a resistant silicone oil and the retina finally tears, it "bypasses" the oil, which thus takes on an hourglass shape.

- Removal of the silicone oil from a traumatized eye should not be rushed. The PVR and retinal detachment can occur as late as several months post-injury. For the removal, silicone oil-BSS exchange is advised, followed by several fluid–air exchanges to reduce the number of silicone oil droplets left behind.[75] Endoscopy-assisted vitrectomy is able to achieve a more complete job (see Chap. 2.20). The oil may also adhere to a silicone ICL, making removal very difficult (see above and Chap. 2.7).
- If the ciliary body sustained irreversible damage, silicone oil is the surgeon's only option to prevent phthisis (see Chap. 2.19). In these eyes the fill must be "100% and some more": the entire globe (i.e., including the AC) is to be filled and the IOP set at ~30 mmHg. The cornea, paradoxically, has a better chance of remaining clear with a complete fill since if any aqueous is produced, it is unable to gain access to the damaged endothelium.[76]

2.9.5.5.4 Use of Retinal Tacks

Although retinal tacks are much less popular than a decade or so ago, they are an excellent intraoperative tool, and they are well tolerated in the eye long term [70].

2.9.6 Small-Gauge Vitrectomy in Ocular Traumatology

Small-gauge vitrectomy[77] is advantageous in many elective conditions for both patient and ophthalmologist. It has, however, certain disadvantages:

---

75 Complete oil removal is not possible because tiny droplets will remain hidden at inaccessible places such as behind the iris.

76 Eventually, the cornea will become cloudy or the silicone oil will emulsify. A corneal specialist must be consulted whether DSAEK or PK is to be performed. The silicone oil should be reimplanted. EDTA may also bring temporary clearing.

77 23 or 25 g

the armamentarium is still not the same as for the standard 20-g systems; the instruments have a tendency to bend, making intravitreal manipulations more difficult; the speed of vitreous removal is slower; and the use of a cannula inherently limits the size of instruments that can be inserted into the eye. Furthermore, the real advantages[78] of the small-gauge system offer no benefit to the patient with a traumatized eye.

2.9.7 Retinal Injury: Prophylactic Measures

In eyes with scleral wounds located in Zone 3, the occurrence of a retinal injury must always be considered. The need to prevent retinal detachment using prophylactic laser treatment, cryopexy, and/or scleral buckling is still debated.

2.9.7.1 Prophylactic Laser Treatment

Endolaser cerclage[79] is a very reasonable recommendation in eyes undergoing vitrectomy for trauma. The procedure creates a new ora serrata (Fig. 2.9.8) with a very low complication rate[80] but offers substantial benefits [63]. This new ora serrata is likely to encompass the entire area where retinal tears develop. It also destroys tissue that may be responsible for the release of inciting agents partially responsible for PVR development. Performing laser cerclage during surgery as a prophylaxis means that subsequent opacification of the media will not interfere with laser delivery if it were to become necessary for a newly developing pathology.

78 There is need neither for lengthy wound preparation nor for wound closure at the end of surgery.

79 A term coined by R. Morris, Birmingham, Alabama.

80 EMP in 1–3% and occasionally mydriasis if the two horizontal meridians received too heavy treatment.

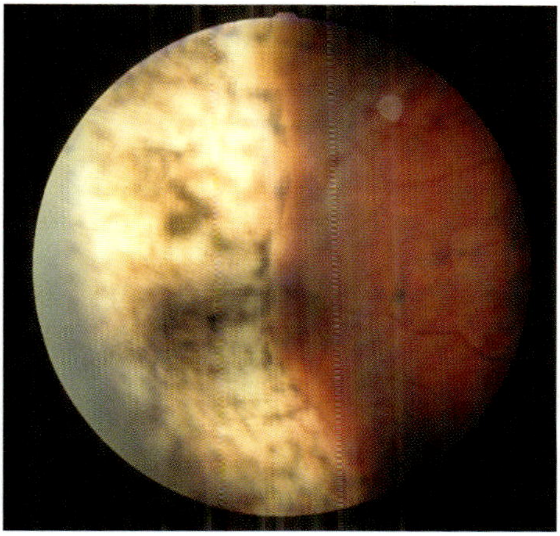

Fig. 2.9.8 Endolaser cerclage. Vitrectomy has been performed in this eye for a contusion-related vitreous hemorrhage. A new ora serrata has been created to prevent retinal detachment from a potential (unidentified) retinal break. Such breaks can occur years after the injury but may also be caused by the surgery itself

2.9.7.2 Prophylactic Cryopexy

The rationale behind the procedure is to seal any retinal break that may have occurred or would subsequently develop underneath the scleral wound. There are several possible scenarios, which are shown in Table 2.9.7.

Cave

Cryopexy to prevent retinal detachment in eyes with a visible retinal break is *not recommended*; laser retinopexy should be used instead. Cryopexy is *contraindicated* if its effect on the retina cannot be monitored due to media opacity.

2.9.7.3 Prophylactic Scleral Buckling

The rationale for placing a scleral buckle over a freshly closed scleral wound is to prophylactically counter any traction that may subsequently originate from the wound area.

Table 2.9.7 Prophylactic retinopexy in eyes with a scleral wound. + Prophylactic (laser) retinopexy is recommended, – prophylactic retinopexy is not recommended

	Retinal break found	Retinal break not found
The peripheral retina[15] *can* be visualized	+	–
The peripheral retina *cannot* be adequately visualized[16]	–[a]	–

[a] A break is not visible, but its presence is reasonably suspected because of the nature of the injury (i.e., vitreous penetration of the agent). Although cryopexy is technically possible in such cases, it is *not* recommended

[15] i.e., underneath a scleral wound that has been closed

[16] i.e., media opacity is present

Controversial

The literature remains divided whether prophylactic buckling of the injured eye brings any benefit or not [33, 80]; worse outcomes with buckling have also been reported [39, 88].

If the media are opaque, the complication risk[81] of placing a prophylactic buckle probably outweighs it potential benefit: blind manipulations over the sclera is a risk factor for PVR development [7]. If the media are clear and the surgeon decides to place a prophylactic buckle, it is ideally done during the initial surgery, not secondarily: within a few days after wound closure, subconjunctival scarring develops, making secondary buckle placement much more difficult. The buckle should be circumferential, not segmental.

81 Too high a buckle and subsequent anterior segment ischemia; furthermore, the buckle may not be placed at where its optimal site would be.

DO:

- try to achieve a complete PVD in each case, consistent with safety
- consider early removal of a vitreous hemorrhage, irrespective of whether open or closed globe trauma was the cause
- explain to the patient that visual symptoms caused by contusion retino(maculo)pathy may spontaneously improve with time, but no specific treatment can be offered
- trauma-related retinal breaks should be treated with laser, especially if they are symptomatic
- the primary goal of vitrectomy for most retinal detachments is the elimination of traction; in a hemorrhagic detachment, the blood needs to be evacuated
- don't compromise in your surgical goals because of visibility problems; most of these problems can be eliminated or at least improved intraoperatively if proper attention is given to them
- if silicone oil use in a traumatized eye is contemplated, the answer is generally "yes"

DON'T:

- accept the preoperative finding that a PVD is present in the injured eye; even intraoperatively, TA use is recommended to confirm this
- assume that retinal detachment is unlikely to occur in an eye with contusion-related vitreous hemorrhage
- forgo treatment of a macular hole just because additional macular pathologies are present; the visual acuity can nevertheless improve
- assume that just because all went well intraoperatively in an eye undergoing surgery with trauma-related PVR, all will go well postoperatively; the recurrence rate is high
- insist on lens preservation if this might compromise the success of retinal surgery
- use PFCL to open a closed funnel: viscoelastic is the right tool
- remove the silicone oil too early from an injured eye
- use prophylactic cryopexy in eyes with scleral wound, especially if this were to be done "blindly"

Summary

The visual outcome of the injured eye is primarily determined by the condition of the macula. Careful evaluation of the posterior segment is mandatory after a serious injury, and timely treatment should be considered if a treatable pathology is identified.

References

[1] Abrams G, Azen S, McCuen B, Flynn H, Lai M, Ryan S (1997) Vitrectomy with silicone oil or perfluorocarbon gas in eyes with severe PVR. Results of additional and long-term follow-up. Arch Ophthalmol 115: 335–344

[2] Alameri A, Baker NS (2005) Successful use of recombinant activated factor VII in the treatment of vitreous haemorrhage: a report of seven cases. Blood Coagul Fibrinolysis 16: 573–578

[3] Allinson RW (2002) Adjuvant 5-FU and heparin prevent PVR. Ophthalmology 109: 829–830; author reply 830

[4] Aralikatti AK, Haridas AS, Smith JM (2006) Delayed Nd:YAG laser membranotomy for traumatic premacular hemorrhage. Arch Ophthalmol 124: 1503

[5] Asaria RH, Kon CH, Bunce C, Charteris DG, Wong D, Khaw PT, Aylward GW (2001) Adjuvant 5-fluorouracil and heparin prevents proliferative vitreoretinopathy: results from a randomized, double-blind, controlled clinical trial. Ophthalmology 108: 1179–1183

[6] Asaria RH, Zaman A, Sullivan PM (1999) Retinitis sclopetaria associated with airbag inflation. Br J Ophthalmol 83: 1094–1095

[7] Bartz-Schmidt KU, Kirchhof B, Heimann K (1996) Risk factors for retinal redetachment by proliferative vitreoretinopathy after episcleral surgery for pseudophakic retinal detachment. Klin Monatsbl Augenheilkd 208: 82–86 [in German]

[8] Burk SE, Da Mata AP, Snyder ME, Rosa RH Jr, Foster RE (2000) Indocyanine green-assisted peeling of the retinal internal limiting membrane. Ophthalmology 107: 2010–2014

[9] Campochiaro PA, Gaskin HC, Vinores SA (1987) Retinal cryopexy stimulates traction retinal detachment in the presence of an ocular wound. Arch Ophthalmol 1567–1570

[10] Capeans C, Lorenzo J, Santos L, Suarez A, Copena MJ, Blanco MJ, Sanchez-Salorio M (1998) Comparative study of incomplete posterior vitreous detachment as a risk factor for proliferative vitreoretinopathy. Graefe's Arch Clin Exp Ophthalmol 236: 481–485

[11] Cardillo JA, Stout JT, LaFree L, Azen SP, Omphroy L, Cui JZ, Kimura H, Hinton DR, Ryan SJ (1997) Post-traumatic proliferative vitreoretinopathy. The epidemiologic profile, onset, risk factors, and visual outcome. Ophthalmology 104: 1166–1173

[12] Charteris DG, Aylward GW, Wong D, Groenewald C, Asaria RH, Bunce C (2004) A randomized controlled trial of combined 5-fluorouracil and low-molecular-weight heparin in management of established proliferative vitreoretinopathy. Ophthalmology 111: 2240–2245

[13] Chaudhry N, Mieler W, Han D, Alfaro V, Liggett P (1999) Preoperative use of tissue plasminogen activator for large submacular hemorrhage. Ophthalmic Surg Lasers 30: 176–180

[14] Cibis P, Yamashita T, Rodriguez F (1959) Clinical aspects of ocular siderosis and hemosiderosis Arch Ophthalmol 62: 46–53

[15] Clarkson JG, Flynn HW, Daily MJ (1980) Vitrectomy in Terson's syndrome. Am J Ophthalmol 90: 540–552

[16] Cleary PE, Ryan SJ (1979) Method of production and natural history of experimental posterior penetrating eye injury in the rhesus monkey. Am J Ophthalmol 88: 212–220

[17] Cleary PE, Ryan SJ (1981) Vitrectomy in penetrating eye injury. Arch Ophthalmol 99: 287–292

[18] Coleman D (1982) Early vitrectomy in the management of the severely traumatized eye. Am J Ophthalmol 93: 543–551

[19] Conway MD, Peyman GA, Recasens M (1999) Intravitreal tPA and SF6 promote clearing of premacular subhyaloid hemorrhages in shaken and battered baby syndrome. Ophthalmic Surg Lasers 30: 435–441

[20] Cowley M, Conway BP, Campochiaro PA, Kaiser D, Gaskin H (1989) Clinical risk factors for proliferative vitreoretinopathy. Arch Ophthalmol 107: 1147–1151

[21] Cox MS, Schepens CL, Freeman HM (1966) Retinal detachment due to ocular contusion. Arch Ophthalmol 76: 678–685

[22] Coyler M, Weber E, Weichel E, Dick J, Bower K, Ward T, Haller J (in press) Delayed intraocular foreign body removal without endophthalmitis during Operations Iraqi and Enduring Freedom. Ophthalmology

[23] De Pool ME, Campbell JP, Broome SO, Guyton DL (2005) The dragged-fovea diplopia syndrome clinical characteristics, diagnosis, and treatment. Ophthalmology 112: 1455–1462

[24] Dellaporta AN (1994) Evacuation of subretinal hemorrhage. Int Ophthalmol 18: 25–31

[25] Desai UR (1995) Spontaneous vitreous base avulsion in a patient with neurofibromatosis. Indian J Ophthalmol 43: 33

[26] Desatnik H, Treister G, Moisseiev J (1999) Spontaneous separation of an idiopathic macular pucker in a young girl. Am J Ophthalmol 127: 729–731

[27] Dong X, Chen N, Xie L, Wang S (2006) Prevention of experimental proliferative vitreoretinopathy with a biodegradable intravitreal drug delivery system of all-trans retinoic acid. Retina 26: 210–213

[28] Dumas C, Bonnet M (1996) Choroidal detachment associated with rhegmatogenous retinal detachment: a risk factor for postoperative PVR?. J Fr Ophtalmol 19: 455–463

[29] Durukan AH, Kerimoglu H, Erdurman C, Demirel A, Karagul S (2006) Long-term results of Nd:YAG laser treatment for premacular subhyaloid haemorrhage owing to Valsalva retinopathy. Eye

[30] Ehrenberg M, Tresher RJ, Machemer R (1984) Vitreous hemorrhage nontoxic to retina as a stimulator of glial and fibrous proliferation. Am J Ophthalmol 97: 611–626

[31] Engelbrecht N, Freeman J, Sternberg PJ, Aaberg TS, Aaberg TJ, Martin D, Sippy B (2002) Retinal pigment epithelial changes after macular hole surgery with indocyanine green-assisted internal limiting membrane peeling. Am J Ophthalmol 89–94

[32] Er H, Turkoz Y, Mizrak B, Parlakpinar H (2006) Inhibition of experimental proliferative vitreoretinopathy with protein kinase C inhibitor (chelerythrine chloride) and melatonin. Ophthalmologica 220: 17–22

[33] Ersanli D, Sonmez M, Unal M, Gulecek O (2006) Management of retinal detachment due to closed globe injury by pars plana vitrectomy with and without scleral buckling. Retina 26: 32–36

[34] Fraser EA, Cheema RA, Roberts MA (2003) Triamcinolone acetonide-assisted peeling of retinal internal limiting membrane for macular surgery. Retina 23: 883–884

[35] Girard P, Mimoun G, Karpouzas I, Montefiore G (1994) Clinical risk factors for proliferative vitreoretinopathy after retinal detachment surgery. Retina 14: 417–424

[36] Glatt H, Machemer R (1982) Experimental subretinal hemorrhage in rabbits. Am J Ophthalmol 94: 762–773

[37] Guigon-Souquet B, Salaun N, Macarez R, Bazin S, De La Marnierre E, Mazdou M (2004) Subhyaloid hemorrhage following a Valsalva maneuver. J Fr Ophtalmol 27: 1159–1162 [in French]

[38] Halberstadt M, Domig D, Kodjikian L, Koerner F, Garweg JG (2006) PVR recurrence and the timing of silicon oil removal. Klin Monatsbl Augenheilkd 223: 361–366

[39] Hermsen V (1984) Vitrectomy in severe ocular trauma. Ophthalmologica 189: 86–92

[40] Hesse L, Bodanowitz S, Kroll P (1996) Retinal necrosis after blunt bulbus trauma. Klin Monatsbl Augenheilkd 209: 150–152 [in German]

[41] Horio N, Horiguchi M (2004) Retinal blood flow analysis using intraoperative video fluorescein angiography combined with optical fiber-free intravitreal surgery system. Am J Ophthalmol 138: 1082–1083

[42] Isernhagen RD, Smiddy WE, Michels RG (1988) Vitrectomy for nondiabetic vitreous hemorrhage. Not associated with vascular disease. Retina 8: 81–87

[43] Ismail R, Tanner V, Williamson TH (2002) Optical coherence tomography imaging of severe commotio retinae and associated macular hole. Br J Ophthalmol 86: 473–474

[44] Kennedy C, Parker C, McAllister I (1997) Retinal detachment caused by retinal dialysis. Aust N Z J Ophthalmol 251: 25–30

[45] Kishi S, Hagimura N, Shimizu K (1996) The role of the premacular liquefied pocket and premacular vitreous complex in idiopathic macular hole development. Am J Ophthalmol 122: 622–628

[46] Koh HJ, Kim SH, Lee SC, Kwon OW (2000) Treatment of subhyaloid haemorrhage with intravitreal tissue plasminogen activator and C3F8 gas injection. Br J Ophthalmol 84: 1329–1330

[47] Kuhn F, Kiss G, Mester V, Szijarto Z, Kovacs B (2004) Vitrectomy with internal limiting membrane removal for clinically significant macular edema. Graefe's Arch Clin Exper Ophthal 242: 402–408

[48] Kuhn F, Mester V, Berta A (1998) The Tano diamond dusted membrane scraper: indications and contraindications. Acta Ophthalmol 76: 754–756

[49] Kuhn F, Mester V, Morris R (2004) A proactive treatment approach for eyes with perforating injury. Klin Monatsbl Augenheilk 221: 622–628

[50] Kuhn F, Morris R, Mester V, Witherspoon C (1998) Terson's syndrome. Results of vitrectomy and the significance of vitreous hemorrhage in patients with subarachnoid hemorrhage. Ophthalmology 105: 472–477

[51] Kuhn F, Morris R, Mester V, Witherspoon C (2000) Internal limiting membrane removal for traumatic macular holes. Ophthalmol Surg Laser 31: 308–315

[52] Kuppermann BD, Thomas EL, de Smet MD, Grillone LR (2005) Pooled efficacy results from two multinational randomized controlled clinical trials of a single intravitreous injection of highly purified ovine hyaluronidase (Vitrase) for the management of vitreous hemorrhage. Am J Ophthalmol 140: 573–584

[53] Kuriyama S, Ohuchi T, Yoshimura N, Honda Y, Hiraoka M, Abe M (1990) Evaluation of radiation therapy for experimental proliferative vitreoretinopathy in rabbits. Graefe's Arch Clin Exp Ophthalmol 228: 552–555

[54] Lemor M, Yeo JH, Glaser BM (1986) Oral colchicine for the treatment of experimental traction retinal detachment. Arch Ophthalmol 104: 1226–1229

[55] Li K, Wong D, Hiscott P, Stanga P, Groenewald C, McGalliard J (2003) Trypan blue staining of internal limiting membrane and epiretinal membrane during vitrectomy: visual results and histopathological findings. Br J Ophthalmol 87: 216–219

[56] Liggett P, Gauderman W, Moreira C, Barlow W, Green R, Ryan S (1990) Pars plana vitrectomy for acute retinal detachment in penetrating ocular injuries. Arch Ophthalmol 108: 1724–1728

[57] Lincoff H, Madjarov B, Lincoff N, Movshovich A, Saxena S, Coleman DJ, Schubert H, Rosberger D McCormick S (2003) Pathogenesis of the vitreous cloud emanating from subretinal hemorrhage. Arch Ophthalmol 121: 91–96

[58] Machemer R, Sugita G, Tano Y (1979) Treatment of intraocular proliferations with intravitreal steroids. Trans Am Ophthalmol Soc 77: 171–180

[59] Majid MA, Hussain HM, Haynes RJ, Dick AD (2006) Buckle, no cryo: scleral buckle with no cryotherapy for retinal detachment secondary to commotio retinae. Br J Ophthalmol 90: 1550–1551

[60] Matsumoto C, Arimura E, Okuyama S, Takada S, Hashimoto S, Shimomura Y (2003) Quantification of metamorphopsia in patients with epiretinal membranes. Invest Ophthalmol Vis Sci 44: 4012–4016

[61] Miller-Meeks MJ, Bennett SR, Keech RV, Blodi CF (1990) Myopia induced by vitreous hemorrhage. Am J Ophthalmol 109: 199–203

[62] Morris R, Kuhn F (1998) Surgical treatment of macular surface disorders. Highlights of Ophthalmology International, Panama City, pp 58–64

[63] Morris R, Kuhn F, Mester V (2000) Prophylactic scleral buckle for prevention of retinal detachment following vitrectomy for macular hole. Br J Ophthalmol 84: 673

[64] Morris R, Kuhn F, Witherspoon C (1993) Hemorrhagic macular cysts. Ophthalmology 100: 1

[65] Morris R, Kuhn F, Witherspoon C (1994) Retinal folds and hemorrhagic macular cysts in Terson's syndrome. Ophthalmology 101: 1

[66] Moshfeghi AA, Harrison SA, Reinstein DZ, Ferrone PJ (2006) Valsalva-like retinopathy following hyperopic laser in situ keratomileusis. Ophthalmic Surg Lasers Imaging 37: 486–488

[67] Munir WM, Pulido JS, Sharma MC, Buerk BM (2005) Intravitreal triamcinolone for treatment of complicated proliferative diabetic retinopathy and proliferative vitreoretinopathy. Can J Ophthalmol 40: 598–604

[68] O'Hanley GP, Canny CL (1985) Diabetic dense premacular hemorrhage. A possible indication for prompt vitrectomy. Ophthalmology 92: 507–511

[69] Park SW, Seo MS (2004) Subhyaloid hemorrhage treated with SF6 gas injection. Ophthalmic Surg Lasers Imaging 35: 335–337

[70] Puustjarvi TJ, Terasvirta ME (2001) Retinal fixation of traumatic retinal detachment with metallic tacks: a case report with 10 years' follow-up. Retina 21: 54–56

[71] Richards R, West C, Meisels A (1968) Chorioretinitis sclopetaria. Trans Am Ophthalmol Soc 66: 214–232

[72] Sandner D, Herbrig E, Engelmann K (2007) High-density silicone oil (Densiron) as a primary intraocular tamponade: 12-month follow up. Graefe's Arch Clin Exp Ophthalmol

[73] Schmidt JG (1987) Intravitreal cupriferous foreign bodies: electroretinograms and inflammatory responses. Doc Ophthalmol 67: 253–261

[74] Sebag J (2005) Molecular biology of pharmacologic vitreolysis. Trans Am Ophthalmol Soc 103: 473–494

[75] Shinohara K, Tanaka M, Sakuma T, Kobayashi Y (2003) Efficacy of daunorubicin encapsulated in liposome for the treatment of proliferative vitreoretinopathy. Ophthalmic Surg Lasers Imaging 34: 299–305

[76] Sipperley JO, Quigley HA, Gass DM (1978) Traumatic retinopathy in primates. The explanation of commotio retinae. Arch Ophthalmol 96: 2267–2273

[77] Skorpik C, Menapace R, Gnad HD, Paroussis P (1989) Silicone oil implantation in penetrating injuries complicated by PVR. Results from 1982 to 1986. Retina 9: 8–14

[78] Spraul CW, Grossniklaus HE (1997) Vitreous hemorrhage. Surv Ophthalmol 42: 3–39

[79] Sternberg P Jr, Han DP, Yeo JH, Barr CC, Lewis H, Williams GA, Mieler WF (1988) Photocoagulation to prevent retinal detachment in acute retinal necrosis. Ophthalmology 95: 1389–1393

[80] Stone TW, Siddiqui N, Arroyo JG, McCuen BW 2nd, Postel EA (2000) Primary scleral buckling in open-globe injury involving the posterior segment. Ophthalmology 107: 1923–1926

[81] Tanaka M, Qui H (2000) Pharmacological vitrectomy. Semin Ophthalmol 15: 51–61

[82] Tognetto D, Minutola D, Sanguinetti G, Ravalico G (2005) Anatomical and functional outcomes after heavy silicone oil tamponade in vitreoretinal surgery for complicated retinal detachment: a pilot study. Ophthalmology 112: 1574

[83] Trese MT (2000) Enzymatic vitreous surgery. Semin Ophthalmol 15: 116–121

[84] Ullern M, Roman S, Dhalluin JF, Lozato P, Grillon S, Bellefqih S, Cambourieu C, Baudouin C (2002) Contribution of intravitreal infracyanine green to macular hole and epimacular membrane surgery: preliminary study. J Fr Ophtalmol 25: 915–920 [in French]

[85] van Bockxmeer FM, Martin CE, Thompson DE, Constable IJ (1985) Taxol for the treatment of proliferative vitreoretinopathy. Invest Ophthalmol Vis Sci 26: 1140–1147

[86] Wallace R, McNamara J, Brown G, Benson W, Belmont J, Goldberg R, Federman J (1993) The use of perfluorophenanthrene in the removal of intravitreal lens fragments. Am J Ophthalmol 116: 196–200

[87] Weidenthal D, Schepens C (1966) Peripheral fundus changes associated with ocular contusion. Am J Ophthalmol 62: 465

[88] Wickham L, Xing W, Bunce C, Sullivan P (2006) Outcomes of surgery for posterior segment intraocular foreign bodies-a retrospective review of 17 years of clinical experience. Graefe's Arch Clin Exp Ophthalmol

[89] Wiedemann P, Lemmen K, Schmiedl R, Heimann K (1987) Intraocular daunorubicin for the treatment and prophylaxis of traumatic proliferative vitreoretinopathy. Am J Ophthalmol 104: 10–14

[90] Williams RG, Chang S, Comaratta MR, Simoni G (1996) Does the presence of heparin and dexamethasone in the vitrectomy infusate reduce reproliferation in proliferative vitreoretinopathy? Graefe's Arch Clin Exp Ophthalmol 234: 496–503

[91] Wolf S, Schon V, Meier P, Wiedemann P (2003) Silicone oil-RMN3 mixture ("heavy silicone oil") as internal tamponade for complicated retinal detachment. Retina 23: 335–342

[92] Yamada H, Sakai A, Yamada E, Nishimura T, Matsumura M (2002) Spontaneous closure of traumatic macular hole. Am J Ophthalmol 134: 340–347

[93] Yanoff M (1975) Pathology of cataract. In: Bellows JG (eds) Cataract and abnormalities of the lens. Grune and Stratton, New York, pp 179

[94] Morris R et al. (2006) Prophylactic silicone oil placement for retinal detachments with grades A and B PVR. Association for Research and Vision in Ophthalmology, Fort Lauderdale

2.10 Trauma By Blunt Object: Contusions

Ferenc Kuhn

2.10.1 Introduction

Even if the blunt object's impact was insufficient to cause a full-thickness defect in the eye wall (rupture; see Chaps. 1.1, 2.12), the delivered energy can still seriously damage any tissue of the eye by compressing it and by transferring its energy into "shockwaves" that can reach the posterior pole. The consequences may present acutely or several years later. Chronic problems are especially common if the initial management was inappropriate.

Contusions must be taken seriously, although they do not invoke the same urgency as open globe trauma does: the surgeon has time to evaluate the eye and carefully select the best management option (see Chap. 1.8). The severity of contusions was well demonstrated in a large study, which found the following complication rates: retinal detachment 44%; contusion retinopathy 21%; vitreous hemorrhage 11%; choroidal rupture 8%; evulsion of the optic nerve 1% [2].

Selected consequences caused by a contusion are summarized and compared with damage inflicted by open globe injuries are shown in Table 2.11.1.

2.10.2 Evaluation[1]

If an eye has been hit with a blunt object, the primary goal is the differential diagnosis between a contusion and a rupture.

1 See Chaps. 1.9, 1.10, and 2 12 for further details.

- *History*: lack of severe acute loss of vision makes contusion the more likely diagnosis.
- On *external inspection*, thick subconjunctival hemorrhages and chemosis raise the suspicion of an occult rupture, although they can also occur after a contusion.
- The *slit lamp* examination allows determining the type and severity of most anterior segment pathologies, including the presence (or lack) of a corneal wound. A scleral wound may remain impossible to identify with even the most careful inspection.
- The *ophthalmoscope* permits evaluation of the retina if the media are clear.

Pearl

The lack of a vitreous hemorrhage in an eye that sustained injury from a blunt object makes presence of a rupture unlikely; presence of a vitreous hemorrhage does not make contusion unlikely.

- *Ultrasonography* and various *radiological tests* may be needed to confirm these findings; the most crucial condition to exclude is an occult scleral rupture (see Chap. 2.12).
- If doubt persists regarding the presence of an occult scleral rupture, *exploratory surgery* may become necessary.[2]

2.10.3 Specific Pathologies and Related Management Decisions

There are three crucial decisions to make: Is surgical intervention necessary; and if yes, what type of intervention and when.

2 The gravest error is to leave an occult rupture untreated. This leads to serious medical and legal consequences.

2.10.3.1 Cornea

Bowman's layer/stromal fractures, endothelial cell damage/loss with consequent edema, diffuse endotheliopathy [3], and corneal endothelial rings [13] may occur. Acute surgery is almost never necessary; observation or symptomatic topical treatment is recommended.

2.10.3.2 Anterior Chamber

With regard to the AC:

- If the *hyphema* is large (total) and especially if it is accompanied by significant IOP elevation, early evacuation of the blood is indicated (see Chap. 2.5). If the IOP is normal or can be normalized with medications and there are no signs of corneal blood staining, observation is recommended.
- A *dilated pupil* may cause enough photophobia or dissatisfaction with cosmesis for surgical pupillary constriction to be considered. The intervention is not urgent (see Chap. 2.6).
- In most cases the *iridodialysis* is small. If it is large (see Fig. 2.7.2) and causes visual complaints, suture refixation of the iris root is indicated, especially if surgery is necessary for other indications. The intervention is not urgent (see Chap. 2.6).
- *IOP elevation* seen in association with angle recession or most other pathologies is initially treated medically; if this is unable to normalize the IOP, surgery is indicated. In certain other conditions (e.g., total hyphema, lens swelling), surgery is inevitable, which may be urgent (see Chaps. 2.7, 2.18).

2.10.3.3 Lens

With regard to the lens:

- *Vossius ring:* the imprint of the iris pigments as they were transferred onto the lens capsule at the point of impact.
- *Capsular rupture* (anterior or posterior) may occur as an isolated pathology (see Chap. 2.7).
- *Traumatic cataracts* ("rosette") often require extraction earlier than idiopathic cataracts because of lens swelling with consequent IOP eleva-

tion (see above) or to allow direct inspection of the retina. The surgical technique and the rules of IOL implantation can also differ (see Chap. 2.7).

- *Subluxation* alone rarely justifies surgery; however, if the patient experiences major visual disturbance or the prolapsed vitreous causes corneal touch with consequent endothelial decompensation, timely extraction and anterior vitrectomy are indicated (see Chap. 2.7).
- *Luxation* is an indication for early surgery. If it occurs in the lens in the AC, immediate intervention is recommended. If it is in the vitreous, the intervention may be delayed, but the surgeon should keep in mind that inflammation is a powerful inciting factor for PVR development (see Chaps. 2.7, 2.9).

2.10.3.4 Ciliary Body

With regard to the ciliary body:

- *Cyclodialysis*: If the cleft causes hypotony with anatomical (e.g., macular edema) and functional (decreased visual acuity) consequences, timely treatment is indicated. Surgery should be performed if the conservative approach is ineffective (see Chap. 2.8).
- *Ciliary body shutdown*: Hypotony may be temporary (caused by ciliary body "shock") or permanent (acute necrosis or chronic destruction in the context of PVR). Treatment is indicated early, although surgery is not necessarily the first resort (see Chaps 2.8, 2.9, 2.19, 2.20).

2.10.3.5 Vitreous

With regard to the ciliary vitreous:

- *Vitreous base avulsion* does not require surgery unless accompanying complications (e.g., vitreous hemorrhage, retinal break/detachment) demand it (see Chap. 2.9).

- *Hemorrhage* is one of the most commonly encountered pathologies after a contusion: vitreous or retinal hemorrhages occur in up to three-fourths of contused eyes [8].[3] In one study, 45% of eyes had accompanying retinal pathology, and 79% of eyes had a final visual acuity of worse than 20/40 [15]. Data from the USEIR are further proof that contusion-related vitreous hemorrhage must be considered a serious condition (see below). Unfortunately, it is common in clinical practice to:
  - Observe eyes with vitreous hemorrhage if this was caused by contusion; the patient is usually advised to undergo ultrasonography every 3 months or so to "detect a *retinal detachment* in its earliest phase" or to "identify *vitreous organization* before PVR commences" (see Chap. 2.9).
  - Perform vitrectomy only when either of these two conditions is recognized or the vitreous hemorrhage has not shown signs of spontaneous absorption for several months.
- A safer alternative to this conservative approach is *early vitrectomy* (i.e., within weeks and without waiting for the above-mentioned pathologies to occur). There are risks associated with observation (Table 2.10.1), even if the patient does rigorously adhere to the follow-up schedule.

Controversial

Early vitrectomy should be considered for contusion-related vitreous hemorrhage. Although the bleeding may resolve spontaneously, the advantages of early blood removal are substantial: instant visual rehabilitation; treatment of retinal breaks before they could lead to detachment; prevention of blood-related complications, including PVR; and reduced surgical risks if vitrectomy is performed *before*, rather than *for*, secondary complications. Conversely, there are risks associated with vitrectomy itself.

3 Other pathologies such as hyphema, probably have a higher incidence, but because their visual consequences are usually less severe and more temporary, they go underreported. Conversely, a vitreous hemorrhage is likely to make the patient seek medical attention early. This is reflected in the findings of the USEIR (see below).

Table 2.10.1 Retinal complications in eyes with vitreous hemorrhage in the USEIR database (%)

Pathology	Contusion (*n*=528)	Rupture (*n*=861)	Penetrating (*n*=1311)	IOFB (*n*=530)	Perforating (*n*=258)
Retinal break[a]	16	14	24	31	19
Macular hole	5	0.2	0.2	0.2	0.2
Retinal hemorrhage	30	23	23	28	29
Retinal detachment	16	35	27	33	34

Based on 14,523 injuries

[a]Includes all peripheral lesions (tear, necrotic hole, dialysis). All numbers are rounded

- *Prolapse* alone is rarely an indication for surgical intervention (see above).
- *PVD* is not a surgical indication, unless secondary retinal complications follow (see Chap. 2.9).
- *Syneresis* is not a surgical indication.

2.10.3.6 Retina

With regard to the retina:

- *Contusion retinopathy* or *maculopathy* (see Fig. 2.9.4) is not a surgical indication. If vitrectomy is performed for other pathologies, extreme caution is necessary to avoid tearing the retina at the edge of the contused area (see Chap. 2.9).
- Retinal tears can develop at the border of a contused area weeks or even months later. The patient must be properly informed and followed.
- *Chorioretinitis sclopetaria*: instead of direct contusion, the blunt object's impact is conferred on the globe via shockwaves. Surgery is not indicated for the condition itself, but its consequences may require vitrectomy (see Chap. 2.9).
- *Hemorrhage* is an indication for early vitrectomy if the blood is submacular and thick. Early surgery should also be considered for submembranous hemorrhagic cysts in the macula and when nonsurgical methods have proved ineffective (see Chap. 2.9).

- *Peripheral breaks* are rather common after contusion (Table 2.10.2). Myopic eyes are at especially high risk [5, 10]. The breaks should be treated as soon as possible to prevent retinal detachment. Laser retinopexy is preferred to cryopexy. If vitreous hemorrhage prevents visualization of the retina but a break is suspected/confirmed on ultrasonography, immediate vitrectomy is indicated (see above and Chap. 2.9). Table 2.10.2 provides details on the association between contusion and retinal breaks/detachment.
- *Macular hole*: Observation or early surgery are the two options. Spontaneous hole closure is possible [14], although it is rare, and the prognosis may be better [11] if vitrectomy is not delayed (see Chap. 2.9).
- *Retinal detachment* has been reported to occur in up to 9% of contusions, but may take many years to develop [1]. The risk has reached 16% in the USEIR if the eye also had a vitreous hemorrhage. Immediate surgery is indicated. Unless the break is a dialysis, which is effectively treated with scleral buckling, vitrectomy is preferred because it is able to eliminate all tractions completely and because it allows the treatment of other pathologies (see Chap. 2.9).
- Adding a circumferential buckle to vitrectomy does not increase the success rate [9].
- *Vascular occlusion* in small arterioles may occur, although infrequently. There is no known therapy [6].

Table 2.10.2 Contusion-related retinal breaks and detachment: a literature review

Following a contusion, 12–19% of eyes develop a peripheral retinal break [1, 12]
Following a contusion, 6% of eyes develop a macular hole [1]
Of contusion-related breaks, 9% are posterior to the equator [5]
Of contusion-related breaks, 76% are dialyses [12]
Of contusion-related dialyses, two-thirds are inferotemporal [4]
Of contusion-related necrotic breaks, two-thirds are inferotemporal [8]
Of contusion-related retinal detachments, three-quarters are caused by dialysis [8]
Of traumatic retinal detachments, three-quarters are caused by contusion [7]

2.10.3.7 Choroid

With regard to the choroid:

- *Rupture* can occur in a third of contused eyes [1], but it is not a surgical indication. If, however, the initially good vision subsequently deteriorates because of CNV development, treatment is indicated. Surgical removal is one of the options to consider (see Chap. 2.8).
- *Hemorrhage*: No treatment is necessary.
- *Suprachoroidal hemorrhage*: see Chap. 2.8.

2.10.3.8 Optic Nerve

Although direct contusion of the nerve itself is rare, optic nerve evulsion or TON may be caused by blunt force impacting the eye/orbit (Fig. 2.10.1).

Table 2.10.3 shows data on contusion-related trauma from the USEIR.

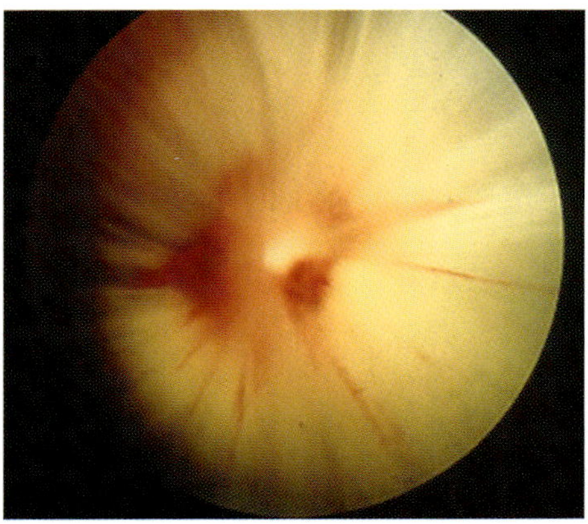

Fig. 2.10.1 Fresh optic nerve evulsion. The typical appearance is the complete loss of the normal optic disc image, loss of retinal blood circulation, and the presence of a few hemorrhages. The injury was caused during basketball by another player's finger accidentally entering the orbit. There was no other visible globe pathology. It is not known whether the pathomechanism of optic nerve evulsion was forward dislocation of the eye, which tore the optic nerve at its insertion into the globe, or the increased IOP "blew" the nerve out

Table 2.10.3 Contusion-related eye injuries: selected data from the USEIR

Variable	Finding (%)
Place of injury	Home 34
	Recreation/sport 15
	Street and highway 17
Assault	18
Incidence of hyphema	32
Incidence of glaucoma	5
Incidence of hypotony	1
Incidence of traumatic cataract	6
Incidence of lens sub/luxation	4
Incidence of vitreous hemorrhage	19
Incidence of retinal break	10
Incidence of retinal detachment	4
Incidence of optic nerve damage	5
Incidence of choroidal rupture	5
Incidence of orbital fracture	7
Prophylactic laser treatment for retinal break	5
Evisceration/enucleation	1
Visual acuity: preoperative/postoperative	NLP: 2 /3
	LP/HM: 14 / 4
	1/200–20/120: 16 / 13
	20/100–20/50: 14 / 13
	20/40 or greater: 37 / 53

Based on cases collected between 1 January 1989 and 31 December 2004. All percentages are rounded

DO:

- make sure that the injury is indeed a contusion, not an occult rupture
- perform a complete evaluation (with special attention paid to the cornea and sclera) of all eyes injured with a blunt object,
- consider the benefits of early intervention; natural history may involve a higher complication risk than surgery does

DON'T:

- assume that a vitreous hemorrhage caused by contusion has identical implications as a vitreous hemorrhage caused by nontraumatic conditions such as diabetes or venous occlusion
- leave retinal breaks untreated; up to 16% of contusions eventually lead to retinal detachment

Summary

Contusions rarely evoke emergency, and the treatment of its complications are usually straightforward. The most common, avoidable error in the management of contused eyes is not to consider early surgery for vitreous hemorrhage.

References

[1] Archer DB, Canavan YM (1983) Contusional eye injuries: retinal and choroidal lesions. Aust J Ophthalmol 11: 251–264

[2] Atmaca L, Yilmaz M (1993) Changes in the fundus caused by blunt ocular trauma. Ann Ophthalmol 25: 447–452

[3] Brooks AM, Grant G, Gillies WE (1987) Reversible corneal endothelial cell changes in diseases of the anterior segment. Aust N Z J Ophthalmol 15: 283–289

[4] Cox MS (1980) Retinal breaks caused by blunt nonperforating trauma at the point of impact. Trans Am Ophthalmol Soc 78: 414–466

[5] Cox MS, Schepens CL, Freeman HM (1966) Retinal detachment due to ocular contusion. Arch Ophthalmol 76: 678–685

[6] Dalma-Weiszhausz J, Meza-de Regil A, Martinez-Jardon S, Oliver-Fernandez K (2005) Retinal vascular occlusion following ocular contusion. Graefe's Arch Clin Exp Ophthalmol 243: 406–409

[7] Dumas JJ (1967) Retinal detachment following contusion of the eye. Int Ophthalmol Clin 7: 19–38

[8] Eagling EM (1974) Ocular damage after blunt trauma to the eye. Its relationship to the nature of the injury. Br J Ophthalmol 58: 126–140

[9] Ersanli D, Sonmez M, Unal M, Gulecek O (2006) Management of retinal detachment due to closed globe injury by pars plana vitrectomy with and without scleral buckling. Retina 26: 32–35

[10] Goffstein R, Burton TC (1982) Differentiating traumatic from nontraumatic retinal detachment. Ophthalmology 89: 361–368

[11] Kuhn F, Morris R, Mester V, Witherspoon C (2000) Internal limiting membrane removal for traumatic macular holes. Ophthalmol Surg Las 31: 308–315

[12] Tasman W (1972) Peripheral retinal changes following blunt trauma. Trans Am Ophthalmol Soc 70: 190–198

[13] van Rij G (1981) Traumatic corneal endothelial rings. Doc Ophthalmol 50: 315–319

[14] Yamada H, Sakai A, Yamada E, Nishimura T, Matsumura M (2002) Spontaneous closure of traumatic macular hole. Am J Ophthalmol 134: 340–347

[15] Yeung L, Chen TL, Kuo YH, Chao AN, Wu WC, Chen KJ, Hwang YS, Chen Y, Lai CC (2006) Severe vitreous hemorrhage associated with closed-globe injury. Graefe's Arch Clin Exp Ophthalmol 244: 52–57

2.11 Open Globe Injury: a Brief Overview

Ferenc Kuhn

2.11.1 Introduction

If the injury caused a full-thickness defect in the eye wall (see Chap. 1.1), the treatment dramatically differs from that in a contusion. The two most important initial factors driving the surgeon's thought process[1] and thus the management are the threat of ECH, which can rapidly cause irreversible loss of vision and eye (see Chap. 2.8), and the risk of endophthalmitis, which occurs in up to 5% of eyes with penetrating injuries[2]. The presence of an IOFB roughly doubles the risk [3, 4].

Depending on the type of injury, some of the damage occurs at the time of the trauma, and other complications develop later. Table 2.11.1 provides an overview; for comparison, contusions are also included. Obviously, the ophthalmologist is unable to undo damage already done, but his intervention[3] has a major impact on subsequent events and thus on the prognosis.

2.11.2 Evaluation

See Chaps. 1.9 and 2.12 for details; only a few useful pearls are noted here:

---

1 i.e., management strategy (see Chap. 1.8).

2 The USEIR found a significantly lower figure (2.6%; see Chap. 2.17 for more details).

3 This holds true for the primary as well as secondary interventions.

- Hypotony is a statistically significantly strong indicator of open globe injury; a low IOP makes the presence of a full-thickness wound likely [2].

Cave

Normal or even elevated IOP does not preclude the possibility that an open globe injury has occurred.

Table 2.11.1 Acute vs late consequences of various types of trauma. + Yes; – no

Injury type	Instant complications	Complications within weeks	Complications after months or years
Contusion	+ / – ("+" includes lens dislocation, vitreous hemorrhage, retinal necrosis, or choroidal rupture)	– / + ("+" is usually glaucoma)	+ / – ("+" includes cataract, retinal tear and detachment)
Rupture	+++ (e.g., tissue extrusion, vitreous hemorrhage)	+ (e.g., cataract progression, retinal tear and detachment)	+ (e.g., PVR)
Penetrating	++ (e.g., cataract, vitreous hemorrhage, retinal laceration)	+ / – ("+" includes cataract, retinal tear and detachment)	– / + ("+" is usually PVR)
IOFB	++ (e.g., cataract, vitreous hemorrhage, retinal laceration)	+ / – ("+" includes cataract, retinal tear and detachment)	– / + ("+" is usually PVR or metallosis)
Perforating	++ (e.g., cataract, vitreous hemorrhage, retinal laceration)	+ / – ("+" includes cataract, retinal tear and detachment, PVR)	++ / – ("+" is usually PVR)

Reflecting typical cases; individual exceptions always occur

- Once it has been determined that the eye has a full-thickness defect (see Chap. 2.10) requiring closure,[4] the standard evaluation process should be limited (Fig. 2.12.2) to obtaining information that affects the timing or the type of the primary intervention:
  - Risk of ECH (Chap. 2.8)
  - Risk of endophthalmitis (see Chap. 2.17)
  - Presence of an IOFB (see Chap. 2.13)
  - Probability of a perforating injury (see Chap. 2.14)
  - The patient's systemic condition as this concerns surgery and anesthesia (see Chap. 1 8)

It is important to also look for adnexal and orbital injuries: they are present in 26% of open globe injuries, increasing the risk of posterior segment injury and poor outcome [1].

2.11.3 Management

In this chapter only a brief overview is given (Table 2.11.2); see Chaps. 1.8, 2.12–2.15, and 2.17–2.20 for details. A few additional issues are discussed below:

- As described in Chap 1.8, treatment of a patient with an open globe injury must not be a mechanical, one-by-one restoration of tissue pathologies. If a corneal wound and a hyphema are present, the goal is *not* to introduce sutures until the wound is watertight and wait until the hyphema clears. The surgeon must first design a strategic plan, which answers the overall questions,[5] and then a tactical plan, which answers

4 i.e., the wound is not self-sealing

5 e.g., Is surgery urgent? Is there a posterior scleral extension of the corneal wound? Is the risk of endophthalmitis high? Is an ECH imminent? Is the IOP high? Is there vitreous prolapse into the AC? Is there a lens injury? Is there injury to the posterior segment?

Table 2.11.2 Management issues in eyes with open globe injury.[1]

Variable	Comment
History	Find out what happened and how (the injury's circumstances)
	Determine whether the agent was likely to have been contaminated
	Find out when the incident occurred
	Determine whether the injury occurred at the workplace, and if so, whether a report has been filed
	Determine if the injury was self-inflicted or the result of assault
	Determine if a witness can be identified[1]
	Determine the object's size, material, and whether it is likely to have been retained intraocularly
	Ask about vision and pain as the injury occurred, and how these symptoms have changed since then
	Determine whether someone has already seen/treated the patient, who that person was, and what therapy has been applied
	Ask when the patient took something orally, and if yes, what and when
Visual acuity	Always take it in the injured eye; there is no need to refract if the patient wears glasses and they are unavailable: use a pinhole and note its use in the patient's chart
	Always take it in the fellow eye
	If a standard visual acuity chart is unavailable, use a near chart or even your fingers (see Chap. 1.8)
External inspection	Using a penlight, compare the two eyes[2] and note all major abnormalities. A shallow AC may be easier to diagnose this way than with a slit lamp where simultaneous visualization of the two eyes (comparison) is not possible

[1] See also Chaps. 1.8 and 1.9.

Table 2.11.2 *(continued)* Management issues in eyes with open globe injury.

Variable	Comment
Slit lamp	Never put pressure on the eye when separating the lids; if the lids are impossible to open because of hemorrhage, delay the examination and keep an icepack over the lids to expedite the resolution of the blood and edema
	Meticulously examine the lids, cornea, conjunctiva, sclera, and the anterior segment
	Be wary of thick subconjunctival hemorrhages, which may hide a scleral wound underneath
	Carefully examine the pupils and their reaction, including the presence or absence of an APD
	Take the IOP unless a large and central corneal wound is present
Ophthalmoscopy	Try to examine as much of the retina as possible (Fig. 2.11.1)
	Do not use scleral indentation
	Dilate the pupil unless there is a contraindication[3]
Ultrasonography and radiological examinations	If felt necessary and if the wound is not leaking, very careful B-scan ultrasonography may be attempted; however, it is usually preferable to perform the examination in the OR after the wound has been closed
	The primary goals of CT are to detect an IOFB or the presence of an occult or posterior scleral wound; it can also show orbital pathologies such a fracture
	If presence of a nonmetallic IOFB is suspected, an MRI may be indicated; it can also supply more detailed information on soft tissue injuries
	Exploratory surgery: if still uncertain whether an occult rupture is present, the conjunctiva over the hemorrhage should be opened

Table 2.11.2 *(continued)* Management issues in eyes with open globe injury.

Variable	Comment
Decision making: questions to be answered by the attending ophthalmologist (strategy; see Chap. 1.8)	Is it certain that a full-thickness wound is present?
	Can an occult rupture be excluded?
	Is an IOFB present?
	Is this a high-risk injury for endophthalmitis?
	Can surgery be delayed until general anesthesia becomes available?
	Are prophylactic intravitreal antibiotics necessary?
	Does this injury require more manipulations during the primary surgery than wound toilette and closure?
	Triple "E": Am I capable to properly deal with the complications that are present or may be found during wound closure and need immediate action (*expertise*, *experience*)? Is the facility I am to operate at able to provide the required OR personnel and materials for me to do an optimal job (*equipment*)?
	Shall I aim for a staged approach or perform comprehensive surgery instead?
	Is it preferable to refer this patient to a colleague who is more likely to do an optimal surgery?
	If yes, would the patient arrive there within a reasonably short time?
	Is the eye's condition likely to worsen[4] during transportation?
	Before referral, try to communicate with the colleague directly
Primary (emergency) surgery[5] (tactics; see Chaps. 2.1–2.20)	Wound toilette: make sure no vitreous is left external to the wound, in-between the wound lips, and, if possible, behind (underneath) the wound (vitrectomy must be accomplished in the AC and at least attempted at a scleral wound)
	Wound closure
	AC cleansing as necessary
	Lens extraction as necessary
	Intravitreal antibiotics/corticosteroids as necessary

Table 2.11.2 *(continued)* Management issues in eyes with open globe injury.

Variable	Comment
Postoperative medical treatment	Triple "I": topical or even systemic medications against *infection*, *inflammation*, *IOP* elevation
Secondary (reconstructive) surgery	Determine how long hospitalization is necessary[6]
	Determine whether, and, if yes, when, a reoperation is required
	Determine whether this second surgery should be performed by you or the patient should be referred (see above)
	If the surgery is to be performed by you, make sure that all conditions are optimal at the time of the operation[7]
	Report the case to the eye injury database
	Make sure that the patient has proper follow-up and that the final data[8] are also registered in the database

[1] This is especially important in children (see Chap. 2.16) or if the injury is likely to lead to a legal claim (see Chap. 1.8).

[2] Look for differences even if both eyes have been injured.

[3] Even the history of an acute angle closure glaucoma in the fellow eye and the lack of prophylactic iridectomy in the injured eye is not an absolute contraindication; give oral acetazolamide before dilating. Conversely, do not dilate the pupil if head injury occurred. The pupillary reaction is crucial for the neurosurgeon to examine.

[4] The condition may worsen on its own or because of the patient's action (e.g., rubbing of the eye).

[5] This reflects a staged approach.

[6] Medical as well as societal and financial considerations must be taken into account.

[7] As mentioned earlier (see Chap. 1.8), this includes, among others, equipment (e.g., vitrectomy machine); materials (e.g., silicone oil, IOL), and personnel (OR nurse, assistant). It is also advisable to schedule the case so that it does not put undue pressure on the OR personnel in terms of overtime and that interference with elective cases be minimized. You should antagonize neither your nurses nor your colleagues.

[8] Six months are often too short for "final" data in eyes with severe injury: years may pass before it can be determined that the eye's condition, as related to the injury, is safely considered permanent.

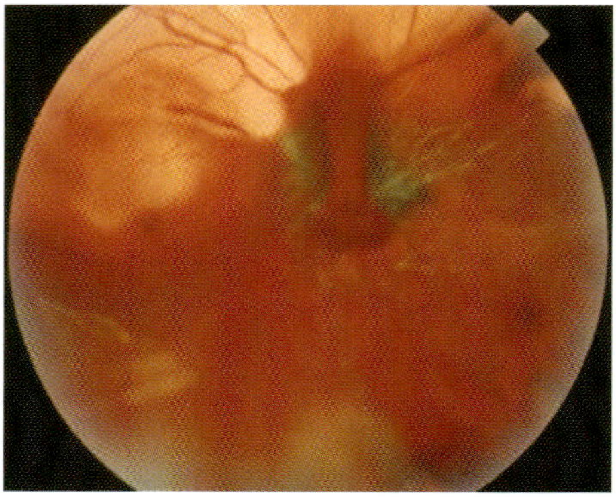

Fig. 2.11.1 Vitreous hemorrhage and retinal inspection. This eye sustained an open globe injury caused by a nail. Despite the vitreous hemorrhage, it is possible to examine much of the retina with the ophthalmoscope

the technical questions[6]. Without such planning, management is bound to be suboptimal.

Pearl

Surgery for an eye with open globe surgery should be delayed for a few minutes so that the most appropriate management plan can be designed. Such a delay does not pose any risk; going to surgery without such a plan does.

- In many institutions it is the OR nurse who prepares the eye for surgery.[7] If the eye has an open globe injury, the eye should always be prepared by the ophthalmologist (Fig. 1.8.16, 2.8.2). The surgeon is more likely to be fully aware of the ECH risk and avoid increasing it by unintentionally exerting pressure on the globe.

6 e.g., How many sutures? What order? How many paracenteses to irrigate the AC?
7 Includes betadine use, draping, even placement of a lid speculum.

- Suturing the cornea and the sclera have very difficult requirements and goals, and demand the use of different tools and technology; these are described in Chaps. 2.2 and 2.3. A brief comparative review of the management of corneal vs scleral wounds is provided in Table 2.11.3.
- The need for antibiotic therapy, the routes of administration, and the type and dose of the drugs must be carefully considered, as must the use of corticosteroids (see Chaps. 1.8, 2.17).

Table 2.11.3 Management of corneal and scleral wounds: a comparison

Variable	Cornea	Sclera
Goal: maintain/restore clarity of tissue	++–	–
Goal: maintain/restore shape of tissue/globe	+++	+ / – ("-" if wound too posterior and closure risks tissue extrusion)
Goal: watertight wound	+++	+++/- ("-" if wound too posterior and closure risks tissue extrusion
Sequence	Inward/halving/running	Antero-posterior/halving
Suture material	Nonabsorbable	Absorbable/nonabsorbable
Suture size	10/0	6/0 to 8/0
Suture removal	After at least a 3-month waiting period	–
Handling of prolapsed tissue	Depending on the type of tissue, reposit, or excise	Depending on the type of tissue, reposit or excise; if wound too posterior, leave
Detailed evaluation if wound easily visible	–	–
Detailed evaluation if wound not visible	+	+++ to determine whether a wound is present (occult rupture)
Best method to evaluate	Slit lamp; fluorescein (rose bengal) staining	Slit lamp; CT; ultrasonography

Table 2.11.3 *(continued)* Management of corneal and scleral wounds: a comparison

Variable	Cornea	Sclera
Injury type	Contusion/concussion common	Contusion/concussion uncommon
	Epicorneal FB very common	Episcleral FB very uncommon;
	Intracorneal FB uncommon	Intrascleral FB uncommon
	Rupture uncommon	Rupture relatively common
	Laceration common	Laceration common
Significance of previous surgery (wound dehiscence/rupture)	+++	+
Symptoms of injury	Pain	Bleeding
	Photophobia	
	Lacrimation	
Wound must always be closed	+++ / –	See above

See Chaps. 2.2 and 2.3 for further details

DO:

- evaluate the eye as dictated by the specific injury, not simply by following a protocol
- design a plan, both in terms of strategy and tactics, before initiating treatment

DON'T:

- let an assistant prepare the eye for surgery; this needs to be done by you, the surgeon
- follow instincts during surgery, but try to think logically and follow-up this logic with your actions

Summary

Open globe injuries present several serious risks not associated with contusion, even if many of the pathologies caused by the two types of trauma are similar or identical. Paradoxically, taking a few minutes to design a management plan is more important for eyes with open than with closed globe injury, despite the relative urgency to close the wound.

References

[1] Hatton MP, Thakker MM, Ray S (2002) Orbital and adnexal trauma associated with open-globe injuries. Ophthal Plast Reconstr Surg 18: 458–461

[2] Lima-Gomez V, Cornejo-Mendoza AM (2004) Value of ocular hypotony as a predictor of open-globe injury in patients with ocular trauma. Circulation 72: 177–181 [in Spanish]

[3] Thompson JT, Parver LM, Enger CL, Mieler WF, Liggett PE (1993) Infectious endophthalmitis after penetrating injuries with retained intraocular foreign bodies. Ophthalmology 100: 1468–1474

[4] Thompson W, Rubsamen P, Flynn H, Schiffman J, Cousins S (1995) Endophthalmitis after penetrating trauma. Risk factors and visual acuity outcomes. Ophthalmology 102: 1696–1701

2.12 Trauma By Blunt Object: Ruptures

Ferenc Kuhn

2.12.1 Introduction

Rupture is the most severe type of injury;[1] partially responsible for the poor prognosis is the instantaneous extrusion of tissues through the wound.[2] Much of the damage occurs at the time of impact (Table 2.11.1) – this is the part of the damage the surgeon cannot influence; however, tissue incarceration and late scarring (Fig. 2.12.1) are significant threats, and here proper and timely intervention is able to positively impact the outcome. Eyes with posterior scleral extension fare much worse than eyes with only a limbal wound [1, 7], especially if primary or secondary retinal incarceration occurs (see Chap. 2.14).

2.12.2 Evaluation

With regard to evaluation, see Chaps. 1.9 and 2.11 for details. Table 2.12.1 provides hints on how to recognize an occult rupture. Artifact may make it difficult on the CT to distinguish between a rupture and an IOFB [5].

1 Stepping on a grape closely approximates what happens to an eye that sustains a rupture.

2 Paradoxically, this also works as a "release" mechanism (see Chap. 2.8). Similarly, optic nerve evulsion is rare in ruptures and much more common with contusions (see Chap. 2.10).

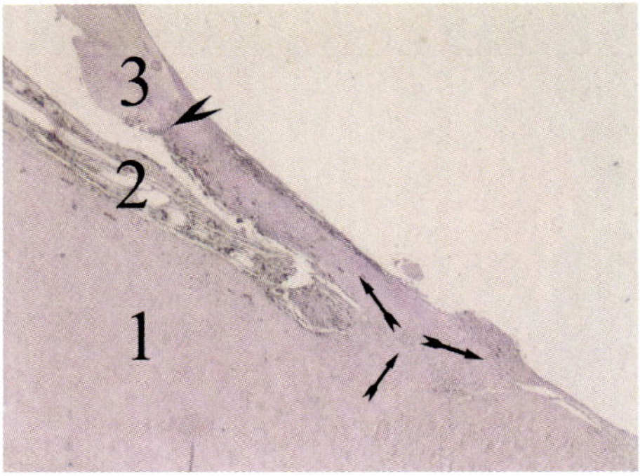

Fig. 2.12.1 Retinal detachment and PVR development following a scleral rupture. This histological specimen is from the enucleated eye of a 17-year-old boy who was injured by fireworks. He had NLP vision, total hyphema, traumatic aniridia and aphakia, and a very severe vitreous hemorrhage. The primary surgery was wound closure and hyphema removal. By day 11 the retina detached; during surgery it was found to have been incarcerated into the scleral wound. Retinectomy was performed with gas tamponade, and the visual acuity temporarily improved to HM. The retina subsequently redetached, the visual acuity became NLP, and by 5 months the eye was painful with an axial length of 17 mm. *1* sclera, *2* choroid, *3* detached retina. The *arrowhead* shows the site of the border of the retinotomy; the *arrows* show the path of the "flow" of proliferative cells, originating from the sclero-choroidal wound (Courtesy of A. Viestenz, Magdeburg, Germany)

Table 2.12.1 Findings that should raise the suspicion of an occult[1] rupture

Variable	Finding and comment
History	Injury caused by large, blunt object hitting the eye with substantial momentum
	Previous ocular surgery [7]
	Eye has high myopia
Visual acuity	Significant loss [11], even NLP [4]
IOP	Usually low [11], although a normal or even increased IOP is also possible

[1] i.e., no eye wall rupture is visible at the lamp.

Table 2.12.1 (*continued*) Findings that should raise the suspicion of an occult rupture

Variable	Finding and comment
APD	Usually present [11]
Slit lamp[2]	Thick subconjunctival hemorrhage (Fig. 2.1.2) should raise suspicion [10] especially if chemosis [6] is also present
	"Step" sign[3,a]
	Presence of an unexplained bulgea under the conjunctiva[4] (Fig. 2.12.2)
	Shallow AC in a phakic or pseudophakic eye [4], usually accompanied by hyphema [6]
	Deep AC in a previously phakic or pseudophakic eye [4]
	Peaked pupil
	Loss of the iris[a]
	Loss of the lens/IOL[a]
	Strands in the anterior vitreous, usually tainted with fresh blood, pointing toward the anterior sclera in one direction (Fig. 2.4.1)
Ophthalmoscopy	Vitreous hemorrhage [4]
	Strands in the vitreous, usually tainted with fresh blood, pointing toward the eye wall in one direction[a]
	Retinal detachment

[a] Pathognomonical signs

[2] Occasionally the anterior segment shows only minor abnormality, yet posterior scleral rupture and vitreous hemorrhage with retinal involvement are present.

[3] The curvature of the bulging conjunctiva abruptly changes.

[4] The crystalline lens

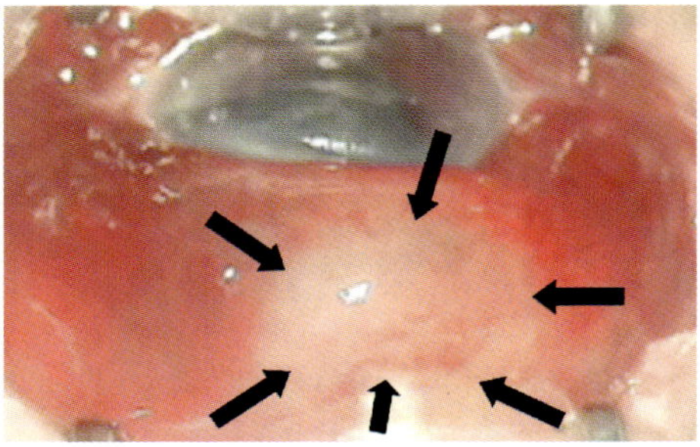

Fig. 2.12.2 Subconjunctival luxation of the crystalline lens in an eye with occult rupture. This 84-year-old woman fell and hit her previously healthy eye with a large, blunt object; the visual acuity instantly became NLP. The lens was not found preoperatively.[1] Intraoperatively, the lens could be discerned under the intact conjunctiva (*arrows*). The 13-mm-long wound was in the limbus, and , by 12 hours post-injury the retina was already detached due to a 360° dialysis. The eye underwent primary comprehensive reconstruction; visual acuity improved to 20/50 within 72 h

[1] Once it was determined that the eye is likely to have suffered an open globe injury, evaluation was stopped, deferring the determination of further details until surgery.

Rupture rarely occurs at the point of impact; the eye wall gives way almost always at its weakest point (see Chap. 1.1). Typically, the rupture, in an eye without prior open globe surgery, is found at the:

- *Limbus*, where the radius of curvature of the cornea and sclera intersect (Fig. 2.12.2)
- *Equator*, behind the insertion of the extraocular muscles, where the sclera is the thinnest
- *Lamina cribrosa*

In eyes with prior open globe surgery (see Table 2.2.2), the wound represents a major hazard for rupture. The risk diminishes with time but never completely disappears [9]. The length of the wound and its construction[3] also influence the risk [9]. In the USEIR database, 6% of *all* eyes with open globe injury had wound dehiscence; among eyes with rupture, the rate was

3 i.e., length and angle of the wound lips.

16%. The greatest danger of wound dehiscence is in an eye that has undergone PK [2].

> **Cave**
> Complete healing of a full-thickness corneal wound takes months, but even then the resistance of the scar never reaches that of the normal cornea [3]; the same is true for limbal wounds [8].

Ruptures may also occur at sites other than described above; they may be radial and extend very posteriorly. Multiple ruptures are often present; the surgeon must make sure that all have been identified.

2.12.2 Management

- Take the patient to surgery as soon as possible. The ECH risk is high until the wound is closed.
- The risk of intraoperative ECH, as the wound is reopened for toilette, increases again; be prepared to immediately close the wound if sudden major tissue prolapse occurs (see Chap. 2.8).
- Decide whether you are going to follow a staged approach or perform primary comprehensive reconstruction; in the latter case, make sure all equipment/materials will be available (see Chap. 1.8). Early vitrectomy in an eye with an unsutured wound always raises the risk of intraoperative retinal extrusion into the orbit; this is discussed in detail in Chap. 2.14.

> **Cave**
> Careful consideration is necessary regarding primary comprehensive reconstruction (see Chap. 1.8) if the rupture is too posterior to close (see Chap. 2.3). Since retinal incarceration is virtually assured, early vitrectomy with prophylactic chorioretinectomy (see Chap. 2.14) will be needed anyway. If vitrectomy is performed before the scleral wound had time to spontaneously close, the threat of intraoperative retinal extrusion is significant.

- Be gentle[4] and careful when opening the conjunctiva. If the wound is radial and posterior, it is always safer to close a smaller section of the scleral wound first, and only then continue with the conjunctival dissection (see Chap. 2.3).
- 360° peritomy may be necessary if the wound cannot initially be located or multiple wounds are suspected.
- Use of traction sutures is very useful in keeping the globe in proper position and/or keeping the extraocular muscle away from the operative field.
- The assistant must be careful in dealing with the traction suture. If too much tension is put on the suture, it can exert substantial pressure on the eye, and risk tissue extrusion or ECH development.
- Excise or reposit all tissues before suture closure (see Chap. 2.4). If there is a large retinal prolapse, the chance of functional improvement is very low. Nevertheless, the condition remains manageable if most of the retina can be reposited and the posterior retina remains relatively intact (see Chaps. 2.4, 2.8). Even extrusion of most of the retina is not an automatic indication for primary enucleation (see Chaps. 1.4, 1.8).
- If the scleral wound is posterior, common sense is necessary to realize that it is time to halt the intervention to avoid further tissue prolapse (see Chap. 2.3).
- If additional surgical manipulations are needed (e.g., hyphema or lens removal), do not use the traumatic wound for access but prepare controlled surgical incisions (see Chap. 2.4).
- If the wound is in Zone III, there is an increased chance of incarcerating vitreous, even retina, in the wound, despite your best efforts. This and the inevitable scarring make PVR development a high risk; consider comprehensive primary surgery or early secondary surgery with prophylactic chorioretinectomy (Fig. 2.14.2D) if appropriate (see above and Chap. 2.14). If the retina does get caught by the developing scar and PVR surgery needs to be performed, the prognosis becomes extremely poor.

4 i.e., avoid exerting pressure on the eye.

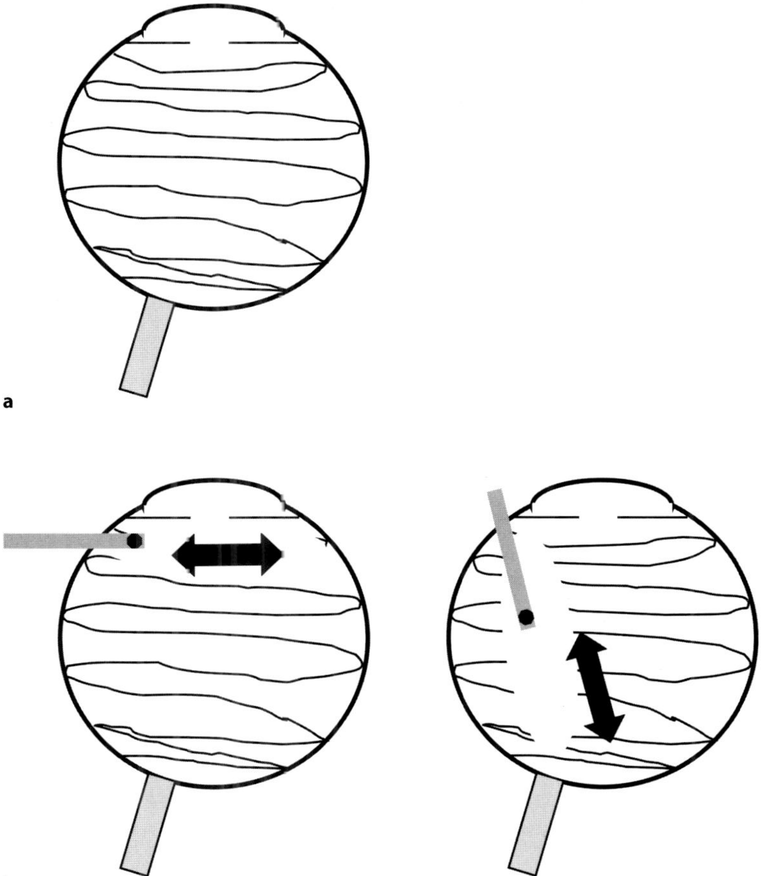

Fig. 2.12.3 Principles of the "well-digging" technique for severe, subacute vitreous hemorrhage. **a** Preoperative condition of the injured eye: severe vitreous hemorrhage. **b** The initial instinct of the surgeon is to" sweep horizontally" with the vitrectomy probe. **c** The recommended technique, however, is to proceed vertically ("well-digging") on the nasal side. This reduces the risk of creating a large iatrogenic retinectomy. The *arrows* show the primary direction of the vitrectomy probe's movements. Table 2.12.2 provides additional details

- If the vitreous hemorrhage is very severe and the injury is at least a few days old, surgery becomes very difficult technically for several reasons.[5]
  - The blood has started to organize, and there are multiple whitish vitreous sheets, layer upon layer, with streaks of red blood on their surface. There is also liquid red blood trapped between these layers as well as subhyaloidally.
  - The sheets resemble white, detached, necrotic retina, which does not bleed when bitten into with the vitreous probe. This makes distinction between the two tissues nearly or truly impossible.[6]
  - Release of the trapped blood may give the impression that an acute hemorrhage (ECH?) is occurring.
  - These difficulties force the surgeon to apply a seemingly paradoxical technique: "vertical digging," instead of "horizontal sweeping" (Fig. 2.12.3; Table 2.12.2).
- Postoperative management (see Chap. 1.8).

Table 2.12.2 Management of eyes with very severe, subacute vitreous hemorrhage

Surgical step	Comment
Select a very long[4] infusion cannula	The risk of subretinal infusion should be minimized
Place the sclerotomies at no more than 3 mm from the limbus[5]	The risk of retinal injury during instrument introduction/exchanges should be minimized
Sacrifice the lens if necessary	The condition of the *retina* determines the outcome

[4] Six or even 7 mm

[5] Scleral transillumination (see Chap. 2.16), but especially the endoscope (see Chap. 2.20), is of great help in selecting a safe site. Transillumination is not able, however, to determine whether the cannula is subretinal.

5 This condition can occur after any injury, but it is most common in ruptures; therefore its management is discussed here.

6 Remember, even the most careful preoperative ultrasonography may not be able to tell with reliable certainty whether the retina is detached.

Table 2.12.2 *(continued)* Management of eyes with very severe, subacute vitreous hemorrhage

Surgical step	Comment
Before actually opening the infusion line, turn the infusion cannula's port toward the center of the pupil, and make sure it is not occluded by vitreous or retina	Proper infusion flow is crucial to maintain the preset IOP. The cannula's port must be in the vitreous cavity, the flow must be free, and the loss of intraocular fluid must not exceed supply; BSS may be lost through the wound, an enlarged sclerotomy, or through aspiration (phacofragmentation; see Chap. 2.7)
Use a wide-angle endoilluminator[6] but at a reduced brightness	Glare from white/light-colored vitreous sheets can be very distracting and hinders fine discrimination of structures
Place the vitrectomy probe nasally	Even if this means using the nondominant hand, the vitrectomy probe should be inserted through the nasal sclerotomy so that its position can be vertical (see next)
Turn the vitrectomy probe vertical (downwards) and start removing the vitreous as if digging a well with a shovel	The surgeon's first instinct would be to carefully "peel" or shave off the vitreous layers horizontally so that as soon as the retina is detected behind the posterior cortical vitreous, cutting can be stopped. In reality, this poses a much greater risk for the retina: there is usually no PVD,[7] and because of the resemblance of the vitreous to the retina (see above), large areas of the retina can be removed before the surgeon realizes what is happening. Proceeding vertically, albeit in a narrow funnel ("well-digging"), does not eliminate the risk of inadvertent retinectomy, but this involves only a small area of the retina and does not threaten the macula. If an inadvertent retinectomy occurs and the vitrectomy probe's port is subretinal, its position is immediately recognized and the exact location of the retina is revealed (Fig. 2.12.3)

[6] A chandelier type of light, which would otherwise allow true bimanual surgery, is not recommended. The light pipe is more useful in these eyes because the surgeon can easily change the angle of illumination to help in tissue differentiation or use it to peep into the depth of the "well" created.

[7] The retina may be detached, but it is still adherent to the posterior cortical vitreous.

Table 2.12.2 *(continued)* Management of eyes with very severe, subacute vitreous hemorrhage

Surgical step	Comment
The "well" can slowly be widened	This allows increasing access to the posterior vitreous; the vitrectomy should proceed very carefully to avoid injury to retina that is still hidden behind layers of vitreous. If fresh blood is encountered, evacuate it with passive extrusion and be patient. Although the blood is most likely not a fresh hemorrhage, it *can* be. The vitreous, which is now quite mobile, often clogs the extrusion needle's port so be prepared to use the vitrectomy probe to do the aspiration: occasional single cuts may be needed to free the port, but be very careful to avoid retinal injury, especially when working on the temporal side
Separate the posterior hyaloid from the retina	If the retina is detached, this may be very difficult; once the cleavage plane has been identified, PFCL can be used. Unless there is a posterior retinal lesion, the PFCL will push the retina back and help dissect the vitreous (PVD). If there is a posterior retinal break, the PFCL will probably leak through[8] and will not help in the creation of the PVD; in such cases detaching the vitreous is either very laborious or may even be impossible at this stage; "viscodelamination" does not work
Complete the vitrectomy anteriorly	Be especially meticulous in the periphery and at the wound site (see Chap. 2.9)
Proceed as needed, based on the actual findings	The most difficult task is now completed; the intraoperative findings determine all subsequent maneuvers (laser, retinectomy, tamponade, etc.)

[8] And must be removed from the subretinal space later

DO:

- try to identify all ruptures; they may be occult and multiple
- consider primary comprehensive reconstruction if the wound was successfully sutured
- when performing vitrectomy in an eye with very severe vitreous hemorrhage where it is uncertain whether a retinal detachment is present, use the "vertical digging", not the "horizontal sweeping" technique
- employ early prophylactic chorioretinectomy as a method of preventing the scar, which develops at the site of the scleral wound, from growing over the adjacent retina and leading to PVR retinal detachment, but be careful to avoid reopening of an unsutured wound

DON'T:

- give up on a ruptured eye just because "it looks really bad" (i.e., there is substantial tissue prolapse) and the visual acuity is very poor; many of these eyes can regain at least some function if comprehensive reconstruction is performed
- force suture closure of scleral wounds that are too posterior for convenient access
- proceed "horizontally" during vitrectomy in an eye with recent, serious vitreous hemorrhage

Summary

Although ruptures remain the type of injury with the poorest prognosis, the visual acuity in many eyes can substantially be improved if timely reconstruction is pursued. The main goal of vitrectomy is PVR prevention, leaving the initial mechanical damage as the main factor limiting the eye's potential.

References

[1] De Juan E, Sternberg P, Michels R (1983) Penetrating ocular injuries: types of injuries and visual results. Ophthalmology 90: 1318–1322

[2] Elder M, Stack R (2004) Globe rupture following penetrating keratoplasty: How often, why, and what can we do to prevent it? Cornea 23: 776–780

[3] Gasset AR, Dohlman CH (1968) The tensile strength of corneal wounds. Arch Ophthalmol 79: 595–602

[4] Kylstra JA, Lamkin JC, Runyan DK (1993) Clinical predictors of scleral rupture after blunt ocular trauma. Am J Ophthalmol 115: 530–535

[5] Lins M, Kopietz L (1985) Foreign body masquerading as a ruptured globe. Ophthal Surg 16: 586–588

[6] Russell S, Olsen K, Folk J (1988) Predictors of scleral rupture and the role of vitrectomy in severe blunt ocular trauma. Am J Ophthalmol 105: 253–257

[7] Sternberg P, de Juan E, Michels RG, al e (1984) Multivariate analysis of prognostic factors in penetrating ocular injuries. Am J Ophthalmol 98: 467–472

[8] Swan KC, Meyer SL, Squires E (1978) Late wound separation after cataract extraction. Ophthalmology 85: 991–1003

[9] Vinger PF (2002) Injury to the postsurgical eye. In: Kuhn F, Pieramici D (eds) Ocular trauma: principles and practice. Thieme, New York, pp 280–292

[10] Wenzel M, Aral H (2003) Indirect traumatic rupture of the globe without conjunctival injury. Klin Monatsbl Augenheilkd 220: 35–38 [in German]

[11] Werner MS, Dana MR, Viana MA, Shapiro M (1994) Predictors of occult scleral rupture. Ophthalmology 101: 1941–1944

2.13 Penetrating Injuries and IOFBs

Ferenc Kuhn

2.13.1 Introduction

Penetrating and IOFB injuries have a lot in common (see Chap. 1.1), but they must be distinguished because of the retained FB's unique management implications. Even though both of these injury types have better prognosis than ruptures, the treatment can be very challenging and the outcome is ultimately determined by the expertise of the surgeon.

2.13.2 Evaluation

The most important question the evaluation should answer is whether an IOFB is present; every effort should be made to confirm its presence or lack thereof.[1] If history and the test results collide, it is safer to presume that an IOFB is present. (See Chaps. 1.9 and 2.11 for details.)

By far CT is the most reliable method of finding an IOFB. For ferrous IOFBs, X-ray usually suffices, but it still has an up to 31% failure rate in detecting the splinter [4]. For nonmetallic IOFBs, the proportion of false-negative tests is much higher.

It is possible that the agent caused an occult penetrating wound in the sclera (Fig. 2.13.1). The length of the wound is, however, usually much smaller than a rupture's length.

1 Failure to do so has severe medical as well as legal consequences.

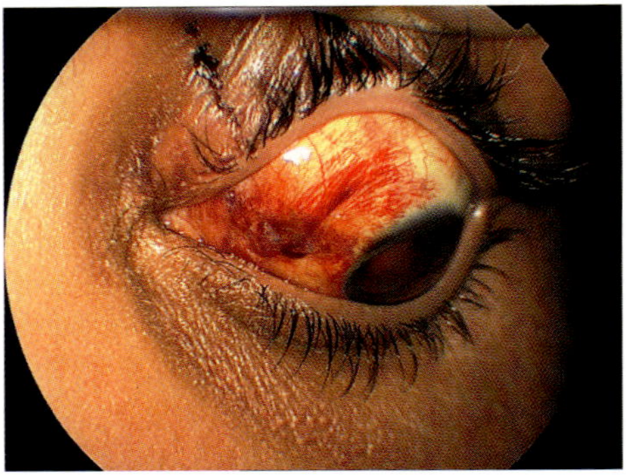

Fig. 2.13.1 Occult penetrating wound of the sclera. The patient felt a minor hit on his eye. On external inspection, a 0.5-mm conjunctival wound was seen. There is mild hemorrhage (as the patient looks down, these hemorrhages appear to be streaking toward the conjunctival wound), but no scleral wound is visible. Because history was also suggestive, a CT was performed, which identified a small IOFB (Courtesy of V. Mester, Abu Dhabi, U.A.E.)

Pearl

The implications of an occult scleral penetrating wound are different from those resulting from a rupture. The ECH risk is much smaller if an occult penetrating wound is present, as opposed to the endophthalmitis risk, which is significant. If the retina has also been injured, it is likely to become incarcerated, and the risk of PVR is high; prophylactic chorioretinectomy (see Chap. 2.14) should be considered.

2.13.3 Management

2.13.3.1 Penetrating Injury

The management follows the steps outlined in Table 2.11.2.

2.13.3.2 IOFB Injury

The risk of endophthalmitis and toxicosis has a great impact on timing, although there are other factors to consider (Fig. 2.13.2[2]; Table 2.13.1). Tables 2.13.2–2.13.4 provide details on several additional, important issues that need to be assessed. Also, a comparison of a large series of eyes with IOFB injury, encompassing a 5-decade interval, is given in Table 2.13.5.

Below is a brief review of the surgical steps in the actual management of eyes with a retained FB. The information is presented according to the location of the IOFB.[3]

Controversial

As a general rule, a fresh IOFB should not be left in the eye; however, if the IOFB is verifiably inert, there is a sign or elevated risk of endophthalmitis, and no intraocular pathology has been caused, surgery may entail more complication than that to which the IOFB might lead. An individual decision must be made regarding management (see Chap. 1.4). The same dilemma arises if an old, symptomless IOFB is accidentally found (see later in this chapter).

2.13.3.2.1 Anterior Chamber

With regard to the anterior chamber:

- With rare exceptions, the entry wound should be closed and a paracentesis prepared for extraction.
- Only occasionally should a direct cut-down be employed, e.g., if the IOFB is very large or stuck in the angle or iris.

2 The understandable anxiety of the patient to have the foreign object removed from the eye as soon as possible adds to the general feeling of urgency.

3 Corneal and scleral FBs are technically not IOFBs; these are discussed in Chaps. 2.2 and 2.3, respectively.

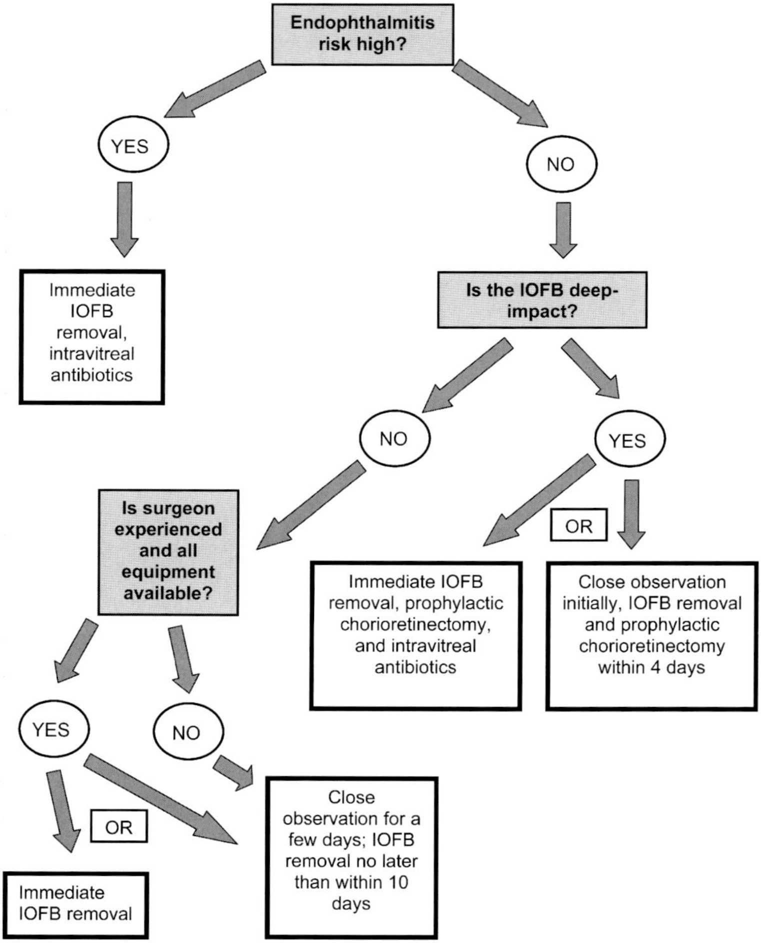

Fig. 2.13.2 Flowchart showing the timing recommendations for eyes with IOFB injury. If the IOFB is in the posterior segment, its removal is almost always performed in the context of a complete vitrectomy (see text for further details)

Table 2.13.1 Timing of intervention in the management of eyes with IOFB injury: literature review

Published finding/recommendation	Comment
"IOFB removal within 24 h may in some clinical situations reduce the endophthalmitis risk" [12]	Triaging the cases was not random but based on surgeon availability; case characteristics were not balanced; the advantages of emergency removal therefore cannot be confirmed
"IOFB removal within 24 hours significantly reduces the endophthalmitis risk" [16]	The endophthalmitis rate was slightly higher in eyes with (7.4%) than without (5.1%) IOFB removal; in 91% of patients the endophthalmitis was already present when the patient presented; delay in wound closure was more important a risk factor than a delay in IOFB removal
Delay in vitrectomy and IOFB removal does not increase the endophthalmitis risk [6, 11, 17]	It is possible that the series were of insufficient power to detect the difference in outcome
Despite an average delay of 21 days from injury to IOFB removal, none of the 79 eyes developed endophthalmitis [8]	War injuries in a dry climate; severe trauma in many eyes and soil contamination may have occurred commonly
Endophthalmitis does not have an adverse effect on the outcome [9]	It is possible that the series was not of sufficient power to detect the difference in outcome; in 100% of patients the endophthalmitis was already present when the patient presented
"IOFB need not be considered an absolute indication for immediate intervention" [13]	The final visual acuity was independent of the interval between injury and IOFB removal – the results were actually better in the delayed-intervention group
"Prompt surgical intervention, the use of intravitreal antibiotics in high-risk-type injuries, and the possible use of vitrectomy surgery may reduce the incidence and severity of endophthalmitis" [18]	Of the 27 eyes, 26% had a positive intraocular culture; 17% of eyes underwent surgery later than 24 h post-injury (as late as 5 months); no case of endophthalmitis

Table 2.13.1 *(continued)* Timing of intervention in the management of eyes with IOFB injury: literature review

Published finding/recommendation	Comment
"There was no significant association between length of time to removal of IOFB and poor visual outcome" [26]	9% of patients presented with endophthalmitis; the median time to removal was 9 days (range 5–18 days)

Table 2.13.2 Important issues influencing the management of eyes with IOFB injury

Issue	Comment
Reliability of history	While most patients notice that an object hit their eyes and caused pain and visual loss, some people experience no adverse effect, and cannot recall any even if asked. Those who were bystanders are more likely not to have noticed the injury
Scleral vs corneal wound	Corneal entry means that the FB lost more of its momentum[1] and is therefore less likely to cause serious damage [3]
Endophthalmitis risk: average vs high	High risk: lens injury [24]; soil contamination/rural setting [2]; and the presence of copper (the impact of timing is discussed in Table 2.13.1)
Prophylactic antibiotics and method of application[2]	Some form of prophylaxis is recommended, even though there is no consensus in the literature as to the route of administration. It appears reasonable to use oral antibiotics (e.g., ciprofloxacin, moxifloxacin) if the risk of endophthalmitis is average; in high risk cases an intravitreal route is recommended (vancomycin, ceftazidine; see Chap. 2.17 for more details)
Wound length	The relation between wound length and the occurrence of retinal lesions due to impact is inversely proportional [15]
Location of retinal impact site	If the wound is corneal and an iris defect has also occurred, they provide trajectory information regarding the likely impact site (see Fig. 2.7.3)

Table 2.13.2 *(continued)* Important issues influencing the management of eyes with IOFB injury

Issue	Comment
Risk of retinal impact site	71% for a single and 21% for two or more [17]. It is always important to carefully weigh the options regarding treatment of the impact site (Fig. 2.13.4)
Toxicosis (Table 2.13.3 shows additional details)	Copper content can lead to an acute, endophthalmitis-like condition or to chronic chalcosis if not removed in time [20]. Because of the danger of acute loss of vision, IOFBs containing copper should be removed as soon as possible [7]. Once the threat of the acute reaction passes, the toxicosis takes longer to develop than with ferrous IOFBs
	Ferrous IOFBs may cause siderosis, but its onset is virtually never instantaneous. If the patient presents with an acute IOFB, it should be removed; if a chronic, symptomless IOFB is encountered, the risk of siderosis development must be weighed against the risk of intervention. If observation is the selected option, serial ERGs[3] and slit lamp examinations should be performed
The importance of accurate preoperative localization of the IOFB	In principle, it is very useful for the surgeon to know the exact location of the IOFB. However, the IOFB may shift position following the test; accepting this possibility can spare the surgeon of a major intraoperative frustration. If the IOFB is not readily found during vitrectomy, its most likely "hiding place" is one of the following: – Inferiorly, behind the iris or in the peripheral vitreous – In the angle[4] – Subretinally, usually in a pool of blood – In the infusion-collecting cassette: it may have been inadvertently removed with the vitrectomy probe if the IOFB was very small or fragile
The need for vitrectomy with a posterior segment IOFB	If the IOFB is in the vitreous and no significant other pathology (media opacity interfering with retinal inspection or major retinal damage) is present, the IOFB can be removed with forceps or an IOM via ophthalmoscopic control[5]

Table 2.13.2 *(continued)* Important issues influencing the management of eyes with IOFB injury

Issue	Comment
Instrumentation	For ferrous IOFBs, a strong IOM is the most ideal instrument; for nonmagnetic IOFBs, several other options are available (Table 2.13.4)
Determining the optimal site and size of the surgical incision for IOFB removal	For most IOFBs in the posterior segment, the pars plana suffices; if the IOFB is very large, a limbal route may be preferred[6] The cross-section of the IOFB must be measured by comparing it to the diameter of the vitrectomy probe;[7] the incision should be slightly larger than what this cross-sectional dimension suggests;[8] the choroid should be incised separately to counter its elasticity

[1] This is due to the lens, not the cornea.

[2] Antibiotics may be a double-edged sword. They may temporarily mask the infection and delay the diagnosis of endophthalmitis; this is a risk especially if less than the full antibiotic dosage has been used (because the patient stopped taking it or the ophthalmologist did not prescribe the recommended strength).

[3] Every 3 months in the first, every 6 months in the next 2, and annually after the third year

[4] Very rarely an IOFB, which has entered the eye from the side when the eye looked the other direction, can take a postero-anterior course intraocularly: it then comes to rest anterior to its entry site.

[5] Because the image is inverted, considerable experience in this technique is necessary.

[6] If the eye is phakic, the lens must obviously be sacrificed.

[7] 0.89 mm if 20 g

[8] Losing the IOFB during extraction can cause a retinal break just posterior to sclerotomy or a retinal laceration in the posterior pole where the IOFB landed.

Table 2.13.3 Factors to consider related to toxicosis[a]

Symptoms	Signs
Chalcosis (chronic) [5]	Deteriorating visual acuity
	Kayser–Fleischer ring
	Sunflower cataract
	Greenish discoloration of the iris
	Chronic uveitis
	Glaucoma
	Vitreous opacities
	ERG changes
Siderosis [19, 25, 27]	Brownish deposits on the corneal endothelium
	Brownish discoloration of the iris (heterochromia[9])
	Dilated, nonreactive pupil[10]
	Yellowish cataract with brown capsular deposits
	Glaucoma
	Pigmentary degeneration of the retina
	Optic disc hyperemia, edema
	ERG changes
Treatment:	*Chalcosis or siderosis*
	Even in advanced cases, IOFB removal and the treatment of complications such as cataract extraction can bring improvement

[9] The difference in color between the two irises is easily appreciated only if the iris had a light color originally. Since heterochromia may have been present since birth and the patient may be unaware, a pre-injury photograph may be needed for comparison.

[10] Dissociation between reaction to light and accommodation, and hypersensitive reaction to weak miotics, may also be present.

[a] Also called metallosis.

Table 2.13.4 Instrumentation for IOFB removal

Instrument	Advantages	Disadvantages
EEM (Fig. 1.6.1)	Simple to use; no need to enter the eye	Effective only in acute cases, before encapsulation of the IOFB occurs The intraocular flight path of the IOFB is beyond the surgeon's control;[11] the outcome is significantly worse if EEM, rather than IOM or forceps, is used [17, 26]
IOM	The extraction is entirely under the surgeon's control[12]	None if the IOM is strong, its working distance is short, the magnetic pull force is directional, and the magnet's power does not diminish with time[13]
Forceps	Suitable for removing non-magnetic IOFBs	Depending on the IOFB characteristics,[14] several different types of forceps may have to be available Extensive intraocular manipulations of the IOFB[15] are often needed, and the threat of iatrogenic retinal injury is not negligible If the extraction incision is not large enough, the IOFB can get lost
Snare [10]	Able to grab even large IOFBs	If the IOFB has a long axis, its position must be adjusted so that the IOFB can be fed into a smaller sclerotomy: this requires considerable intraocular manipulations of the IOFB Considerable intraocular manipulations of the IOFB are often needed, and the threat of iatrogenic retinal injury is not negligible

[11] Complications from unintentional IOFB impact during extraction are fairly common.

[12] Unlike with an EEM, the instrument moves toward the IOFB; the path of the instrument and the IOFB is entirely determined by the surgeon.

[13] If the magnetic pull force does diminish with time, the instrument needs to be remagnetized.

[14] Size, shape, and surface texture

[15] i.e., to ensure a firm grab (the IOFB's position at the initial pickup is rarely a secure one) and to align it with the sclerotomy (so that the IOFB's entry into the sclerotomy is with its smallest cross-section)

Table 2.13.5 Large series of eyes with IOFB injury: a comparison after a 5-decade interval (%). *VA* visual acuity

Variable	555 cases, 1954 [22]	567 cases, 2005 USEIR[a]
Posterior IOFB	35	53
Vitreous hemorrhage	5 (5)	48 (370)
Retinal detachment	2 (10)	20 (23)
VA <20/200	42 (?)	31 (56)
VA 20/200–20/25	34 (?)	55 (39)
VA 20/20	25 (?)	14 (5)
Enucleation	20	8

Preoperative figures are in parentheses

[a] Unpublished data

- The paracentesis should be 90–180° away from the IOFB at a convenient location to increase the ease of manipulations and to provide for maximal flexibility.
- The endothelium and the lens must be protected by injecting viscoelastics before removal.
- The pupil may have to be constricted. This helps protect the lens and bring an IOFB that is lying on the surface of iris (or is buried in it) to a more central location.

2.13.3.2.2 Lens

With regard to the lens:

- Extraction of the lens is not necessary if there is no cataract or the anterior capsule's lesion appears to have healed (Fig. 2.13.3). Early cataract formation is not inevitable just because the capsule has been breached [21].

- The IOFB's enclosure by the lens[4] does not necessarily imply that the eye is protected against siderosis [14].
- If the lens to be removed, lensectomy, ICCE, ECCE, or, in most cases, phacoemulsification, are all valid options; the decision is based on the individual case. The potential for vitreous prolapse should always be kept in mind (see Chap. 2.7).
- Concurrent IOL implantation is encouraged unless there is major damage to the posterior segment or it is impossible to preoperatively determine the correct IOL power.

2.13.3.2.3 Intravitreal

Pearl

If an IOFB is in the midvitreous and has not caused any posterior segment pathology, it may be removed with an IOM or a forceps without performing vitrectomy. If, however, vitreous hemorrhage or a retinal lesion is present, a complete vitrectomy is necessary in conjunction with IOFB extraction.

- Remove as much of the vitreous as needed until the IOFB is clearly visible.
- If the IOFB is visible, bring it into the midvitreous with the IOM or forceps. If the IOFB is hidden by vitreous hemorrhage, carefully remove the vitreous until the IOFB becomes visible.
- Withdraw the light pipe and use the vitrectomy probe to severe any vitreous attachment to the IOFB.
- Prepare the removal site (Table 2.13.2).
- Make sure that no vitreous remains attached to the IOFB.
- Remove the vitrectomy probe, put a plug in this sclerotomy, and gape the extraction sclerotomy with a tooth forceps.
- Slowly remove the IOFB.
- Put a suture in the sclerotomy to restore it to its original size.

4 i.e., the FB is completely intralenticular, not protruding.

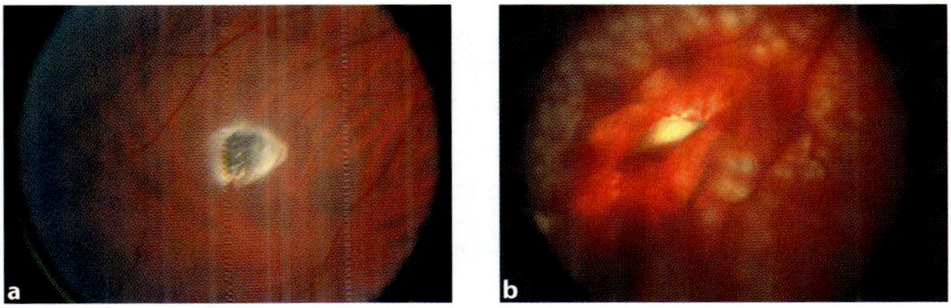

Fig. 2.13.4 Retinal impact sites. **a** The IOFB is lying on the retina surface. It has caused a fibrinous reaction, which must not be mistaken for endophthalmitis. Nevertheless the finding does require close observation for the first 24 h. A much larger area of retinal opacification is also seen. This may eventually develop into a contusion retinopathy. A tiny amount of retinal hemorrhage is visible at 12 o'clock from the IOFB. Since a retinal break (laceration) has not occurred, laser prophylaxis does not appear to be indicated around the current position of the IOFB, and neither is it likely to be needed at the margin of the opaque area. **b** A typical deep-impact IOFB with chorioretinal bleeding. The lesion has been surrounded by laser spots; these may be helpful in keeping the retina attached as far as the retinal break is concerned, but they take several weeks to reach full strength. The real danger, however, is scar formation, against which the laser does not offer protection. Prophylactic chorioretinectomy, performed within a few days, should be considered (see Chap. 2.14)

- Complete the vitrectomy.
- Search for retinal impact site(s) and determine whether they require laser treatment (Fig. 2.13.4).

Controversial

Laser treatment for an impact that is purely[5] retinal is unnecessary if all the vitreous has been removed and the traction potential has been eliminated [1].[6] Conversely, properly executed laser retinopexy does not increase the risk of complications and may help the surgeon sleep better. ("I've done all that's possible to prevent retinal detachment.") An individual decision should be made (see Chap. 2.9).

5 i.e., not involving the choroid and the sclera, and not causing a subretinal hemorrhage.
6 Such complete vitreous removal is possible posterior to the equator but not anteriorly.

- Examine the peripheral retina with scleral indentation;[7] obviously, the equator must also be inspected, especially in young people.
- Consider endolaser cerclage even in the absence of a visible retinal break (see Chap. 2.9).
- Carefully weigh the benefits and disadvantages of gas tamponade.

2.13.3.2.4 Retinal

With regard to retinal IOFB injury:

- Complete the vitrectomy first; it is especially important no to leave any vitreous at the IOFB site. If the vitreous is impossible to detach, circumscribe it at the impact site, leaving only a "stump" over the IOFB (see Chap. 2.9).
- Make sure that the IOFB is free and mobile. If it is not, use a *sharp* instrument to break all its connections from the retina and/or to open the fibrous capsule if one has already formed. Never use a magnet or blunt dissection to break the IOFB free.

Pearl

The danger during sharp tissue dissection is hemorrhage, which can be prevented with diathermy. The danger during blunt dissection is that it is the tissue the "decides" where to separate: it is much less under the surgeon's control than during sharp dissection (see Chap. 2.5).

- The remaining steps of surgery have been described above.

2.13.3.2.5 Subretinal

With regard to subretinal IOFB injury:

- Complete the vitrectomy first; it is especially important not to leave any vitreous at the IOFB site.

---

7 Even if extreme caution has been used, it is not unusual to find a break just posterior to the extraction sclerotomy.

- If the retina is *detached*, create a retinotomy in the midperiphery in an area where a PVD exists or has been created. If possible, select one of the superior quadrants. The retinotomy should be as far away from major vessels as possible, and it should not be too large. Retinal elasticity permits passage of an IOFB whose cross-section is larger than the area of the retinotomy itself.[8] Use an IOM if the IOFB is ferrous; insert it through the retinotomy and carefully remove the IOFB.
- If the IOFB is under an *attached* retina, the ideal retinotomy site is right on top of the IOFB. No fibrous capsule is expected to occur, and the IOFB is usually quite free: if pushed from one side through the retina, it will actually move.[9] If subretinal blood is present, it may have to be irrigated first. The retinotomy should be large enough[10] to comfortably let the IOFB pass through[11].
- If the IOFB must be moved in the subretinal space before extraction,[12] a small retinal detachment, incorporating the IOFB and the retinotomy site, must be created first. It is preferable to use viscoelastics than BSS for this purpose: the viscoelastic provides protection for the photoreceptors and the size of the detached area is easier to control. The viscoelastic can be aspirated after IOFB removal to reattach the retina.
- In most cases, the IOFB has entered the subretinal space through the retina, not from the scleral side. The site of this retinal lesion should be identified; this and the extraction retinotomy may have to be treated with laser (see above).
- The remaining steps of surgery have been described above.

8 i.e., in cases of a detached retina., the retinotomy can be slightly smaller than the size of subretinal IOFB.

9 Not that this is recommended: the photoreceptors and RPE would be injured in the process.

10 This larger retinotomy reduces the risk of causing a iatrogenic retinal detachment.

11 i.e., in cases of an attached retina, the retinotomy should be slightly larger than the size of subretinal IOFB.

12 e.g., because it is under a major blood vessel or is subfoveal.

2.13.3.2.6 Choroidal/Scleral (Deep-impact IOFBs)

In most acute cases, there is subretinal/choroidal bleeding and the retina is initially attached. There are two majors risks associated: first, the creation of an iatrogenic retinal detachment and reopening the posterior wound intraoperatively; and second, severe PVR developing postoperatively. Careful surgery is needed to avoid the first risk; prophylactic chorioretinectomy is recommended for the second (see below and Chap. 2.14). If prophylactic chorioretinectomy is not performed, the rate of PVR in eyes with the IOFB injuring the choroid ("deep impact") reaches 38%.[13]

- If the IOFB causes a major retinal impact and especially if deeper tissues (choroid, retina) are also involved, the vitreous may be "burned" into this impact site, making its detachment impossible. In such cases the vitreous must be circumcised here, rather than forcefully detached, which would risk creating a retinal break and detachment (see Chap. 2.9).

> **Controversial**
>
> It may be technically difficult to remove an IOFB that is embedded deeply ("stuck") in the sclera. Leaving a ferrous IOFB behind presents a siderosis risk, even if the IOFB is encapsulated [23]. Conversely, if the IOFB has perforated the sclera, forced removal can reopen the wound, which is a difficult-to-control complication (see Chap. 2.14). An individual decision must be made.

- If the IOFB is very difficult to mobilize, the surgeon probably has to leave it in situ for the time being and address the problem later. The risks vs benefits of *observation* with the potential of siderosis development vs *reoperation* at a later date must be discussed in detail with the patient, from whom the decision preferably comes (see Chap. 1.4). The probability of successful IOFB removal is not necessarily higher during a subsequent attempt, but the risk of wound reopening may be smaller.

---

13 Unpublished study, Gregory L., Birmingham, Alabama, based on USEIR data.

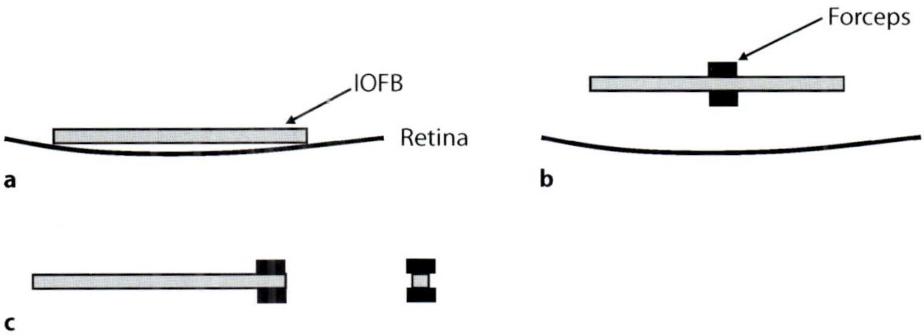

Fig. 2.13.5 The need to adjust the IOFB's position if a forceps or a snare is used. **a,b** The initial grab: the IOFB is grasped in its mid section to allow for maximal stability and control. **c** For the actual extraction, the IOFB has to be grabbed at its end. This means that the grab is insecure, but the length of the extraction sclerotomy can be short

- As in all eyes with choroidal and scleral involvement, the risk of PVR is sufficiently great to warrant at least consideration of prophylactic chorioretinectomy to prevent a developing scar from incarcerating the retina and lead to tractional retinal detachment (see Chap. 2.14).
- The remaining steps of surgery have been described above.

2.13.3.3 Nonmagnetic IOFBs

For the roughly 20% of IOFBs that are not ferrous, the forceps or the snare are available as extraction tools (see above; Fig. 2.13.5). An epiretinally located IOFB can also be floated up by PFCL and then removed.

Pitfall

If PFCL is used to bring an epiretinal object closer to the sclerotomy, there is always a danger that the heavy liquid will be layered on top of, rather than underneath, the object (see Chap. 2.7). If an IOFB with a sharp edge must be removed, an additional danger is that the PFCL will first push it sideways, causing a retinal lesion.

DO:

- despite a negative slit lamp examination, assume that a wound is present if the injury was caused by a sharp object; even if the visual acuity is good and the media are clear, a retinal injury may be present, making it certain that a scleral wound has occurred
- consider immediate surgery to remove the IOFB and the infected medium if the injury poses a high risk of endophthalmitis; otherwise, an individual decision regarding the timing of the intervention must be made
- consider prophylactic chorioretinectomy if the IOFB has caused a deep impact

DON'T:

- forgo ordering a CT if the slightest doubt exists about the possibility of a retained FB
- let the magnet's power to rip the IOFB free from a capsule or even to "cut through" the choroid; controlled opening of the capsule and choroid with a sharp instrument is much less traumatic or risky
- use an EEM to extract a ferrous IOFB; a strong IOM provides complete surgeon control and reduces the risk of iatrogenic damage substantially

Summary

Penetrating and JOFB injuries have a lot in common, but the latter cause vastly more concern to the patient – and to the ophthalmologist – because of the presence of a foreign object in the eye. Although these injuries have an increased risk of endophthalmitis their prognosis is relatively good, presumed the recommended rules of management are followed.

References

[1] Ambler J, Meyers S (1991) Management of intraretinal metallic foreign bodies without retinopexy in the absence of retinal detachment. Ophthalmology 98: 391–394

[2] Boldt H, Pulido J, Blodi C et al. (1989) Rural endophthalmitis. Ophthalmology 101: 332–341

[3] Brown I (1968) Nature of injury. Int Ophthalmol Clin 8: 147–152
[4] Bryden FM, Pyott AA, Bailey M, McGhee CNJ (1990) Real time ultrasound in the assessment of intraocular foreign bodies. Eye 4: 727–731
[5] Budde WM, Junemann A (1998) Chalcosis oculi. Klin Monatsbl Augenheilk 212: 184–185
[6] Camacho H, Mejia LF (1991) Extraction of intraocular foreign bodies by pars plana vitrectomy. Ophthalmologica 202: 173–179
[7] Cooling RJ, McLeod D, Blach RK, Leaver PK (1981) Closed microsurgery in the management of intraocular foreign bodies. Trans Ophthalmol Soc UK 181–183
[8] Coyler M, Weber E, Weichel E, Dick J, Bower K, Ward T, Haller J (in press) Delayed intraocular foreign body removal without endophthalmitis during Operations Iraqi and Enduring Freedom. Ophthalmology
[9] De Souza S, Howcroft MJ (1999) Management of posterior segment intraocular foreign bodies: 14 years' experience. Can J Ophthalmol 34: 23–29
[10] Eckardt C, Eckert T, Eckardt U (2006) Memory snare for extraction of intraocular foreign bodies. Retina 26: 845–847
[11] El-Asrar AM, Al-Amro SA, Khan NM, Kangave D (2000) Visual outcome and prognostic factors after vitrectomy for posterior segment foreign bodies. Eur J Ophthalmol 10: 304–311
[12] Jonas JB, Budde WM (1999) Early versus late removal of retained intraocular foreign bodies. Retina 19: 193–197
[13] Karel I, Diblik P (1995) Management of posterior segment foreign bodies and long-term results. Eur J Ophthalmol 5: 113–118
[14] Keeney AH (1971) Intralenticular foreign bodies. Arch Ophthalmol 86: 499–501
[15] Kuhn F, Mester V, Morris R (2002) Intraocular foreign bodies. Thieme, New York, pp 1201
[16] Lansing M, Glaser B, Liss H, Hanham A, Thompson J, Sjaarda R, Gordon A (1993) The effect of pars plana vitrectomy and transforming growth factor-beta 2 without epiretinal membrane peeling on full-thickness macular hole. Ophthalmology 100: 868–872
[17] Mester V, Kuhn F (2000) Ferrous intraocular foreign bodies retained in the posterior segment: management options and results. Int Ophthalmol 22: 355–362
[18] Mieler WF, Ellis MK, Williams DF, Han DP (1990) Retained intraocular foreign bodies and endophthalmitis. Ophthalmology 97: 1532–1538
[19] Monterio ML, Ulrich RF, Imes RK, Fung WE, Hoyt WF (1984) Iron mydriasis. Am J Ophthalmol 97: 794–796
[20] Neubauer H (1979) The Montgomery Lecture, 1979. Ocular metallosis. Trans Ophthalmol Soc UK 99: 502–510
[21] Pieramici D, Capone AJ, Rubsamen P, Roseman R (1996) Lens preservation after intraocular foreign body injuries. Ophthalmology 103: 1563–1567

[22] Roper-Hall MJ (1954) Review of 555 cases of intra-ocular foreign bodies with special reference to prognosis. Br J Ophthalmol 38: 65–99
[23] Sneed SR (1988) Ocular siderosis. Arch Ophthalmol 106: 997
[24] Thompson W, Rubsamen P, Flynn H, Schiffman J, Cousins S (1995) Endophthalmitis after penetrating trauma. Risk factors and visual acuity outcomes. Ophthalmology 102: 1696–1701
[25] Weiss MJ, Hofeldt AJ, Behrens M, Fisher K (1997) Ocular siderosis. Diagnosis and management. Retina 17: 105–108
[26] Wickham L, Xing W, Bunce C, Sullivan P (2006) Outcomes of surgery for posterior segment intraocular foreign bodies-a retrospective review of 17 years of clinical experience. Graefe's Arch Clin Exp Ophthalmol
[27] Yamaguchi K, Tamai M (1989) Siderosis bulbi induced by intraocular lens implantation. Ophthalmologica 198: 113–115

2.14 Perforating Injuries

Ferenc Kuhn

2.14.1 Introduction

Eyes with a perforating injury[1] pose unique challenges for the surgeon because access to, and therefore closure of, the posterior (exit) wound is usually impossible, making retinal incarceration in the wound likely. This incarceration may occur primarily (i.e., at the time of the injury or during wound closure if it was possible to suture it) or secondarily (i.e., as the scar forms at the wound). Presence of a posterior (exit) wound therefore has important management but also prognostic implications: in a metaanalysis of 15 published reports, the anatomical success rate was only 69%, the functional[2] only 56% [4].

2.14.2 Evaluation

The possibility of an exit wound should be suspected based on information gained from history; objects that are sharp, short in one diameter but long in the other, and have significant momentum are more likely to perforate the eyeball than objects that are large and blunt. Detailed knowledge of the

1 An injury with internal scleral (although not full thickness) or at least choroidal involvement may have similar consequences to a trauma that is truly perforating, and should be treated accordingly.

2 Defined as a final visual acuity of 5/200 or better.

object's characteristics (e.g., size and shape) along with the circumstances of the injury (e.g., the force of the strike, the patient's distance from the event) must be sought – information of the object *and* the injury is necessary to make an intelligent prediction.[3] (See Chaps. 1.9 and 2.11 for details on evaluation.)

2.14.3 Management

In general, the steps outlined in Table 2.11.1 should be followed; there are, however, additional factors to consider:

- Wound closure. The exit wound is rarely located anteriorly enough to allow convenient access and suturing. Forceful inspection and suturing of the wound must be avoided (see Chap. 2.3).
- Spontaneous closure of the wound. This starts by an outside-in mechanism[4] within hours [2], and clinical experience shows that in 24 h most wounds are sealed with sufficient strength so as to withstand the typical IOP values employed during vitrectomy.
- Timing of reconstruction. Whether a staged approach or a primary comprehensive surgery is performed depends on factors described previously (see Chaps. 1.8, 2.11, 2.12). As a general rule, it is much less urgent to indicate primary comprehensive surgery in an eye with a perforating injury compared with a ruptured eye.[5]
- The PVR threat remains significant (Table 2.14.1), even with early vitrectomy and laser treatment, and despite the use of scleral buckling [5].

3 A good example is one of the author's latest cases: an 11-year-old boy was injured while sharpening a stick with a knife. He was pulling the pocket knife toward himself, the knife slipped, and caused a 9-mm-long corneal laceration; the iris and lens were also injured. To cause such a long wound, the blade had to penetrate deep into the eye. A perforating injury was therefore suspected, and confirmed during vitrectomy.

4 i.e., from the episclera inward.

5 The wound is smaller; therefore, the incarceration is more likely to be secondary (see above).

Table 2.14.1 The PVR rates and visual outcomes in different types of injury (%).

Injury type	PVR rate [1]	Final visual acuity[a]	
		<20/200	>20/40
Rupture[b]	21	80	11
Penetrating	15	34	46
IOFB[c]	11	34	44
Perforating	43	72	16

Both ruptures and IOFB injuries show a lower PVR incidence and better functional outcome here than they would if data had been collected only on ruptures with a posterior scleral wound or IOFBs with deep impact. In the USEIR, the PVR rate was 38% among eyes with deep-impact IOFB injury (see Chap. 2.13)

[a] Data from the USEIR database 2003.

[b] Includes eyes with *anterior* rupture (i.e., no chorioretinal injury or retinal incarceration; see Chap. 2.12).

[c] Includes eyes *without a deep impact* (i.e., no chorioscleral injury; see Chap. 2.13).

Irrespective of whether the scar results from the normal episcleral scar tissue growing intraocularly (see Fig. 2.12.1) or developing internally from the injured RPE/choroid, this scar is prone to incarcerate the retina and continue its growth (PVR).

- Even if scar formation stops in its early phase (i.e., it does not continue growing onto the retinal surface and lead to full-fledged PVR), the condition is still much more severe than an EMP. The deep scar involves the retina full thickness; scar contraction often creates radiating retinal folds (Fig. 2.14.1), which can reach into areas far away, including the macula, causing severe visual disturbance (Fig. 2.14.2).
- If the scar continues to grow, a typical PVR develops, although the origination site (i.e., the exit wound) almost always remains discernible.
- The best chance of dealing with the PVR problem appears to be early and proactive surgery (prophylactic chorioretinectomy [3]; Fig. 2.14.3; Table 2.14.2). It appears that this procedure is able to dramatically lower the PVR rate, prevent the formation of retinal folds, and improve the

prognosis. Dealing with the posterior wound (impact site) is always the last step of surgery.

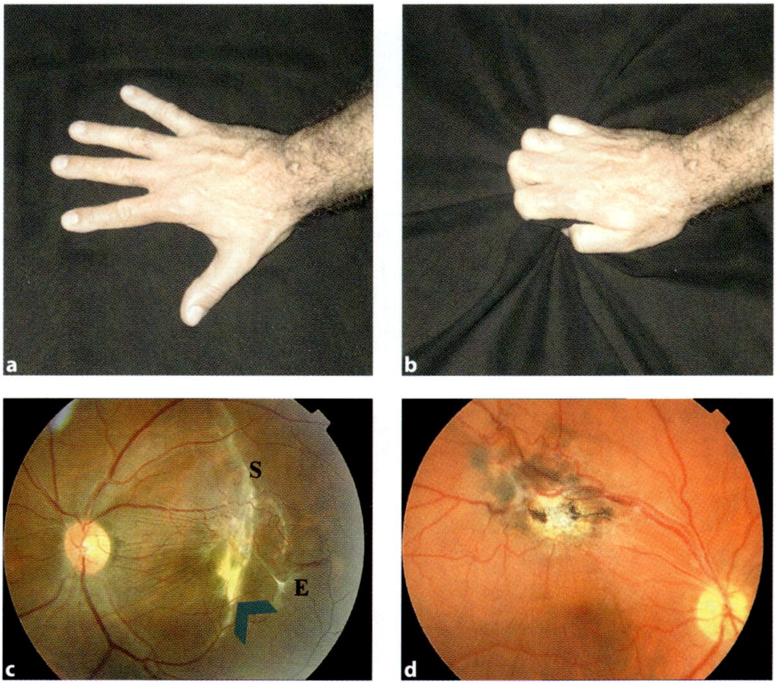

Fig. 2.14.1 Full-thickness retinal folds radiating from the exit wound in an eye with perforating injury. **a** The table cloth, representing the retina, is smooth; the scar, represented by the hand, has not yet grabbed it. **b** The scar is now fully developed, the table cloth has become the epicenter of full-thickness folds that radiate from this spot, reaching far into the distance. **c** Clinical example of scar growing subretinally (*S*) and epiretinally (*E*) from a juxtafoveal exit wound (*yellow area*; *arrowhead*). The scar causes radiating, full-thickness retinal folds in the maculopapillary bundle. The patient's visual complaints far exceed those that the scar alone would have caused: he is complaining more about the distortion[1] than about the scotoma. **d** In this case, the exit wound is rather far from the fovea, but the scar tissue causes major distortion of the superotemporal blood vessels and produces full-thickness retinal folds reaching into the fovea (Photographs C and D courtesy of V. Mester, Abu Dhabi, U.A.E.)

[1]The patient actually has to cover this eye so that "it does not bother his good eye."

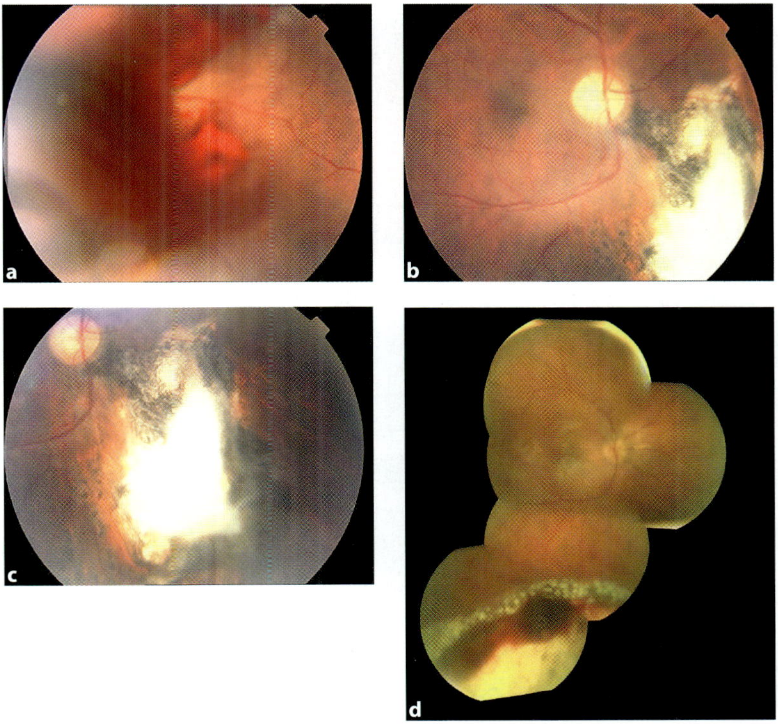

Fig. 2.14.2 Prophylactic chorioretinectomy for perforating injury. **a** Preoperative image showing intravitreal and subhyaloid hemorrhage. The exit wound is blocked from view. The patient underwent prophylactic chorioretinectomy, laser retinopexy, and silicone oil implantation. **b,c** Postoperative images after silicone oil removal. Bare sclera is visible at and around the exit wound, with RPE hypertrophy along the retinal edge; this is partially the result of the body's inflammatory response to the chorioretinectomy and partially due to the laser treatment. There is development of neither PVR nor retinal folds; the macula shows completely normal anatomy. (Courtesy of V. Mester, Abu Dhabi, U.A.E.). **d** This young boy sustained a posterior scleral rupture with retinal incarceration into a 12-mm wound. Prophylactic chorioretinectomy was performed 2 days post-injury; only SF_6 gas was used as tamponade. This photograph was taken on the first postoperative day[1]; the bare sclera and the laser spots are clearly visible. Six months post-injury, there is no PVR or retinal fold formation, and the visual acuity is 20/20

[1]Hence, the haziness of the image

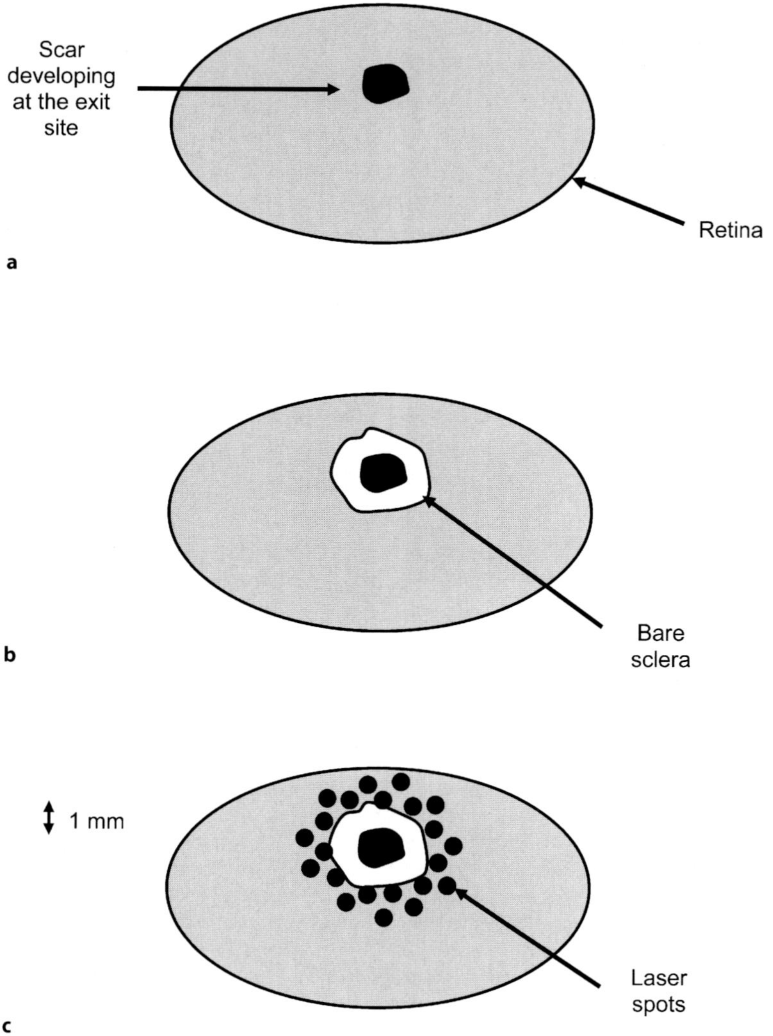

Fig. 2.14.3 Schematic representation of a prophylactic chorioretinectomy. **a** The exit wound and the developing scar. **b** After treatment (complete vitrectomy, followed by diathermy destruction of the choroid and retina), the scar remains intact, but it is now ringed by bare sclera. **c** Laser is applied on the remaining retinal edge

Table 2.14.2 Proactive treatment (prophylactic chorioretinectomy) in eyes with high-PVR-risk injury

Variable	Comment
Injury type	
Rupture	Especially dangerous is a wound too posterior to suture
	Even if the rupture is anterior, it may be impossible to suture it without retinal or at least vitreous incarceration
Penetrating injury	If the wound is large and posterior, the condition is similar to that described with rupture, or a direct chorioretinal injury may occur[1]
IOFB, deep impact	The impact causes damage to the RPE and choroid; in addition to bleeding, a heavy inflammatory response is induced
Perforating injury	A combination of what is presented here with rupture and deep-impact IOFB trauma
Incidence	Shown in Table 2.14.1
Consequence/pathophysiology	After it effectively closed the wound or healed the impact site, the emerging scar commonly does not stop but continues to grow on the retinal surface[2]. It may turn into a full-blown PVR or arrest itself and cause only radiating retinal folds; the latter is a much less severe problem, yet it may also lead to major visual impairment since these folds can reach into the macula even if the original site is at considerable distance
Historic treatment	The primary surgery is wound closure
	The secondary surgery is primarily for vitreous hemorrhage; the site of the wound/deep impact is usually lasered; should a retinal detachment already have occurred, it is also treated in the usual fashion
	If PVR develops, this is managed by repeat vitrectomy with or without scleral buckling; retinectomy and repeat laser are performed around the scar site
	The PVR commonly recurs, requiring re-repeat vitrectomies, often with re-retinectomy

[1]This should always be suspected if the injury was caused by a strong wire or scissors.

[2]Occasionally even subretinally

Table 2.14.2 (continued) Proactive treatment (prophylactic chorioretinectomy) in eyes with high-PVR-risk injury

Variable	Comment
Results with traditional treatment	Shown in Table 2.14.1
Results with proactive treatment[3]	In the author's pilot study, none of the five eyes developed PVR [3][4]
Timing of surgery and its primary goal	Early vitrectomy to prevent the scar from growing onto/from the undersurface of the scleral wound and onto the retina. The retina and choroid must be removed in a ring-like fashion around the wound/impact site, leaving an area of bare sclera to act as a barrier between the scar and the remaining retinal edge
Surgical steps	
Complete the vitrectomy	Partially illustrated in Fig. 2.14.3
Identify the site of the scleral wound or impact/exit site	See Chap. 2.9 The entire area must be visualized; use scleral indentation if necessary
Use the diathermy's highest power and completely surround the area[5]	The goal is not just to prevent bleeding but to destroy, necrotize, and burn away the retina and choroid.[6] Use of a diathermy probe with a blunt, rather than a sharp, tip is recommended. A 1-mm ring of bare sclera should be left behind,[7] but the scar itself remains intact. If the area of destruction were to involve the fovea, optic disc, or a major blood vessel, a sensible compromise regarding choroidal/retinal destruction would have to be sought
Surround the remaining retinal edge with laser	See Chap. 2.13 whether this is always necessary
Use gas or silicone oil tamponade	If complete vitreous removal has been achieved in the vicinity[8] and bare sclera surrounds the scar, gas tamponade may be sufficient

[3] A prospective, multicenter study (as suggested by W. Schrader, Würzburg, Germany) is now underway to evaluate the effectiveness of prophylactic chorioretinectomy in a much larger patient population (www.weironline.org). The study found that among its first 21 eyes, only 2 (10%) developed PVR; both were mild cases that were successfully treated.

[4]The idea of prophylactic chorioretinectomy came to the author upon observing no PVR in eyes undergoing vitrectomy with removal of the choroid and retina in eyes with malignant melanoma. It appears that the proliferative cells do not bridge the bare sclera to seed the retina if the scleral bridge is wide enough.

[5]Numerous small gas bubbles form during the procedure. In phakic eyes, these bubbles collect behind the lens if there is still vitreous there, making it easier and less risky for the surgeon to remove both the bubbles and the retrolental vitreous. In pseudophakic eyes the bubbles usually migrate away from the visual center.

[6]The goal is not to cut the retina and choroid with scissors or the vitrectomy probe, but to use the diathermy's heat to actually destroy the entire tissue here.

[7]i.e., the debris should be collected

[8]The lesion is posterior to the equator.

Pearl

The urgency to perform primary comprehensive surgery in an eye with *rupture* lies in the risk of retinal incarceration at the time of wound closure; the more posterior the wound, the higher this risk. In a *perforating* injury, the exit wound is rarely large enough to incarcerate the retina; the danger lies in events occurring postoperatively.

2.14.3.1 Intraoperative Wound Reopening

2.14.3.1.1 Risk Factors

The risk factors are as follows:

- Large wound
- Very fresh injury
- Older patient
- Significantly raised IOP (e.g., to stop an intraoperative hemorrhage).

2.14.3.1.2 Prevention

Prevention consists of:

Fig. 2.14.4 Schematic representation of IOP control during vitrectomy. **a** Traditional setup: the infusion bottle is directly connected to the eye through the infusion line. The IOP is regulated by up-or-down movements of the bottle, either electronically via the vitrectomy machine[1] or manually. The problem with this setup is that the true IOP value is never known since there is no adjustment based on the distance of the patient's head (eye) from the floor. **b** If (a) the air pump of the vitrectomy machine is used to drive the pressure inside the infusion bottle, and (b) the drip chamber of the infusion bottle is at the same distance from the floor as the patient's eye, the air pressure set on the vitrectomy machine gives an accurate, digital reading of the actual IOP [6].

[1] Newer machines even translate the bottle's distance from the floor to mmHg.

- Delaying vitrectomy until the posterior wound is firmly closed[6]
- Controlling and monitoring the IOP very closely during vitrectomy (Fig. 2.14.4)

2.14.3.1.3 Recognition

The pathognomic signs are:

- Full-thickness sclero-chorio-retinal folds radiating from the wound
- Rapidly collapsing globe due to increased intraorbital pressure exerted on the posterior sclera

2.14.3.1.4 Management

With regard to management:

- In the unlikely event that a posterior wound reopens during vitrectomy, the infusion must be turned off or at least significantly lowered so that additional fluid loss into the orbit is stopped.
- Silicone oil injection should be started as fast as possible, which reconstitutes the IOP and prevents further collapse of the eyeball. The amount of silicone oil implanted is usually half to two-thirds of the volume the eye would normally take.

6 As mentioned previously, the risk of wound reopening is much smaller if the injury is perforating, rather than a rupture.

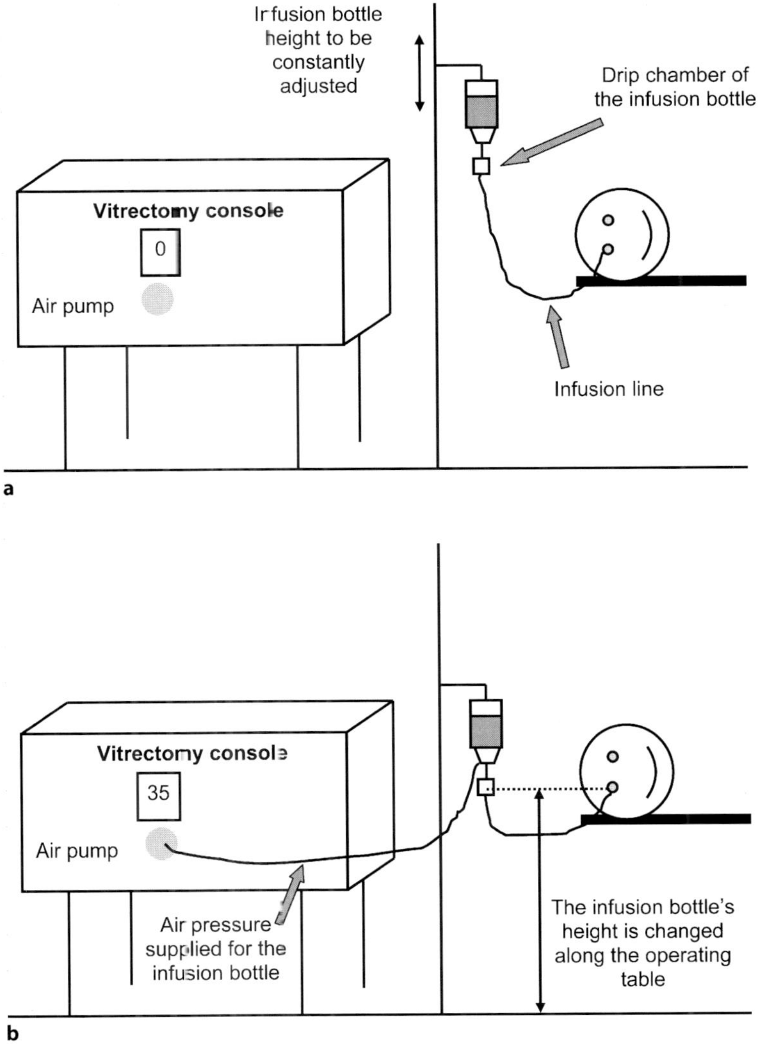
Infusion bottle height to be constantly adjusted
Drip chamber of the infusion bottle
Vitrectomy console
0
Air pump
Infusion line
a
Vitrectomy console
35
Air pump
Air pressure supplied for the infusion bottle
The infusion bottle's height is changed along the operating table
b

- The orbital volume may be so greatly increased by the BSS (even silicone oil may be extruded into the orbit) that occasionally it is difficult to close the lids. In these rare cases the eye is treated as if temporary lagophthalmos were present.
- The orbital fluid rapidly reabsorbs, and a reoperation can be performed in a few days. It is also possible to suture the exit wound using an *ab interno* approach (J. Schmidt et al., unpublished data).

DO:

- try to verify whether the injury was penetrating or perforating
- if you are uncertain or if the injury is likely/definitely perforating, consider vitrectomy with prophylactic chorioretinectomy within the first few days post-injury

DON'T:

- try to suture-close an exit wound that is too posterior for convenient access
- panic in the unlikely case of intraoperative reopening of the exit wound: silicone oil implantation allows controlling the situation and the abandoned procedure can be completed in a subsequent surgery within days

Summary

Perforating injuries typically have very poor prognosis. Fortunately, in most eyes the outcome is poor not because the injury caused irreversible damage upon impact but because of subsequent scarring originating from the exit wound. Early prophylactic chorioretinectomy is a very promising procedure in preventing this complication and improving the functional outcome.

References

[1] Cardillo JA, Stout JT, LaBree L, Azen SP, Omphroy L, Cui JZ, Kimura H, Hinton DR, Ryan SJ (1997) Post-traumatic proliferative vitreoretinopathy. The epidemiologic profile, onset, risk factors, and visual outcome. Ophthalmology 104: 1166–1173

[2] Cleary PE, Ryan SJ (1979) Experimental posterior penetrating eye injury in the rabbit. II. Histology of wound, vitreous, and retina. Br J Ophthalmol 63: 312–321

[3] Kuhn F, Mester V, Morris R (2004) A proactive treatment approach for eyes with perforating injury. Klin Monatsbl Augenheilk 221: 622–628

[4] Schwartz S, Mieler WF (2002) management of eyes with perforating injury. In: Kuhn F, Pieramici D (eds) Ocular trauma: principles and practice. Thieme, New York, pp 273–279

[5] Vatne HO, Syrdalen P (1985) Vitrectomy in double perforating eye injuries. Acta Ophthalmol (Copenh) 63: 552–556

[6] Witherspoon CD, Morris R, Goggans WE (1986) Automated regulation of fluid infusion pressure during vitrectomy. Arch Ophthalmol 104: 1551

2.15 Injury Involving the Entire Globe

Ferenc Kuhn, Robert Morris, C. Douglas Witherspoon

2.15.1 Introduction

Open globe injuries[1] may cause substantial damage to the eye, making the situation akin to that of a polytraumatized person: the condition of one pathology influences the condition and treatment of another (Fig. 2.2.14). The most serious of the potential scenarios is when the retina requires major surgery urgently but the cornea has become opaque and interferes with visibility. Such an injury represents one of the most challenging indications for the ocular traumatologist, and the number of viable options is limited.

2.15.2 Evaluation

The cornea is so badly damaged that even the color of the iris may be impossible to determine at the slit lamp (Fig. 2.2.14). The condition of the cornea may be due to the presence of multiple wounds with excessive edema and/or blood staining. The lens, if present at all (Fig. 2.12.2), is rarely clear. The vitreous hemorrhage is usually very severe, and the retina is often incarcerated in the wound. Early retinal detachment and the development of PVR are frequent complications. The visual acuity is typically in the NLP to HM range. The treatment should not be based on whether the visual acuity is NLP or greater (see Chap. 1.8).

1 Occasionally, a contusion can also inflict such damage.

2.15.3 Management Options

The outcome of the injury is primarily determined by the condition of the postequatorial retina.[2] The main question is to what extent the traumatized cornea interferes with posterior segment surgery. The following management options are available:

- *No surgery.* Abandoning the eye is equal to a death sentence: spontaneous improvement is unreasonable to expect. Early phthisis is likely.
- *Delayed surgery.* Vitrectomy is performed only when the cornea's interference with visibility is sufficiently reduced. Unfortunately, this is usually very late, and the prognosis of the injury is extremely poor.
- *Timely but limited surgery.* Vitrectomy is performed within the first 2 weeks, but it is not carried to completeness because the condition of the cornea does not permit it. The prognosis is very poor.
- *Incremental surgeries.* Posterior segment surgery is done in several surgical sessions. Even though performed early, each vitrectomy is incomplete, depending on the condition of the cornea. The disadvantages far outweigh the benefits; the prognosis is very poor.
- *Endoscopy-assisted vitrectomy.* The endoscopic approach has the advantage of bypassing the corneal interference (see Chap. 2.20). It also makes corneal transplantation potentially avoidable.[3] Endoscopy-assisted vitrectomy has its own, significant technical difficulties, mainly that is performed without stereoscopy and surgery is not bimanual, and it requires considerable experience. Another factor to consider is the inability to postoperatively inspect the retina until the media opacity clears. Nevertheless, EAV is a viable option and should be high on the surgeon's consideration list. In summary, the main advantage of the endoscope over the TKP is that the patient is spared the risks associated with PK if the corneal opacity is temporary.

---

2 Presuming that the optic nerve is not injured, the tissue (other than the postequatorial retina) with decisive impact on the outcome is the ciliary body (see Chap. 2.8).

3 Not all eyes sustain irreversibly damage; with time some corneas recover.

Cave

Use of the endoscope in an eye that has sustained major damage to both the anterior and posterior segments demands a surgeon who has great experience in both ocular traumatology and endoscopy (see Chap. 2.20).

- *Temporary keratoprosthesis vitrectomy.* Considering all options this is the most promising alternative. Most trauma specialists have sufficient experience in vitrectomy as well as in corneal grafting; if not, two specialists should operate in a joint procedure (see below). In summary, the main advantage of the TKP over the endoscope is that it provides early vision restoration to the patient and retinal inspection to the surgeon.

Pearl

There is no justification for abandoning eyes with serious anterior- and posterior segment trauma. Both the endoscope and the TKP allow the surgeon to perform uncompromising vitrectomy in the subacute period.

2.15.3.1 TKP Vitrectomy

The TKP is an artificial, temporary graft, replacing the patient's nontransparent cornea for the duration of posterior segment surgery (Fig. 2.15.1). Independent of design and material (Table 2.15.1), the TKP provides a crystal-clear view during vitrectomy while providing for the necessary closed globe environment. Ideally, a standard PK is performed at the conclusion of vitrectomy, replacing the TKP with donor tissue (Fig. 2.15.2). If a donor tissue is unavailable, two temporary solutions[4] are available: the TKP is left in the cornea or the patient's own damaged cornea is used as a graft.

4 Both are acceptable for a few days, and either of these solutions is preferred to delaying the vitrectomy

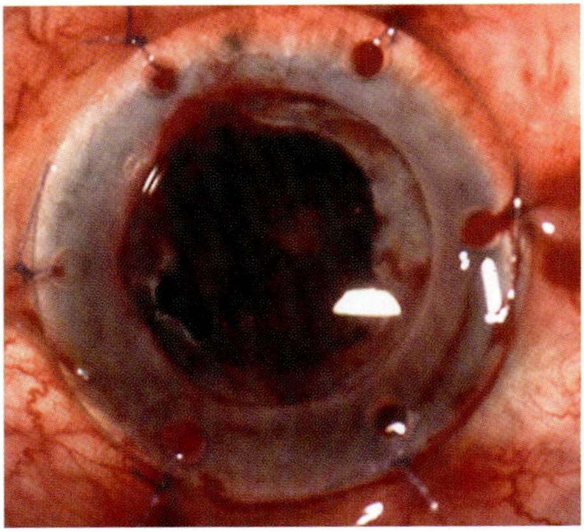

Fig. 2.15.1 The temporary keratoprosthesis (TKP) device intraoperatively. As opposed to a completely nontransparent cornea (see Fig. 2.2.14), the Landers TKP provides unhindered viewing of the retina. Use of a wide-angle system or a contact lens for fine epiretinal work are both possible

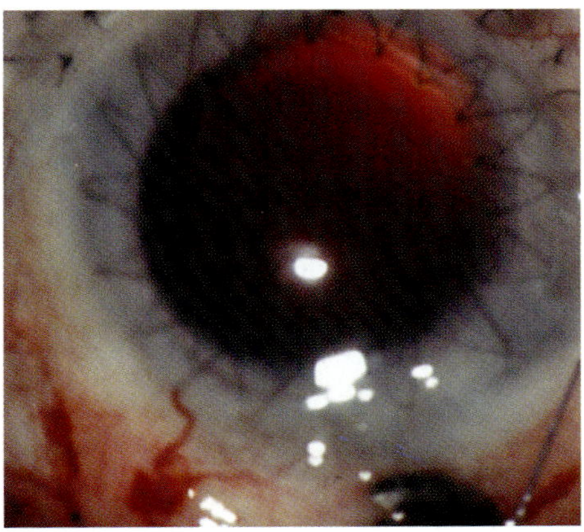

Fig. 2.15.2 PK to complete the procedure. At the end of surgery, a corneal graft is placed. There is excellent red reflex and the retina is attached

Table 2.15.1 A comparison of two temporary keratoprosthesis designs

Variable	Eckardt [1]	Landers [10]
Diameter	7 or 8 mm	7.2 or 8.2 mm[a]
Phakic version available	Yes	Yes
Suture placement	Up to surgeon	Predetermined holes
Reusable	Yes[b]	Yes
Material	Silicone	PMMA
Manufacturer	DORC[1]	Ocular instruments[2]

A third device, the Aachen keratoprosthesis, has also been used on a temporary basis [3]

[a] Provides 2.3× magnification and 30° field of static view

[b] Limited because the sutures eventually destroy the rim of the device

[1] Zuidland, The Netherlands

[2] Bellevue, Washington

Pitfall

Timing is a critical issue. There is no rational reason to delay TKP vitrectomy for weeks; if intense topical corticosteroid therapy is employed after the initial surgery (see Chap. 1.8), surgery can be scheduled as early as a few days post-injury. The ideal time to perform TKP vitrectomy is within a few days, *not* after 3 weeks.

2.15.3.1.1 The Surgeon

Depending on how (sub)specialized ophthalmology in the particular country is, TKP vitrectomy may be performed by a single individual from start to finish, or by two teams, an "anterior" and a "posterior" (Table 2.15.2). If a single surgeon performs the entire operation, he or she must be a vitrectomy specialist who is also experienced in anterior segment surgery, not the other way around: the major difficulty of surgery lies in dealing with

Table 2.15.2 Approaches to TKP vitrectomy. *AS* anterior segment surgeon, *PS* posterior segment surgeon

	Single surgeon	Teamwork: AS and PS
Advantage	Surgical decisions, which could otherwise fall under the competence of the other surgeon, are easier to make	All pathologies, whether in the anterior or posterior segment, receive expert treatment
	Less time is wasted as there is no need to repeatedly switch between AS and PS	Both surgeons have a "break" during the operation
	The responsibility for a surgical problem is easy to determine	
	The experience gained from the case is complete[3]	
Disadvantage	Surgery is long and exhausting; it requires hours of uninterrupted concentration and brings many difficult challenges	Occasionally, decisions would need to be made by the other surgeon, who may not be readily available
	The PS is less knowledgeable about all aspects of PK than an AS would be	Conflicts regarding certain maneuvers may arise as the other surgeon would prefer a different solution
		The overall time of surgery may be longer

[3] If two surgeons are involved, neither is likely to stay in the OR throughout the entire procedure; thus, neither gains from the knowledge of the other surgeon.

the retinal problems. It is the condition of the macula that primarily determines the functional success.[5]

5 A corneal graft that subsequently becomes opaque can usually be replaced; conversely, damage to the postequatorial retina (e.g., detachment with severe PVR) often cannot be reversed.

2.15.3.1.2 The Procedure

The surgical steps are summarized in Table 2.15.3.

Table 2.15.3 A brief overview of the surgical steps during TKP vitrectomy

Procedure	Comment	Surgeon[a]
Designing the surgical plan	All factors, such as history, evaluation results, equipment availability, patient desire, etc., must be carefully weighed; if two teams are involved, a mutually agreeable plan and a clear understanding of "who does what, when, and how" must be established	PS, or PS and AS
Placement of the pars plana infusion	3 mm from the limbus; a long cannula[4] should be used; the infusion should not be turned on until the position of its tip is verified (see Chap. 2.9)	PS
Preparation of the working sclerotomies	This can alternatively be done later; if done at this stage, the sclerotomies should be plugged until vitrectomy commences. As in almost all cases, the two incisions should be ~170° apart to allow for maximum intraocular maneuverability. It is advisable to consider using a bimanual technique: a fourth sclerotomy may have to be prepared for the independent light source. The exact location for this sclerotomy is best determined after the initial intraocular examination	PS
Placement of a Flieringa ring	Its use is highly recommended to provide stability during the corneal maneuvers. The size must be carefully selected to avoid interference with the sclerotomies, and it must be securely fixed to the sclera, not to the conjunctiva	PS or AS
Selection of the keratome of proper size	The diameter of the trephine for the corneal bed should be either 1/4 mm larger than or equal to the diameter of the TKP. This allows easy TKP placement yet prevents leakage during vitrectomy. A relatively large button is advised: if the PK needs to be repeated later, this should be smaller than the size of the first one	AS

[a] If a "team", rather than a single surgeon, performs the operation; otherwise, as mentioned above, a posterior segment specialist should be the surgeon

[4] 6 or even 7 mm

Table 2.15.3 *(continued)* A brief overview of the surgical steps during TKP vitrectomy

Procedure	Comment	Surgeon[a]
Removal of the button	The standard PK rules are followed	AS
Suture fixation of the TKP	If the Eckhard model is used, the number and type of sutures are entirely at the surgeon's discretion. The Landers model has six predetermined holes; however, two (instead of six) limbus-parallel sutures, partial thickness in the cornea, suffice: each suture encompasses two holes [8]. The use of 8-0 nylon sutures is recommended	AS
Anterior segment reconstruction as needed	Removal of blood, iris, and pupillary membranes, injured lens, even IOL if deemed necessary; freeing the angle, etc. If the pupil is narrow, adrenalin drops can be instilled directly or iris retractors can be used (see Chap. 2.9). The time the eye is open should be minimized to reduce the ECH risk; the iris diaphragm must not be reconstructed at this point to allow unhindered view of the posterior segment	AS
Placement of an AC infusion	This is unavoidable if the pars plana infusion cannula's position could not be reliably verified; once it is, the AC maintainer can be removed	PS
Vitreoretinal surgery (see Chaps. 2.4–2.9 and 2.10–2.14 for details)	All necessary and possible steps must be taken to achieve retinal attachment, including silicone oil tamponade. Freeing the ciliary body from membranes and reattaching it if it is detached are crucial. If silicone oil is injected,[5] this should be done either at the conclusion of vitrectomy once the AC has been filled with viscoelastics[6], or the BSS–air–silicone oil exchanges are performed after the corneal graft is in place. In either case, the sclerotomies are only plugged, not sutured, and the infusion cannula also remains in place	AS

[5] Which is the vast majority of the cases

[6] The AS is asked not to irrigate in the AC with BSS after this point.

Table 2.15.3 *(continued)* A brief overview of the surgical steps during TKP vitrectomy

Procedure	Comment	Surgeon[a]
Removal of the TKP and completing reconstruction of the anterior segment	The sutures are cut, the AC is rechecked for depth, fresh bleeding, fibrinous membranes, etc. An IOL may be implanted in those exceptional cases when the retina was not detached and silicone oil is not injected. If silicone oil is used, the viscoelastics should be either left behind[7] or replaced with air, not BSS.[8] The iris diaphragm should be reconstituted if the pupil is mydriatic and sufficient amount of the iris is left. If the iris needs to be sutured, the pupil must not be made too small so that it does not interfere with postoperative inspection of the retina or hinder any future posterior segment surgery	AS or PS
Grafting	The standard PK rules are followed. The graft diameter should be 0.5 or 0.75 mm larger than the trephined button's diameter	AS
Final check on the posterior segment	To determine whether any additional manipulation needs to be made (e.g., adjusting the silicone oil level, removal of fresh hemorrhage)	PS or AS
Closure of the sclerotomies	The infusion cannula is finally removed and all sclerotomies are closed	PS
Removal of the Flieringa ring	Alternatively, this may precede the closure of the sclerotomies	PS or AS

[7] In which the IOP must be very closely monitored during the first few postoperative days

[8] If air is left in the AC in an aphakic eye with silicone oil implantation, the patient should not be in a face-down position for a few days to prevent silicone oil prolapse.

2.15.3.1.3 Outcomes

With regard to outcome:

- In the vast majority of the cases, the donor cornea is not rejected and remains clear. In one large study with long-term follow-up, the graft remained clear at 1 year in 65% of eyes [7]. Another large study with an average follow-up of 25 months showed that the retina was attached and the graft remained clear in 73% of eyes.
- Postoperative graft failure may or may not be caused by the fact that the transplantation was done on an acutely injured eye, but the potential risk of graft failure must not serve as a justification for not performing timely TKP vitrectomy.
- Risks for graft failure include silicone oil implantation, multiple surgeries, and retinal detachment [7]. The TKP vitrectomy offers reasonable hope to achieve functional improvement for eyes with NLP vision [4, 12] or endophthalmitis [9].

2.15.3.1.4 Eyes with Irreparable Anterior segment Damage

The TKP is useful in eyes with combined anterior- and posterior segment trauma to allow vitreoretinal surgery to be performed in a timely manner. If the cornea does not to remain clear because of major anterior segment ischemia, a permanent keratoprosthesis can be implanted instead of repeated PK procedures.[6]

Permanent keratoprostheses (see Chap. 3.1) are well tolerated long term, offering vision in otherwise hopeless situations; the device even allows carrying out subsequent vitrectomy procedures [2, 6, 11]. It is crucial, however, to perform the initial TKP vitrectomy early, before the retina suffers irreversible damage.

6 Careful anterior segment reconstruction, however, may alleviate the need for PK or the permanent keratoprosthesis (Fig. 2.5.4).

DO:

- carefully consider whether EAV or TKP vitrectomy is more beneficial for eyes with severe combined anterior and posterior segment trauma; if the corneal opacity is not likely to resolve within a few weeks or months, perform TKP vitrectomy
- do meticulous surgery based on a well-designed plan; this is especially important if two surgeons operate and it is questionable which surgeon should perform which maneuvers and at what time during the operation
- try to accomplish all surgical goals in a single operation; conditions may be unfavorable for another major procedure in the next few days or weeks

DON'T:

- delay vitrectomy or perform suboptimal vitrectomy because of reduced corneal clarity; the window of opportunity to address a serious retinal condition is very narrow
- use too small a graft; if regrafting is necessary, the new button should be smaller than the previous one

Summary

Severe posterior segment trauma and a coexisting corneal injury incompatible with intraoperative visualization of the retina should not serve as justification for abandoning the eye. Both EAV and TKP vitrectomy offer surgery without dangerous compromise on timing or completeness. The TKP allows virtually instantaneous visual rehabilitation due to corneal grafting.

References

[1] Eckardt C (1987) A new temporary keratoprosthesis for pars plana vitrectomy. Retina 7: 34–37

[2] Jahne MG (2000) 25 years Cardona keratoprosthesis after severe chemical eye burns: long-term outcome of 4 eyes. Klin Monatsbl Augenheilkd 216: 191–196

[3] Langefeld S, Kompa S, Redbrake C, Brenman K, Kirchhof B, Schrage NF (2000) Aachen keratoprosthesis as temporary implant for combined vitreoretinal surgery

and keratoplasty: report on 10 clinical applications. Graefe's Arch Clin Exp Ophthalmol 238: 722–726

[4] Morris R, Kuhn F, Witherspoon CD (1998) Management of the recently injured eye with no light perception vision. In: Alfaro V, Liggett P (eds) Vitrectomy in the management of the injured globe. Lippincott Raven, Philadelphia, pp 113–125

[5] Park S, Marcus D, Duker J, Pesavento R, Topping P, Frederick A, D'Amico D (1995) Posterior segment complications after vitrectomy for macular hole. Ophthalmology 102: 775–781

[6] Ray S, Khan BF, Dohlman CH, D'Amico DJ (2002) Management of vitreoretinal complications in eyes with permanent keratoprosthesis. Arch Ophthalmol 120: 559–566

[7] Roter S, Szurman P, Hermes S, Thumann G, Bartz-Schmidt K, Kirchhof B (2003) Outcome of combined penetrating keratoplasty with vitreoretinal surgery for management of severe ocular injuries. Retina 23: 48–56

[8] Smith RJ, Bhavsar AR (1998) Simplified technique for suturing a temporary keratoprosthesis for pars plana vitrectomy. Am J Ophthalmol 125: 251–252

[9] Steiner M, Steinhorst UH, Winter R (1996) Temporary keratoprosthesis, vitrectomy and autokeratoplasty in endophthalmitis treatment. Ophthalmologe 93: 729–731 [in German]

[10] Toth CA, Landers MB III (1993) A new wide-field temporary keratoprosthesis. Retina 13: 353–355

[11] Fischern T von, Langefeld S, Yuan L, Volcker N, Reim M, Kirchhof B, Schrage NF (1998) Development of a surface modified silicone-keratoprosthesis with scleral fixation. Acta Chir Hung 37: 219–225

[12] Yan H, Cui J, Zhang J, Chen S, Xu Y (2006) Penetrating keratoplasty combined with vitreoretinal surgery for severe ocular injury with blood-stained cornea and no light perception. Ophthalmologica 220: 186–189

2.16 Ocular Trauma in Children and in Elderly Patients

Ferenc Kuhn

2.16.1 Introduction

Injuries occurring to children and elderly people[1] have some unique features that deserve special attention. A brief overview of these distinctive features are provided below; otherwise, see the relevant chapters for more information.

2.16.2 Pediatric Injuries[2]

2.16.2.1 General

- The younger the child, the more different the injury's characteristics are from those occurring in the adult population. This is compounded by the eye's different anatomy (see Sect. 2.16.2.6.1).

Children are at a higher risk of an eye injury than adults due to:

- Immature motor skills, paired with a tendency to imitate adult behavior
- Reduced "common sense" control over behavior and emotions
- Strong motivation from peer pressure and natural curiosity to "just do it"

1 In this chapter, children are defined as those under 19 and elderly as those 60 years of age or older.

2 The author is greatly indebted to JM Rohrbach, Tübingen, Germany for his invaluable contributions to this chapter.

- Increased levels of male hormones in adolescent boys.
- The child usually has a long life expectancy; permanent visual loss therefore represents a greater burden for individual, family, and society.
- Amblyopia is a major concern in the appropriate age group;[3] every effort should be made to restore the normal anatomy and the eye's refractive power as early as possible, and to instigate anti-amblyopia (orthoptic) treatment as necessary. The threat of amblyopia is somewhat smaller in children who are myopic since they have relatively preserved near vision.
- Posttraumatic stress disorder is common in children and may require professional help to treat [50].

2.16.2.2 History

With regard to history:

- Wearing a white coat during the examination may be frightful to the child; wearing "civilian" clothes is recommended instead.
- Explaining what is going to happen and that the examination will be painless is much more important in children than in adults.
- The child may refuse to cooperate with the ophthalmologist's efforts to elicit exactly how the injury occurred. The child may be afraid of the parent's[4] retribution (e.g., because abuse has occurred; see Chap. 3.3) or of punishment for an illegal activity[5]. To escape responsibility or accountability, the child may give no information, false information, or even fabricated information [40]. The reliability of history is greatly enhanced if a witness can be identified.[6]
- Injuries that rarely occur in adults, such as an animal bite to the face and eyes (Fig. 1.1.5), are much more common in children. Such injuries have systemic implications,[7] which must not be neglected.

---

3 Typically, under 7 years.

4 Throughout this chapter, the "parent" may be a legal guardian or a caretaker.

5 i.e., fighting with a sibling.

6 Unless, of course, the witness is the adult responsible for the injury.

7 e.g., tetanus or rabies prophylaxis.

2.16.2.3 Epidemiology[8] and Prevention

With regard to epidemiology and prevention:

- Children suffer 27–52% of all ocular trauma [18, 26, 39], a disproportionate rate. One-quarter of open globe injuries occurred in children in one study [16].
- Up to a third of persons hospitalized for trauma in the U.S. are children [30, 46, 59], with a hospitalization rate of 9 per 100,000 persons per year among those aged 20 years or less [8].
- Injury is the leading cause of monocular blindness in children [28].
- In a population-based report from the U.S., the estimated incidence rate of ocular trauma for those under 16 years of age was 15 per 100,000 persons per year [53].
- The risk of eye injury is measurably increased for children from a socio-economically challenged population [13].
- Injuries to children (and to the elderly) are especially common at the home (39% and 59% in the USEIR, respectively). In one study, 15 cases of eye injury caused by pointed door handles were treated at a single facility over a 2-year period [10]. The trauma was very severe: the rate of optic nerve evulsion reached 93%.
- In developing countries, children are disproportionally represented among those injured. An unpublished study[9] from Mali found that 40% of all eye injury cases involved children. The most common activity was play.[10] One-third of the injured children did not arrive at the ER within 24 h.
- Needle injury is surprisingly frequent among children: in one study 1% of all pediatric cataracts undergoing surgery were caused by a needle [42]. Of the 42 eyes, 29% developed endophthalmitis; the rate reached 50% if the object was a hypodermic needle.

8 The data are from the USEIR unless otherwise indicated.
9 KF Sylla, Bamako, Mali
10 Included using sharp needles that women use to plait their hair.

- Trauma sustained during play in general and playing sports in particular is predominant. Using proper protective eyewear during sports is effective and should be encouraged [1, 14].
- The average age of the victim of air-gun-related ocular trauma was 11 years in one study, and 51% of the victims were shot by a friend or sibling [7]. The rate of injury is 14% among children but only 0.8% among adults. A third of the injured eyes were enucleated, another half remained NLP [48].
- Paintball, with the popularity of nonorganized (unofficial) games where the wearing of full facemasks is not enforced, represents an increasingly common source. In a 4-year survey from New Jersey, 75% of the 79 injuries involved children [56]. The outcome is poor: in one study only 43% of eyes had 20/40 or greater final visual acuity [37].
- The rate of children among those injured by fireworks is very high: 75% in Sweden [54], 49% in Austria [43], and 69% in the USEIR, with a bystander being injured in 67% [34].
- Abuse to children is of major importance; this is discussed in Chap. 3.3 (shaken baby syndrome).

2.16.2.4 Evaluation

With regard to evaluation:

- The child may physically resist the examination, and may have to be restrained. Having the parent/guardian to assist in this is very helpful [32].
- To characterize visual performance in children aged 8 years and above, the use of a standardized reading text[11], rather than charts measuring distance vision (i.e., Snellen, EDTRS), may be preferable [57].
- If impacted by a blunt object, a young child's orbital bones fracture but also bend, with a decreased tendency to shatter. As a result, muscle entrapment is much more common than in adults [17]; examining the ocular motility is therefore crucial.

11 MNREAD chart, available in English, Japanese, and Italian.

- Gentle palpation is often able to identify subcutaneous foreign bodies and crepitus as well as finding bone dislocation (see Chap. 1.9).

2.16.2.5 Counseling

For most parents, having their child sustain an eye injury has major psychological implications, and the parents' sensitivity must be appreciated by the ophthalmologist. It is entirely different to discuss "the case" with the very same person if he is the patient vs the parent. In addition, based on the injured child's age (and maturity),[12] it is the parent, rather than the injured child, who must give consent to the procedure(s) to be performed.[13] Occasionally, the ophthalmologist must initiate legal proceedings to save the child's sight, should the parent be negligent or deny consent.

2.16.2.6 Surgical Decision-Making and Surgical Tips

2.16.2.6.1 Anatomical Differences and Their Management Implications

In addition to differences already mentioned, the following must be kept in mind:

- The eye continues to grow after birth, well past age 10 years.[14]
- The younger the child, the less convenient it is to operate on the eye.[15]
- The younger the child, the more difficult it is to predict the correct power of the IOL.
- The cornea is less rigid in children; sutures therefore may become loose much faster than in adults.
- The anterior lens capsule is thinner and more elastic, making capsulorhexis more difficult to perform.

---

12 The country's legal requirements must also be respected.

13 Nevertheless, it is also important to engage the child and gain his confidence. This, as already discussed helps overcome the child's initial resistance.

14 The growth is especially strong in the first 4 years.

15 This is true both for physical access to the eye through a narrow palpebral fissure and the room available for intraocular manipulations.

Table 2.16.1 The recommended distance from the limbus of the sclerotomy in children

Age	Distance (mm)
<6 months	1.5
7–12 months	2
1–2 years	2.5
2–6 years	3
>6 years	3.5

- The vitreous is more adherent to the retina and to the posterior capsule than in adults. This adherence has important implications for management: maneuvers that do not usually lead to complications in adults (i.e., PVD or removal of the posterior capsule) do pose a fairly high risk in children.
- The pars plana region is located more anteriorly in children. The younger the child, the closer to the limbus should the site of the sclerotomy be (Table 2.16.1). An accurate method to determine the site is to use the light pipe: transscleral illumination shows a dark ring representing the pars plana area.

2.16.2.6.2 General Comments

In eyes with IOFB injuries, the presenting visual acuity is lower and the rate of retinal detachment is higher in children than in adults; both differences are statistically significant [58].

Trauma is the most important cause of rhegmatogenous retinal detachment and was the indication for 30% of pediatric vitrectomies in one study, and it appears to be statistically significantly less effective in children under 10 years than in the adult population (35 vs 73%, respectively [24]).

In children, unlike in adults, the etiology of Terson syndrome is almost exclusively traumatic subdural, rather than spontaneous subarachnoidal, hemorrhage (see Chap. 3.3) [33].

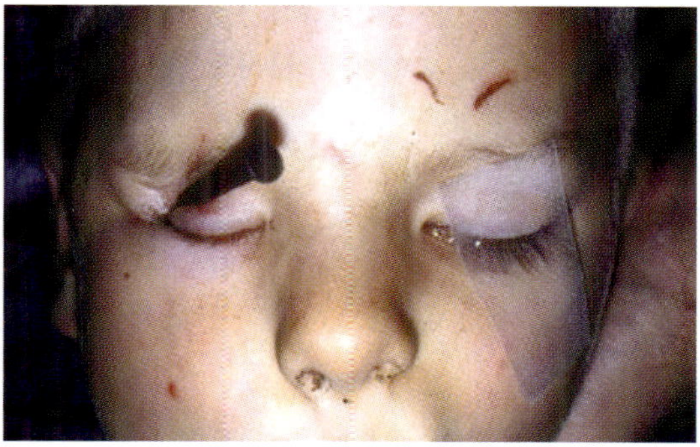

Fig. 2.16.1 Protruding IOFB in a child. A protruding IOFB represents a unique management challenge. The risks associated with keeping the IOFB in situ until optimal conditions for removal are available (see Chap. 1.8) must be balanced against the risks of suboptimal removal conditions. In a cooperating adult, it is possible to refer the patient if the attending ophthalmologist decides not to intervene. It must be thoroughly explained to the patient that no physical pressure must be applied on the eye, and a proper shield[1] must be placed over the eye before transportation. In a young child, such a referral may be very risky unless the child can be securely restrained. If such a restraint is not feasible, it is probably advisable to remove the IOFB acutely, even if the conditions are not optimal[2], and then refer the child for secondary reconstruction

[1] If the standard shield cannot be applied because the protruding object is too long, a shield can be fashioned from a Styrofoam cup.

[2] The removal must still take place in the controlled and sterile environment of an OR.

2.16.2.6.3 Management Pearls

- Closure of corneal (even scleral) wounds *before* referral is much more important in the young: the risk of the child rubbing the eye while in transit, and cause tissue extrusion or ECH, is higher. For the same reason, children with a protruding IOFB (Fig. 2.16.1) must not be referred until the object has been removed in an emergency procedure.
- If the anterior lens capsule is violated, the IOP may rapidly rise to very high levels; the younger the child, the greater the risk. The con-

dition may be so severe as to make emergency surgery necessary (see Chaps. 2.7, 2.18).

- If a child has bilateral traumatic cataracts, consideration should be given to performing lens removal in both eyes in the same surgical session: general anesthesia is technically difficult and potentially dangerous. The eyes must be prepared separately.
- Capsulorhexis is risky if there is capsular fibrosis; the vitrectomy probe is the safest method of creating an anterior (or posterior) capsulectomy.
- Since the nucleus is soft in children, simple aspiration for a traumatic cataract without posterior capsule injury is adequate.
- If a posterior capsular lesion is present, the vitrectomy probe should be used for lens removal (lensectomy; see Chap. 2.7) to avoid traction on the anterior vitreous [35]. Whether a limbal or pars plana approach is chosen, is based on the surgeon's preference [2] and on the accompanying pathologies.
- Since both the anterior and the posterior capsules are prone to opacify – the rate of postoperative opacification of the posterior capsule can reach as high as 100% [11] – and to opacify early [6], a large capsulectomy is recommended [60].
- The creation of a posterior capsulectomy must be preceded by anterior vitrectomy or performed with the vitrectomy probe. Posterior capsulorhexis must not be performed in children.
- Because of the strong connections between the posterior lens capsule and the anterior vitreous,[16] ICCE should never be attempted in children.
- Several methods are available to restore the eye's refractive power after lens removal: prescription glasses; contact lenses; epikeratophakia; and IOL implantation [27]. The IOL implantation is the preferred option method [6], but the age at which this becomes feasible has not been determined.

16 And the peripheral retina.

Controversial

IOL implantation is probably safe in children older than 1 year. It is not clear how the IOL power should be calculated/predicted in an eye that is still growing, especially if primary implantation is planned [15].

- The standard method of calculating the IOL power results in overcorrection if the child is under 8 years, due to the myopic shift with the eye's normal growth [31]. Undercorrection, gradually decreasing from +6 D at age 1 year to plano at age 7 years, has been suggested as a resolution to the controversy [19]. Patients must undergo appropriate contact lens fitting and anti-amblyopia therapy until emmetropia ensues.
- Because children are at a higher risk of additional injury, scleral fixation of the IOL should be considered if the zonules are not completely intact.
- The most common early complication after IOL implantation is severe fibrinous anterior uveitis (51%), especially prominent in patients with dark iris [23].
- In eyes with secondary IOL implantation, the IOL is usually placed onto the capsule[17] because the capsules have scarred together. In-the-sulcus IOL placement does not appear to have adverse consequences [6, 60].
- The IOL should be acrylic or PMMA (heparin surface-modified), with a rather large (6.5 mm) optic.
- In a major study, trauma was the cause in 73% of children presenting with vitreous hemorrhage [49]. Contusion was slightly more common than open globe trauma (30 vs 25%, respectively).
- The risk of the formation of anterior and/or posterior synechia is higher in the young than in adults. Postoperative anti-inflammatory treatment is even more important in children than in adults. In certain cases the inflammation may have to be fought even intraoperatively[18] (see Chap. 2.17).

17 Even if the capsular bag has originally been preserved.
18 i.e., fibrin formation.

- If vitrectomy is performed, the creation of a PVD is crucial. This is a much more difficult (and potentially risky) maneuver in a child's eye than in that of an adult. Intraoperative injection of 0.4 IU autologous plasmin may be helpful [36], but the surgeon has to be ready to abandon the procedure (see Chap. 2.9) if separation of the posterior hyaloid is very difficult.

Pearl

Tenting of the retina[19] during surgical PVD is a sign of very strong vitreoretinal adherence; it signals to the surgeon that the maneuver may have to be stopped.

- The microbiological spectrum of endophthalmitis is slightly different in children, with various *Streptococcus* species being the most common organism. If early and "aggressive" therapy (i.e., as complete as possible vitrectomy; see Chap. 2.17) is performed, most eyes regain at least ambulatory vision [3].
- In children presenting with proptosis, orbital, or ocular[20] trauma should be high on the differential diagnosis list [5].
- The consequences of serious injury are often more complex in children than in adults, due to increased postoperative inflammation and scar formation [21, 28, 38, 47]. PVR may be more pronounced in children [22, 25], presenting earlier and possibly in a more fulminant fashion. Scarring is a risk regardless of the intraocular tissue involved, with secondary complications such as corneal opacity, glaucoma, posterior capsule opacification, and retinal detachment. In one report, 28% of eyes with posterior segment injury developed PVR [28]. Vitrectomy performed within 2 weeks may prevent PVR development [28].

19 An advancing white line is visible as the detaching vitreous elevates the retina.

20 e.g., endophthalmitis.

Controversial

Clinical impression and a few reports suggest that PVR is more prevalent and severe in children [38, 44]; however, no study has conclusively confirmed this, and some authors found no such link [51].

- Enucleation should be even more of a last resort in children than in adults: removal of the eye may arrest facial growth. If enucleation is unavoidable, an implant 2 mm smaller in diameter than the axial length of the removed eye should be used [29].

2.16.2.6.4 Prognosis

With regard to prognosis:

- The visual outcome changes based on the age of the child. It is especially informative to analyze the visual acuity values if these are compared with those in adult eyes (Table 2.16.2).

Table 2.16.2 Visual outcomes in the USEIR database (%). A comparison between the final visual acuities of seriously injured eyes of pediatric vs adult patients

Visual acuity	Children aged 0–4	Children aged 5–14	Children aged 15–18	Children aged 0–18	Adults 19 and older
NLP	10	7	9	8	11
LP to HM	10	8	7	8	12
1/200 to 19/200	12	7	8	8	10
20/200 to 20/50	13	22	25	22	20
20/40 or greater	55	56	51	54	47
Total no. (%)	156 (100%)	1227 (100%)	608 (100%)	1991 (100%)	4286 (100%)

Based on 6168 injuries. The ages are in years

- Amblyopia and PVR development remain the two most important factors in the prognosis [12, 55].
- Fireworks-related trauma, injury caused by a missile, open globe injuries in general and ruptures in particular, presence of a retinal detachment, and age under 4 years have been found to be prognostic factors for poor outcome [4, 20, 28, 43, 60].
- Closed globe injuries have a statistically significantly better outcome than those with open globe trauma [45]. Among open globe injuries, the more posterior the trauma, the worse the outcome [41].
- The risk of poor final visual acuity is 12 times higher if PVR develops. The PVR risk has been reported to be 186 times greater after a perforating injury and 23 times greater after a rupture than after a contusion [9].
- If meticulous primary and secondary reconstruction is performed, the prognosis is relatively good, with 44% of eyes reaching 20/40 or greater vision in one study [28].

2.16.3 Injuries in Elderly Patients[21]

It is not uncommon for elderly patients to have difficulty understanding the nature of the injury, its implications, the significance of each treatment option, or the instructions given for postoperative posturing or treatment. Prescription glasses are much more likely to cause eye injury in the elderly than in young people (see Chap. 1.7).

Male preponderance is seen below the age of 70 years, with the male: female ratio varying between 2.5 to 1 and 7.4 to 1. The ratio declines after age 60 years, and it actually reverses over 80 years.

- A disproportionally high rate of injuries are ruptures (see Chap. 1.7), caused mostly by fall at home (Table 2.16.3). Fall is over ten times more common in those over 60 years than in those who are under 60 years.

21 All data are from the USEIR unless otherwise noted.

It appears that an eye has a lower threshold to rupture from the same impact if the person is old vs young.

- "Fall at home" is so typical an injury in the elderly that prevention naturally comes to mind. Simple but very useful ideas include rearranging the furniture,[22] making the bathtub less slippery, or fixating the rugs to the floor.
- Age is an independent risk factor for the development of glaucoma in eyes with contusion or open globe injury (see Chap. 2.18).
- Compared with younger people, significantly more of the injured eyes in the elderly population have a preexisting condition,[23] which had adversely affected the visual acuity before the injury. The history of open globe surgery (see Chap. 2.12) is an additional, independent risk factor for poor outcome[24].
- Even if controlled for a preexisting condition adversely affecting vision, the outcome of a serious injury is statistically significantly worse in the adult population (Table 2.16.4). This finding is especially striking since the number of surgeries was higher in the elderly cohort than in those under 60 years of age.
- Elderly people have a higher risk for endophthalmitis development, especially if the lens is injured (see Chaps. 2.13, 2.17).
- The risk of eye injury in an MVC, whether or not the air bag has deployed, is about double for a serious eye injury if the person is 65 years old vs those between 16 and 35 years [52].

Cave

Age must not be a deciding factor in whether reconstructive surgery is performed for a serious eye injury[25] and cannot serve as justification for abandoning the eye.

22 e.g., moving objects out of the path connecting the bed and the bathroom door.
23 e.g., age-related macular degeneration, diabetic retinopathy.
24 Unpublished data by the author.
25 This author recently operated on an 84-year-old woman who fell and ruptured her eye, which became NLP. The visual acuity improved rapidly after the operation, reaching 20/50 within 3 days (Fig. 2.12.2).

Table 2.16.3 Selected epidemiological data (%) from the USEIR on eye injuries occurring in persons over 60 years

Place		Source	
Home	59	Blunt objects	34
Public building	11	Fall	22
Work	9	Sharp objects	16
Recreation/sport	5	MVC	9
Farm	4	Hammering	4
		Explosion	4
		Firearm	3
		Lawn equipment	3
		Fireworks	0.5

Based on 561 injuries

Table 2.16.4 Comparsion of presenting and final visual acuities between young and elderly patients from the USEIR database

Visual acuity	Aged 0–59 years		Aged 60 years and older	
	Presenting	Final	Presenting	Final
NLP	399	449	71	94
LP	816	174	168	66
HM to 4/200	1208	472	155	99
5/200 to 19/200	259	187	259	32
20/200 to 20/50	248	200	18	22
20/40 to 20/20	1684	3118	116	227
Total no. of cases	4614	4600	787	540

Based on 5140 injuries

- Surgical treatment of the "aging eye" does not differ from that performed in younger people.[26]

DO:

- try to obtain a witness's description of the injury if the child is not helpful during history-taking
- remember that the same trauma can incite a more pronounced ocular reaction, and do so more rapidly, in a child vs an adult
- keep in mind that the risk of ruptures is much higher in the elderly

DON'T:

- apply the same management strategy in dealing with a pediatric cataract as you would in an adult patient: because of the different anatomy and the future growth of the eye, both the timing and method of extraction, and the timing and power calculation of the IOL, are markedly different in a young child
- try to force removal of the nondetached posterior cortical vitreous in a child; although it is just as much a surgical goal during vitrectomy as it would be in an adult, the strong retinal adherence may make PVD dangerous in the pediatric patient
- give up on a ruptured eye even if it has poor vision and major tissue extrusion just because the patient is elderly

26 Tissue tolerance to certain surgical maneuvers may be decreased, but these observation is based more on anecdotal than scientific evidence.

Summary

The treatment of children with a serious eye injury is quite different from that in an adult patient; the younger the child, the more pronounced these differences. Some of the differences may be overcome by the ophthalmologist (e.g., noncooperativeness of the child), others require recognition of the difference (e.g., a smaller eye to operate on) and adoption of the management strategy and tactics. The characteristics and implications of eye injury are also different if an elderly patient sustained the trauma, mostly because of the increased severity of the injury and the greater vulnerability of the eyeball.

References

[1] American Academy of Ophthalmology (2004) Protective eyewear for young athletes. Pediatrics 113: 619–622

[2] Ahmadieh H, Javadi M, Ahmady M, Karimian F, Einollahi B, Zare M, Dehghan M, Mashyekhi A, Valaei N, Soheilian M, Sajjadi H (1999) Primary capsulectomy, anterior vitrectomy, lensectomy, and posterior chamber lens implantation in children: limbal versus pars plana. J Cat Refr Sur g 25: 768–775

[3] Alfaro DV, Roth DB, Laughlin RM, Goyal M, Liggett PE (1995) Paediatric posttraumatic endophthalmitis. Br J Ophthalmol 79: 888–891

[4] Apt L, Sarin L (1962) Causes for enucleation of the eye in infants and children. J Am Med Assoc 181: 948–953

[5] Belmekki M, el Bakkali M, Abdellah H, Benchrifa F, Berraho A (1999) Epidemiology of orbital processes in children. 54 cases. J Fr Ophtalmol 22: 394–398 [in French]

[6] Ben Ezra D, Cohen E, Rose L (1997) Traumatic cataract in children: correction of aphakia by contact lens or intraocular lens. Am J Ophthalmol 123: 773–782

[7] Bratton S, Dowd M, Brogan T, Hegenbarth M (1997) Serious and fatal air gun injuries: more than meets the eye. Pediatrics 100: 609–612

[8] Brophy M, Sinclair S, Hostetler S, Xiang H (2006) Pediatric eye injury-related hospitalizations in the United States. Pediatrics 117: 1263–1271

[9] Cardillo JA, Stout JT, LaBree L, Azen SP, Omphroy L, Cui JZ, Kimura H, Hinton DR, Ryan SJ (1997) Post-traumatic proliferative vitreoretinopathy. The epidemiologic profile, onset, risk factors, and visual outcome. Ophthalmology 104: 1166–1173

[10] Chaudhry IA, Al-Sharif AM, Shamsi FA, Elzaridi E, Al-Rashed W (2005) Severe ocular injuries from pointed door handles in children. Ophthalmology 112: 1834–1837

[11] Crouch EJ, Pressman S, Crouch E (1995) Posterior chamber intraocular lenses: long-term results in pediatric cataract patients. J Pediatr Ophthalmol Strab 32: 210–218

[12] Dana M, Schaumberg D, Moyes A, Gomes J, Laibson P, Holland E, Sugar A, (1995) Outcome of penetrating keratoplasty after ocular trauma in children. Arch Ophthalmol 113: 1503–1507

[13] Dandona L, Dandona R, Srinivas M, John R, McCarty C, Rao G (2000) Ocular trauma in an urban population in southern India: the Andhra Pradesh Eye Disease Study. Clin Exp Ophthalmol 28: 350–356

[14] Danis R, Hu K, Nell M (2000) Acceptability of baseball face guards and reduction of oculofacial injury in receptive youth league players. Inj Prev 6: 232–234

[15] DeVaro JM, Buckley EG, Awner S, Seaber J (1997) Secondary posterior chamber intraocular lens implantation in pediatric patients. Am J Ophthalmol 123: 24–30

[16] Dunn E, Jaeger E, Jeffers J, Freitag S (1992) The epidemiology of ruptured globes. Ann Ophthalmol 24: 405–410

[17] Egbert J, May K, Kersten R, Kulwin D (2000) Pediatric orbital floor fracture: direct extraocular muscle involvement. Ophthalmology 107: 1875–1879

[18] Elder M (1993) Penetrating eye injuries in children of the West Bank and Gaza strip. Eye 7: 429–432

[19] Enyedi L, Peterseim M, Freedman S, Buckley E (1998) Refractive changes after pediatric intraocular lens implantation. Am J Ophthalmol 126: 772–781

[20] Farr A, Hairston R, Humayun M, Marsh M, Pieramici D, MacCumber M, de Juan EJ (2001) Open globe injuries in children: a retrospective analysis. J Pediatr Ophthalmol Strab 38: 72–77

[21] Ferrore P, McCuen IB, de Juan EJ, Machemer R (1994) The efficacy of silicone oil for complicated retinal detachments in the pediatric population. Arch Ophthalmol 112: 773–777

[22] Glaser B, Michels R, Kupperman B (1991) Medical and surgical retina. Mosby, St. Louis, pp 241–243

[23] Gradin D, Yorston D (2001) Intraocular lens implantation for traumatic cataract in children in East Africa. J Cat Refr Surg 27: 2017–2025

[24] Gribomont AC, Ledoux A (2005) Vitreo-retinal pediatric surgery: epidemiologic factors, etiology and prognosis. Bull Soc Belge Ophtalmol 61–65 [in French]

[25] Guillaume J, Godde-Jolly D, Haut J (1991) Surgical treatment of traumatic retinal detachment in children under 15 years of age. J Fr Ophthalmol 14: 311–319

[26] Hemo Y, Ben Ezra D (1987) Traumatic cataracts in young children; correction of aphakia by intraocular lens implantation. Ophthalmic Paediatr Genet 8: 203–207

[27] Hiatt RL (1998) Rehabilitation of children with cataracts. Trans Am Ophthalmol Soc 96: 475–477

[28] Jandeck C, Kellner U, Bornfeld N, Foerster M (2000) Open globe injuries in children. Graefe's Arch Ophthalmol 238: 420–426

[29] Kaltreider S, Peake L, Carter B (2001) Pediatric enucleation: analysis of volume replacement. Arch Ophthalmol 119: 379–384

[30] Klopfer J, Tielsch J, Vitale S et al. (1992) Ocular trauma in the United states, eye injuries resulting in hospitalization, 1984 through 1987. Arch Ophthalmol 110: 838–842

[31] Kora Y, Shimizu K, Inatomi M, Fukado Y, Ozawa T (1993) Eye growth after cataract extraction and intraocular lens implantation in children. Ophthalmic Surg Las 24: 467–475

[32] Kuhn F, Morris R, Mester V (2005) Pediatric trauma. In: Hartnett ME (eds) Pediatric retina. Lippincott Willams Wilkins, Philadelphia, pp 467–489

[33] Kuhn F, Morris R, Mester V, Witherspoon C (1998) Terson's syndrome. Results of vitrectomy and the significance of vitreous hemorrhage in patients with subarachnoid hemorrhage. Ophthalmology 105: 472–477

[34] Kuhn F, Morris R, Witherspoon CD, Mann L, Modis L, Berta A (2000) Serious fireworks-related eye injuries. Ophthal Epidemiol 7: 139–148

[35] Malukiewicz-Wisniewska G, Kaluzny J, Lesiewska-Junk H, Eliks I (1999) Intraocular lens implantation in children and youth. J Pediatr Ophthalmol Strab 36: 129–133

[36] Margherio A, Margherio R, Hartzer M, Trese M, Williams G, Ferrone P (1998) Plasmin enzyme-assisted vitrectomy in traumatic pediatric macular holes. Ophthalmology 105: 1617–1620

[37] Mason Jr, Feist R, White MJ (2002) Ocular trauma from paintball-pellet war games. South Med J 95: 218–222

[38] Moisseiev J, Vidne O, Treister G (1998) Vitrectomy and silicone oil injection in pediatric patients. Retina 18: 221–227

[39] Nelson L, Wilson T, Jeffers J (1989) Eye injuries in childhood: demography, etiology, and prevention. Pediatrics 84: 438–441

[40] Olver J, Hague S (1989) Children presenting to an ophthalmic casualty department. Eye 3: 415–419

[41] Patel B (1989) Penetrating eye injuries. Arch Dis Child 64: 317–320

[42] Rabiah PK (2003) Penetrating needle injury of the eye causing cataract in children. Ophthalmology 110: 173–176

[43] Sacu S, Segur-Eltz N, Stenng K, Zehetmayer M (2002) Ocular firework injuries at New Year's eve. Ophthalmologica 216: 55–59

[44] Sadeh A, Dotan G, Bracha R, Lazar M, Loewenstein A (2001) Characteristics and outcomes of paediatric rhegmatogenous retinal detachment treated by segmental scleral buckling plus an encircling element. Eye 15: 31–33

[45] Saxena R, Sinha R, Purohit A, Dada T, Vajpayee R, Azad R (2002) Pattern of pediatric ocular trauma in India. Indian J Pediatr 69: 863–867

[46] Schein O, Hibberd P, Shingleton B (1988) The spectrum and burden of ocular injury. Ophthalmology 95: 300–395

The definition of the "Controversial" on page 373 is incorrect, and the sentence should read "As a general rule, a fresh IOFB should not be left in the eye; however, if the IOFB is verifiably inert, there is **no** sign or elevated risk of endophthalmitis, and no intraocular pathology has been caused, surgery may entail more complication than that to which the IOFB might lead."

The dosages presented in Table 2.17.3 are incorrect and the corrected version is given below.

Table 2.17.3 Pharmacotherapy for eyes with bacterial traumatic endophthalmitis

Route of application	Drug	Dose
Intravitreal injection	Ceftazidime	2.2 mg/0.1 ml
	Vancomycin	1–2 mg/0.1 ml
	Dexamethasone	0.4 mg/0.1 ml
Vitrectomy infusion fluid[a]	Ceftazidime	2.2 · 25 mg/100 ml
	Vancomycin	25 mg/100 ml
	Dexamethasone	0.4 · 25 mg/100 ml
Subconjunctiva	Ceftazidime	100 mg in 0.5 ml
	Vancomycin	25 mg/0.5 ml
	Dexamethasone	15 mg/1 ml
Topical	Fortified topical antibiotics (e.g., ciprofloxacin [15])	Hourly
	Prednisolone acetate	1%, several times a day
Oral[b]	Moxifloxacin	400 mg/day
Intravenous	Ceftazidime	1 g/12 h
	Vancomycin	1 g/12 h

The initial ("blind") choice; must be modified as resistance test results become available from culturing

[a]The drug concentrations are identical to those of an intravitreal injection

[b]Because of its excellent penetration into the eye, oral moxifloxacin is usually sufficient; if not, intravenous therapy can be chosen

ERRATUM

Ocular Traumatology

Ferenc Kuhn

ISBN 978-3-540-33824-6

Unfortunately Figure 1.9.1 was presented incorrectly, and the corrected version is given below.

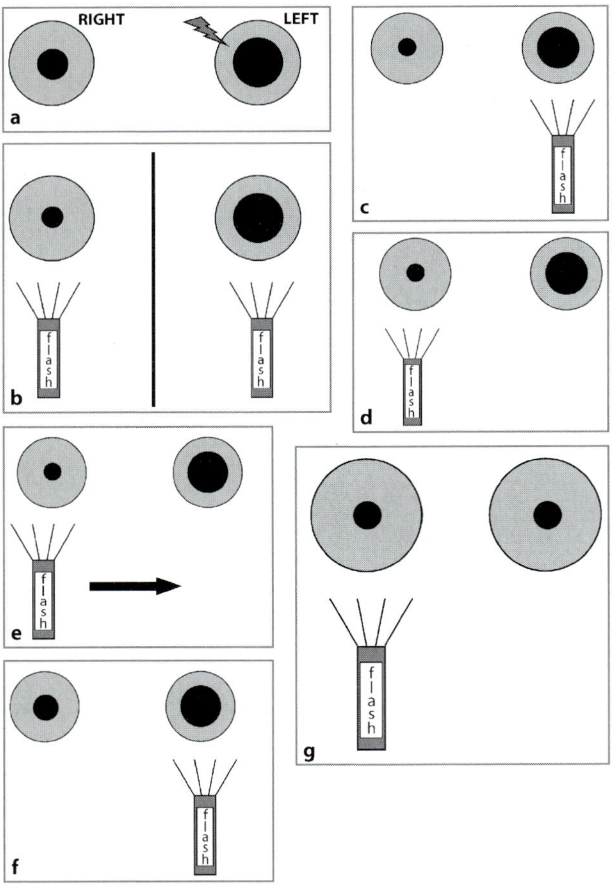

[47] Scott I, Flynn HJ, Azen S, Lai M, Schwartz S, Trese M (1999) Silicone oil in the repair of pediatric complex retinal detachments: a prospective, observational, multicenter study. Ophthalmology 106: 1399–1407

[48] Smith G, Knapp J, Barnett T, Shields B (1996) The rockets' red glare, the bombs bursting in air: fireworks-related injuries to children. Pediatrics 98: 1–9

[49] Spirn MJ, Lynn MJ, Hubbard GB III (2006) Vitreous hemorrhage in children. Ophthalmology 113: 848–852

[50] Steiner G, Peterson L (1992) Severe emotional response to eye trauma in a child: awareness and intervention. Arch Ophthalmol 110: 753

[51] Sternberg PJ, de Juan EJ, Michels R (1984) Penetrating ocular injuries in young patients. Initial injuries and visual results. Retina 4: 5–8

[52] Stitzel JD, Hansen GA, Herring IP, Duma SM (2005) Blunt trauma of the aging eye: injury mechanisms and increasing lens stiffness. Arch Ophthalmol 123: 789–794

[53] Strahlman E, Elman M, Daub E, Baker S (1990) Causes of pediatric eye injuries. A population-based study. Arch Ophthalmol 108: 603–606

[54] Sundelin K, Norrsell K (2000) Eye injuries from fireworks in Western Sweden. Acta Ophthalmol Scand 78: 61–64

[55] Umeh R, Umeh O (1997) Causes and visual outcome of childhood eye injuries in Nigeria. Eye 11: 489–495

[56] Vassilev ZP, Marcus SM (2004) Paintball injuries in children: the cases managed out of hospitals. Pediatrics 113: 1468

[57] Virgili G, Corcaro C, Bigoni A, Crovato S, Cecchini P, Menchini U (2004) Reading acuity in children: evaluation and reliability using MNREAD charts. Invest Ophthalmol Vis Sci 45: 3349–3354

[58] Williams DF, Mieler WF, Abrams GW (1990) Intraocular foreign bodies in young people. Retina 10: S45–S49

[59] Zagelbaum B, Tostanoski J, Kerner D, Hersh P (1993) Urban eye trauma. A one-year prospective study. Ophthalmology 100: 851–856

[60] Zwaan J, Mullaney P, Awad A, al-Mesfer S, Wheeler D (1998) Pediatric intraocular lens implantation. Surgical results and complications in more than 300 patients. Ophthalmology 105: 112–118

2.17 Endophthalmitis

Ferenc Kuhn

2.17.1 Introduction

The development of a purulent infection is the second most dreaded complication[1] of an open globe injury. The risk of endophthalmitis varies with injury type (Table 2.17.1), but it is also greatly influenced by the circumstances of the injury. In a 14-year survey on IOFB injuries from Canada in a civilian environment, a 17% rate was found [5], as opposed to a 0% rate in Iraq among military IOFB cases [4].

Early recognition and proper treatment of endophthalmitis are crucial to save vision, save the eyeball, and reduce the risk of litigation against the ophthalmologist.

2.17.2 Basic Principles Guiding the Management of Endophthalmitis

Endophthalmitis is not a microbiological but a *clinical* diagnosis. If the clinical picture is compatible with endophthalmitis, the condition should be interpreted and treated as such:

- A *negative* culture yield means not that an infectious organism is not present but that it could not be identified [12].

1 After an ECH

Table 2.17.1 The endophthalmitis incidence in different types of open globe injury in the USEIR database

Injury type (no. of cases)	Endophthalmitis incidence (%)
Rupture (2117)	1
Penetrating (4220)	3
IOFB (1235)	5
Perforating (464)	0.6

- Conversely, a *positive* culture is not synonymous with the diagnosis of endophthalmitis: IOFBs have routinely been cultured positive without the development of an infection [11].
- The traditional *staging* of endophthalmitis ("mild" vs "severe") does not force the ophthalmologist to appreciate the infection as a continuum. In a real-life scenario it is counterproductive to artificially classify an ongoing infection as "mild" as if the process could not rapidly turn into a "severe" one.
- Endophthalmitis should be classified as *early* if there is minimal anterior segment involvement and the red reflex is preserved.
- Endophthalmitis should be classified as *advanced* if the infection caused significant anterior segment or vitreoretinal pathologies [12].
- A *macular hypopyon* (Fig. 2.17.1) is often present in an eye with endophthalmitis. In this condition pus settles on the macula [12]. Such a macular pathology explains why only half of the eyes regained 20/40 or greater vision in the EVS [6] and why it is so important to create a PVD during vitrectomy [10]. Complete vitreous removal is especially crucial if the endophthalmitis is trauma related (see below).

2.17.3 Evaluation and Recognition

The examination is carried out in the usual manner (see Chap. 1.9). If an open globe injury is found (see Chap. 2.11), the possibility of endophthalmitis development should always be on high the ophthalmologist's list.

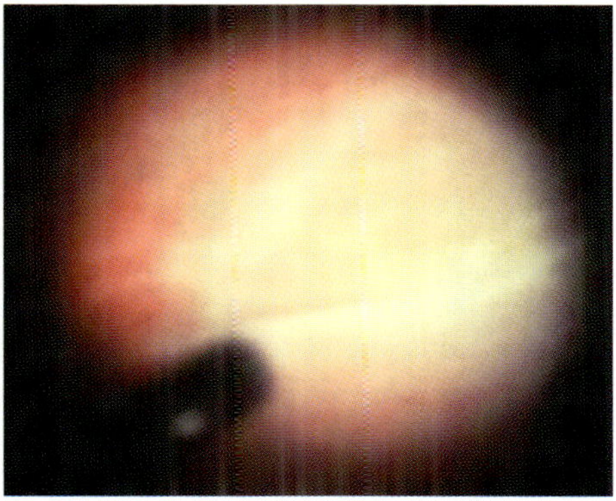

Fig. 2.17.1 Macular hypopyon in endophthalmitis. This intraoperative photograph[1] shows a severe accumulation of pus over the macula. A fibrinous membrane can form on top of the pus, making its appearance similar to that of a cyst. The membrane may have to incised before careful passive aspiration can remove the pus entirely or at least reduce its amount. If the pus is not extracted, there is little hope for recovering useful macular vision. Use of TPA (see Chap. 2.9) greatly aids in detaiching the fibrinpus complex from the macular surface.

[1]The light pipe is visible in the lower left corner.

Specific questions during history-taking should be directed toward determining whether the injury was of average or increased risk.

2.17.3.1 Risk Factors

The risk factors are as follows:

- Delay in wound closure exceeding 24 (36) h [7, 18].
- Injury with soil contamination, whether this happened on a farm or in the home garden.[2]
- Even indirect contact with soil represents an increased risk: open globe trauma caused by barbed wire has been reported to involve a 38% endophthalmitis incidence [16].

2 The term "rural setting" is misleading since soil contamination may occur in urban settings as well.

- Presence of an IOFB (see Chap. 2.13), especially if it is of organic matter.
- Lens injury [7], especially if associated with older age [18, 19].
- Presence of a “dirty” wound [7].
- Presence of a filtering bleb (Fig. 2.18.1).

2.17.3.2 Symptoms

The patient may experience pain that exceeds what a similar injury without endophthalmitis might cause; however, this is not a reliable indicator, nor is the presence or absence of photophobia or decreased visual acuity. Similar complains may be caused by the injury irrespective of whether endophthalmitis is present.

2.17.3.3 Clinical Signs

On slit lamp examination, the signs of an early infection may be impossible to discern from those that the injury would have caused anyway. With time – and progression can be rapid, especially if caused by *Bacillus* species – the diagnosis becomes easier.

> **Pearl**
>
> The ease of recognizing a traumatic endophthalmitis and the prognosis of the condition are inversely proportional.

The clinical signs of an early (**e**) or advanced (**a**) bacterial endophthalmitis include:

- Lid edema and erythema, chemosis, (**e** / **a**), proptosis (**a**).
- Corneal edema (**e**), purulent corneal infiltration (**a**), or abscess (**a**). The presence of a ring ulcer (**a**) is a sign of *Bacillus* infection (Fig. 2.17.2).
- Accumulation of white blood cells in the AC (**e**); they form a hypopyon (**a**) if the patient is in the erect position.
- Fibrinous membrane in the AC (**e** / **a**), blanketing the iris, lens/IOL, and extending into the angle.
- Loss of retinal details (**e** / **a**; Fig. 2.17.3) or of red reflex (**a**).
- If the anterior vitreous can be visualized, it often shows cellular infiltration (**e**) or abscess (**a**). The nondetached posterior vitreous may con-

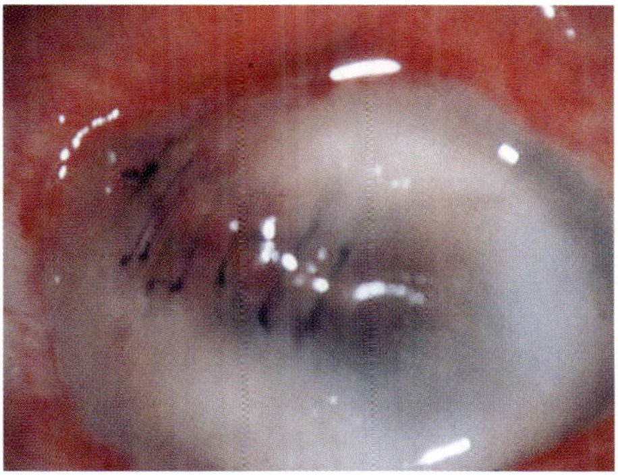

Fig. 2.17.2 Ring ulcer in *Bacillus* endophthalmitis. A ring-like peripheral corneal infiltration is typical of an endophthalmitis caused by *Bacillus* species. It is extremely unlikely that an eye with such an advanced infection can be saved

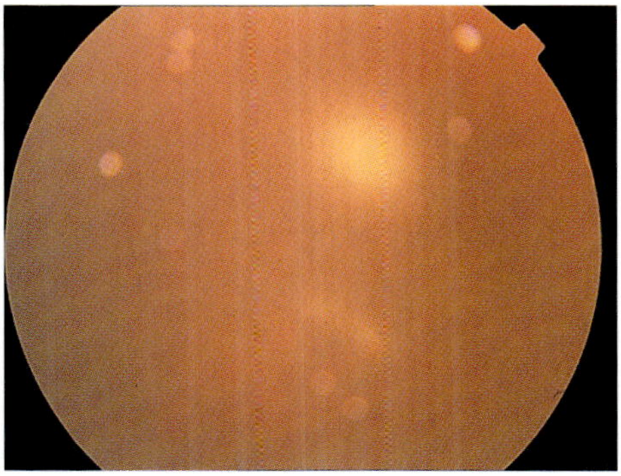

Fig. 2.17.3 Loss of retinal details in an eye with preserved red reflex in endophthalmitis (Courtesy of V. Mester, Abu Dhabi, U.A.E.)

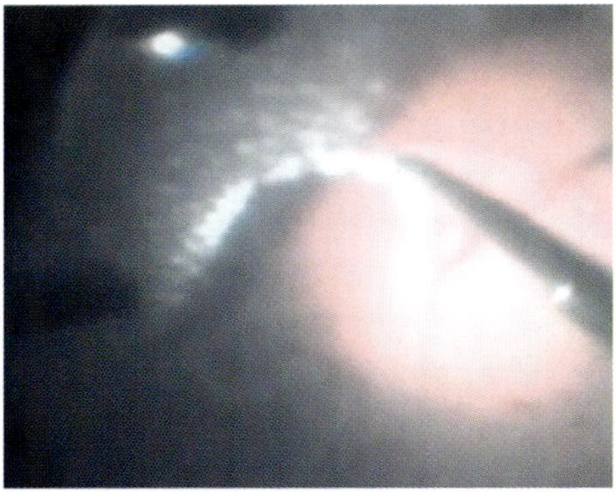

Fig. 2.17.4 Colonization of a nondetached posterior cortical vitreous in endophthalmitis. This intraoperative photograph shows a forceps carefully detaching the posterior hyaloid face in an eye that has had endophthalmitis for over a week. Despite the long duration of the infection, no spontaneous PVD has occurred, and the cortical vitreous is heavily colonized by bacteria, as shown here by the numerous *white dots*

tain multiple colonies of bacteria in the form of white-yellowish dots (**a**; Fig. 2.17.4).

- Endophthalmitis retinopathy (**a**), characterized by perivascular infiltration (periphlebitis), stress hemorrhages, areas of edema, exudative retinal detachment, and necrosis.[3]
- Panophthalmitis (**a**), characterized by proptosis and fever.

Fungi may cause a clinical picture that is in many ways similar to that described above, but usually such an infection:

- Has a history of soil contamination
- Is caused by an organic IOFB
- Shows a more chronic course

3 The retina is rarely seen until vitrectomy is performed and the cloudy media have been cleared.

- Demonstrates "snowball" or "string of pearls" appearing opacities in the vitreous [14].

2.17.3.4 Culturing

The bacterial spectrum is different if the endophthalmitis is trauma related and not postoperative. The organisms involved are typically more virulent and multi-organism infections are also more common. Frequently encountered bacteria causing traumatic endophthalmitis with poor prognosis include *Bacillus* species ([2], *Clostridium perfringens* [1], and Gram-negative rods [3].

Culturing is important to identify the organism and determine the in-vitro antimicrobial profile;[4] initiation of the therapy, however, must not be delayed until the lab report is received. Multiple culture media should be used (blood and chocolate agar, Sabouraud's, thioglycollate broth, anaerobic blood, as well as various stains (Gram, Giemsa, fungal), but the most accurate and rapid identification comes from polymerase chain reaction [20]. Bactec broth[5] is another medium with a high and fast yield [9].

2.17.4 Treatment

A two-pronged attack is necessary for eyes with traumatic endophthalmitis: surgery and medications.

Pearl

Traumatic endophthalmitis is a surgical indication; pharmaceutical treatment is to be employed in addition to, not instead of, vitrectomy.

Vitrectomy for endophthalmitis, especially if it is of traumatic origin, is technically one of the most challenging indications. The difficulty is due to the often hazy media and to the intricacy in distinguishing between yellowish layers of vitreous, which may have blood streaks mimicking retinal

4 Even though the in-vivo sensitivity may be different.
5 Bactec Peds Plus F, Becton Dickinson, Sparks, Maryland.

blood vessels, and a detached, necrotic, nonperfused retina, which may not bleed when injured. It is mandatory for the surgeon to take a slow, cautious approach, similar to that described in Chap. 2.12. The surgical steps are outlined in Table 2.17.2.

Table 2.17.2 Vitrectomy for traumatic endophthalmitis: surgical steps

Surgical step	Comment
Scrape the corneal epithelium	Most of the corneal edema resides in the epithelium; removing this layer is alone sufficient to dramatically increase visibility
Drying the corneal stroma	If the stroma is also hazy, applying a shield wetted with 40% glucose for a few minutes usually reduces the edema (see Chap. 2.9 for further options)
Cleaning of the AC	An AC maintainer is necessary to prevent hypotony. Gentle aspiration through a paracentesis is sufficient to remove white and red blood cells and most of the debris. The angle should also be irrigated. In the vast majority of eyes a fibrinous membrane is covering the angle, iris, and lens; this must be removed, using forceps, or aspiration with a blunt cannula or the vitrectomy probe. Irrigation of the AC may have to be repeated during surgery because the inflammatory debris may reaccumulate. The fibrinous membrane may also reform, especially in children; this must be removed as often as needed
Enlarging the pupil	Unless the sphincter has been damaged, the pupil is small; if not dilated, visibility of the posterior segment remains poor, even if wide-angle viewing is employed. If adrenaline does not achieve dilatation, iris retractors must be used (see Chap. 2.9)
Preparing the sclerotomies	These are made using the standard method.[1] The infusion must not be opened until the cannula's proper location is confirmed. A long cannula[2] should be considered

[1] Currently it is not recommended to use small-gauge vitrectomy for traumatic endophthalmitis.

[2] 6 or even 7 mm

Table 2.17.2 *(continued)* Vitrectomy for traumatic endophthalmitis: surgical steps

Surgical step	Comment
Dealing with the lens	Even if uninjured, the lens may have to be extracted to allow unhindered vitrectomy.[3] If an IOL is present, a large posterior capsulectomy should be created to allow irrigation of the bag. The surfaces of the IOL may have to wiped repeatedly
Performing vitrectomy	A careful antero-posterior approach is used, keeping the vitrectomy probe close to the visual axis[4] but nasal to it. Very slow progression is necessary, and it is crucial to go deep before going wide (see Chap. 2.12)
	The posterior hyaloid should be separated from the retina if possible.[5] If the retina is necrotic or if the vitreous is very adherent, this surgical goal must be abandoned
	The peripheral vitreous is carefully shaved, but a complete vitreous removal must not be attempted since this significantly raises the risk of creating a retinal break
Consider using silicone oil tamponade	Organisms do not proliferate in the oil [13]. Silicone oil use, however, is not a must; it should be preserved for those cases with major retinal pathology such as a break, detachment, or widespread necrosis, and then only if the vitreous cavity has been adequately cleaned.[6] Antibiotics and corticosteroids should be placed into the infusion fluid (Table 2.17.3) and the vitreous/capsular bag/AC irrigated, then silicone oil injected

[3] The capsules may be "dirty" from debris that settled on their surface; their "vacuuming" with the vitrectomy probe may be impossible without causing a capsular break.

[4] i.e., not close to the eye wall/retina

[5] Even in eyes with endophthalmitis persisting for several days, a vitreoschisis is more likely to be present than a true PVD. Leaving vitreous on the retinal surface increases the risk of macular injury from the organism's toxins, enzymes, and the body's inflammatory/immune response.

[6] All pus and vitreous, except in the periphery, have been removed.

Cave

A methodical, anterior-to-posterior sequence must be followed during vitrectomy for endophthalmitis; any attempt to bypass a step threatens with decreased visualization and thus increases the risk of iatrogenic retinal damage. If visibility is so poor as to make tissue identification impossible, surgery must be stopped.

If the cornea is in such poor shape that it does not allow visualization of deeper structures, the surgeon has three options:

- *Foregoing surgery* until the cornea clears. More than likely this results in loss of vision and probably even loss of the eye.
- *EAV* (see Chap. 2.20). It is a technically difficult surgery, and one of its major advantages, the complete cleansing of the vitreous base, should not be utilized; however, EAV does reduce the amount of pus in the eye and alleviates the need for PK.
- *TKP vitrectomy* (see Chap. 2.15). Currently, this appears to be the most effective, albeit complex, option. Even in these highly inflamed eyes, the graft rejection rate is very low.[6]

Silicone oil (Table 2.17.2) can be employed if the retina is injured and detachment is present or threatens. It has the following advantages:

- It maintains retinal attachment.
- It prevents pus reaccumulation.
- It maintains a clear retinal view even in the early postoperative period.

The details of pharmaceutical treatment are shown in Table 2.17.3. It must be mentioned that the efficacy of subconjunctival antibiotics has not been proven [17]. Recently there is an increase in the resistance of the organisms to vancomycin [21]. If an eye is filled with silicone oil, one-quarter of the

6 R. Morris, Birmingham, Alabama, unpublished data

Table 2.17.3 Pharmacotherapy for eyes with bacterial traumatic endophthalmitis

Route of application	Drug	Dose
Intravitreal injection	Ceftazidime	2.2 mg/0.1 ml
	Vancomycin	1–2 mg/0.1 ml
	Dexamethasone	0.4 mg/0.1 ml
Vitrectomy infusion fluid[a]	Ceftazidime	2.2×25 mg/100 ml
	Vancomycin	25 mg/100 ml
	Dexamethasone	0.4×25 mg/100 ml
Subconjunctival	Ceftazidime	100 mg in 0.5 ml
	Vancomycin	25 mg/0.5 ml
	Dexamethasone	15 mg/1 ml
Topical	Fortified topical antibiotics (e.g., ciprofloxacin [15])	Hourly
	Prednisolone acetate	1%, several times a day
Oral[b]	Moxifloxacin	400 mg/day
Intravenous	Ceftazidime	1 g/12 h
	Vancomycin	1 g/12 h

The initial ("blind") choice; must be modified as resistance test results become available from culturing

[a] The drug concentrations are identical to those of an intravitreal injection

[b] Because of its excellent penetration into the eye, oral moxifloxacin is usually sufficient; if not, intravenous therapy can be chosen

normal dose of the intravitreal regimen (Table 2.17.3) can be injected into the oil at the conclusion of surgery [8].

In addition to the treatment described above, the patient must be constantly reminded not to be in the supine position. The patient should stay in bed as little as possible, but if he does, he should turn to either side. Such posturing helps to prevent settling of the pus on the macula.

2.17.5 Prophylaxis

There is no consensus in the literature regarding the type of prophylactic antibiotics in eyes with open globe injury. Oral, topical, and subconjunctival antibiotics are always recommended. Whether intravitreal antibiotics should be used in every case of open globe injury or just in high-risk eyes [11] is an individual decision the surgeon has to make.

Pearl

Although no scientific study has proven that prophylactic antibiotics reduce the risk of endophthalmitis development, common sense tells us that they do. Antibiotic prophylaxis also makes sense from a medicolegal point of view.

DO:

- always think about the possibility of endophthalmitis if the eye sustained an open globe injury, and especially if the risk is high (e.g., IOFB, soil contamination, lens injury)
- proceed with as complete as possible vitrectomy and proper pharmaceutical therapy as soon as possible

DON'T:

- perform vitrectomy as if the condition of the eye were similar to a postoperative endophthalmitis; intraocular injuries make this operation, which is not an easy one even in the postoperative setting, even more complex and difficult
- leave infected vitreous behind unless visualization is poor and cannot be improved by a meticulous anterio-posterior approach; cleansing of the vitreous cavity should be as complete as possible

Summary

Endophthalmitis is one of the most dreaded complications of an open globe injury. Recognition is not as straightforward as in most cases of postoperative endophthalmitis, due to masking by the injury. The selection of treatment for a posttraumatic endophthalmitis, however, is noncontroversial: prompt vitrectomy with intravitreal, systemic, and topical antibiotics offers the best prognosis. Corticosteroids should also be employed to reduce the deleterious effects of the accompanying inflammation.

References

[1] Abu el-Asrar AM, al-Amro SA, al-Mosallam AA, al-Obeidan S (1999) Post-traumatic endophthalmitis: causative organisms and visual outcome. Eur J Ophthalmol 9: 21–31

[2] Affeldt J, Flynn H, Forster R et al. (1987) Microbial endophthalmitis resulting from ocular trauma. Ophthalmology 94: 407–413

[3] Boldt HC, Pulido JS, Blodi CF, Folk JC, Weingeist TA (1989) Rural endophthalmitis. Ophthalmology 96: 1722–1726

[4]Coyler M, Weber E, Weichel E, Dick J, Bower K, Ward T, Haller J (in press) Delayed intraocular foreign body removal without endophthalmitis during Operations Iraqi and Enduring Freedom. Ophthalmology

[5] Souza S de, Howcroft M J (1999) Management of posterior segment intraocular foreign bodies: 14 years' experience. Can J Ophthalmol 34: 23–29

[6] Endophthalmitis Vitrectomy Study Group (1995) Results of the Endophthalmitis Vitrectomy Study. Arch Ophthalmol 113: 1479–1496

[7] Essex RW, Yi Q, Charles PG, Allen PJ (2004) Post-traumatic endophthalmitis. Ophthalmology 111 2015–2022

[8] Hegazy HM, Kivilcim M, Peyman GA, Unal MH, Liang C, Molinari LC, Kazi AA (1999) Evaluation of toxicity of intravitreal ceftazidime, vancomycin, and ganciclovir in a silicone oil-filled eye. Retina 19: 553–557

[9] Kratz A, Levy J, Belfair N, Weinstein O, Klemperer I, Lifshitz T (2006) Broth culture yield vs traditional approach in the work-up of endophthalmitis. Am J Ophthalmol 141: 1022–1026

[10] Kuhn F, Gini G (2005) Ten years after... Are findings of the Endophthalmitis Vitrectomy Study still relevant today? Graefe's Arch Clin Exp Ophthalmol 243: 1197–1199

[11] Mieler WF, Ellis MK, Williams DF, Han DP (1990) Retained intraocular foreign bodies and endophthalmitis. Ophthalmology 97: 1532–1538

[12] Morris R, Witherspoon CW, Kuhn F, Bryne JB (1995) Endophthalmitis. Williams and Wilkins, Baltimore, pp 560

[13] Ozdamar A, Aras C, Ozturk R, Akin E, Karacorlu M, Ercikan C (1999) In vitro antimicrobial activity of silicone oil against endophthalmitis-causing agents. Retina 19: 122–126

[14] Pflugfelder SC, Flynn HW Jr, Zwickey TA, Forster RK, Tsiligianni A, Culbertson WW, Mandelbaum S (1988) Exogenous fungal endophthalmitis. Ophthalmology 95: 19–30

[15] Rao SK, Madhavan HN, Sitalakshmi G, Padmanabhan P (2000) Nocardia Asteroides keratitis: report of seven patients and literature review. Indian J Ophthalmol 48: 217–221

[16] Schrader WF (2004) Epidemiology of open globe eye injuries: analysis of 1026 cases in 18 years. Klin Monatsbl Augenheilkd 221: 629–635 [in German]

[17] Smiddy WE, Smiddy RJ, Ba'Arath B, Flynn HW Jr, Murray TG, Feuer WJ, Miller D (2005) Subconjunctival antibiotics in the treatment of endophthalmitis managed without vitrectomy. Retina 25: 751–758

[18] Thompson JT, Parver LM, Enger CL, Mieler WF, Liggett PE (1993) Infectious endophthalmitis after penetrating injuries with retained intraocular foreign bodies. Ophthalmology 100: 1468–1474

[19] Thompson W, Rubsamen P, Flynn H, Schiffman J, Cousins S (1995) Endophthalmitis after penetrating trauma. Risk factors and visual acuity outcomes. Ophthalmology 102: 1696–1701

[20] Varghese B, Rodrigues C, Deshmukh M, Natarajan S, Kamdar P, Mehta A (2006) Broad-range bacterial and fungal DNA amplification on vitreous humor from suspected endophthalmitis patients. Mol Diagn Ther 10: 319–326

[21] Vedantham V, Nirmalan PK, Ramasamy K, Prakash K, Namperumalsamy P (2006) Clinico-microbiological profile and visual outcomes of post-traumatic endophthalmitis at a tertiary eye care center in South India. Indian J Ophthalmol 54: 5–10

2.18 Posttraumatic Glaucoma

Ferenc Kuhn

2.18.1 Introduction

Secondary elevation of the IOP is a frequent complication after a serious eye injury. If proper treatment is not instigated, the consequences are just as devastating as in eyes with primary open angle glaucoma. A vicious circle can also develop: an eye injury can lead to glaucoma, which in turn increases the risk of sustaining another (eye) injury through a fall or an MVC (see Chap. 1.7) [14].

Cave

An almost infinite number of pathologies may be caused by a serious eye injury, all of which require proper attention and treatment. Failure to detect IOP elevation and bring the values down into the normal range is not uncommon.

The definition of posttraumatic glaucoma is not straightforward;[1] in this chapter glaucoma is defined as IOP elevation that is high or long-lasting enough to warrant treatment to avoid functional loss.

2.18.2 Evaluation

A careful slit lamp examination is necessary to recognize the presence of risk factors for IOP elevation after trauma (see below). Taking the IOP with a to-

1 Should a one-time IOP reading of 26 mmHg qualify?

nometer may be impossible or misleading if the cornea is severely injured. An estimate via palpation by an experienced ophthalmologist is preferred over not taking the IOP at all. The fellow eye should serve as control.

2.18.3 Treatment[2]

Primarily, the underlying cause of the IOP elevation must be resolved; this is detailed below. In addition, topical agents (beta blockers, prostaglandin analogs[3], carbonic anhydrase inhibitors, and, occasionally, alpha agonists) are used, occasionally supported by oral carbonic anhydrase inhibitors.

If the IOP remains elevated despite maximal medical treatment, laser (argon laser iridectomy and trabeculoplasty, YAG trabeculopuncture, diode laser cyclodestruction [2, 3, 15, 17, 18, 22, 26, 28, 41]), cyclocryopexy [24], and surgery (iridectomy, trabeculectomy with or without antimetabolites [20, 30, 36], shunt implantation [31]) are the next weapons in the ophthalmologist's armamentarium. The most commonly used antimetabolites are mitomycin-C (0.2–0.4 mg/ml) and 5-FU 5-fluorouracil (50 mg/ml) [38]. Eyes that have undergone a filtering procedure are at a higher risk of endophthalmitis (Fig. 2.18.1): if an antimetabolite has been used, the annual incidence reaches 1.3% [9]. For eyes with intractable glaucoma, retinectomy remains a viable therapeutic option [16].

2.18.4 Specific Conditions

2.18.4.1 Mechanical Globe Trauma

2.18.4.1.1 Contusion

A blunt object with insufficient momentum to cause rupture initially compresses the eye antero-posteriorly; this is followed by a rebound effect and

2 Detailed description of the management is beyond the scope of this book; the reader is referred to glaucoma textbooks.

3 Should not be administered in the acute, only in the chronic, phase because they may increase the inflammation.

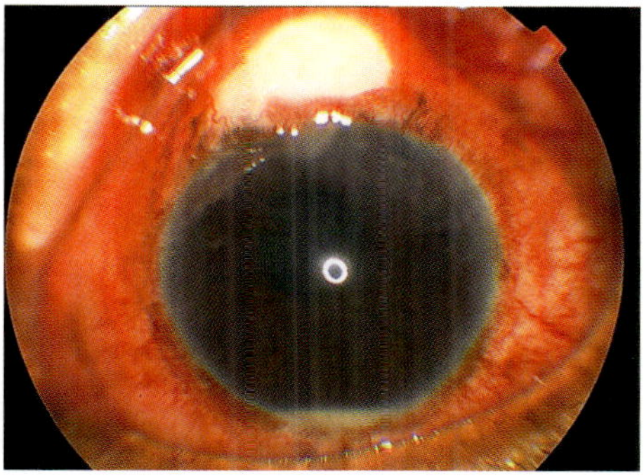

Fig. 2.18.1 Endophthalmitis following trabeculectomy for trauma-related glaucoma. Trabeculectomy was able to lower the IOP in this eye, but years later a bleb-related infection developed. The bleb has purulent material in it and there is also a 1-mm hypopyon (Courtesy of V. Mester, Abu Dhabi, U.A.E.)

subsequent oscillations with decreasing frequency (see Chap. 2.10). Several consequences of such an injury can lead to IOP elevation. Data from the USEIR [10] show that 3.4% of contused eyes develop glaucoma, and that the independent risk factors[4] are:

- Hyphema
- Lens injury (dislocation more so than cataract)
- Initial visual acuity of <20/200
- Angle recession
- Iris injury
- Older age

2.18.4.1.1.1 Early-onset Glaucomas

2.18.4.1.1.1.1 Inflammatory Debris Obstructing the Trabecular Meshwork

The outflow from the AC is decreased due to blockage by inflammatory cells and material; there may also be edema of the trabecular meshwork. The IOP elevation is self-limiting.

4 In decreasing order

Regarding *therapy*, topical corticosteroids, without antiglaucoma medications, usually suffice.

2.18.4.1.1.1.2 Damage to the Trabecular Meshwork

The trabecular meshwork is ruptured. A trabecular flap, hinged at the scleral spur, may also be present. There may be blood in Schlemm's canal, and cyclodialysis is a common additional finding.

Regarding *therapy*, anti-glaucoma medications or filtering surgery are used.

2.18.4.1.1.1.3 Hyphema

Blood in the AC may coexist with damage to the trabecular meshwork or may obstruct it in a fashion similar to that described above (inflammatory debris). Total hyphema and repeat hemorrhage represent elevated risk for glaucoma development, increasing the incidence from 0–25% [27] to 25–67% [34, 39]. The risk of glaucoma is directly proportional with the size of the hemorrhage: 14% if the hyphema is one-quarter, 27% if half, and 52% if the hyphema is total.

Regarding *therapy*, see Chap. 2.5.

2.18.4.1.1.1.4 Lens Swelling (Phacomorphic)

This condition is much more likely to occur in children than in adults, and occur in a very short period of time (see Chap. 2.16). Aqueous enters the lens through a capsular break, and the lens rapidly becomes a space-occupying lesion, causing pupillary block or pushing the iris forward to prevent aqueous access to the angle.

Regarding *therapy*, if a cataract is present, the best option is lens extraction (see Chap. 2.7). An iris bombans may be treated with peripheral iridectomy (laser or surgical; see above), but medical treatment often needs to be added.

2.18.4.1.1.1.5 Postinflammatory

Uveitis often leads to an IOP elevation [12], due mostly to trabecular meshwork obstruction, although other mechanisms are also possible (see below).

Regarding *therapy*, unless another specific cause exists (e.g., synechia, sympathetic ophthalmia), corticosteroids and cycloplegics are the primary weapons.

2.18.4.1.1.2 Delayed-onset Glaucomas

2.18.4.1.1.2.1 Angle Recession

The ciliary body is widened due to a split between its longitudinal and circular muscles.[5] The iris may be displaced posteriorly and the ciliary processes may become visible. Irido- and/or cyclodialysis may also be present. The IOP elevation typically occurs if at least a 180° separation is present, and even then it may be delayed by years since scarring and thus chronic obstruction of aqueous outflow are important in the pathogenesis. The recession is more likely to be an indicator, rather than cause, of the glaucoma [40]. Genetic predisposition to diminished trabecular function, present in both eyes, may partially be responsible [32]. Fewer than 10% of eyes with angle recession develop glaucoma [4], even though in eyes with contusion-related hyphema, angle recession occurs in 70–100% [6, 23, 35].

2.18.4.1.1.2.2 Blood-related

2.18.4.1.1.2.2.1 Hemolytic

Blood-breakdown products and macrophages that have phagocytized them obstruct the trabecular meshwork.

Regarding *therapy*, AC lavage is used if medication proved unable to cure this self-limiting IOP rise.

2.18.4.1.1.2.2.2 Hemosiderotic

The endothelial cells in the trabecular meshwork are responsible for the phagocytosis of hemoglobin. Iron is released in the process, causing siderosis, which usually affects other tissues of the eye as well (see Chap. 2.13).

Regarding *therapy*, removal of all iron particles from the eye, but antiglaucoma medications or even filtration surgery, may become necessary.

---

5 The longitudinal muscle remains attached to the scleral spur, but the circular muscle is displaced posteriorly.

2.18.4.1.1.2.2.3 Ghost Cell

In eyes with vitreous hemorrhage, red blood cells occasionally undergo a degenerative process and their cell wall is altered so that these khaki-colored cells become rigid and oval. If the anterior hyaloid face is disrupted or absent, these cells can enter the AC but are unable to exit through normal outflow channels, obstructing the trabecular meshwork. The condition can occur after closed or open globe trauma [5].

Regarding *therapy*, vitrectomy is necessary to remove the reservoir of the ghost cells and AC lavage to cleanse the outflow channels [1].

> **Pearl**
>
> Irrigation of the AC for eyes with glaucoma secondary to ghost cells will not permanently reduce the IOP if the resupply of such cells from the vitreous cavity has not been addressed.

2.18.4.1.1.2.3 Lens-related[6]

2.18.4.1.1.2.3.1 Subluxation and Luxation

The displaced lens can cause pupillary[7] or angle block. In the former case, iris bombans may also be seen (see below); in the latter case, closure of the angle is easy to recognize on gonioscopy or with the UBM.

Regarding *therapy*, a pupillary block can be managed with (laser or surgical) iridectomy; otherwise, the lens needs to be removed.

2.18.4.1.1.2.3.2 Phacolytic

Lens proteins, recognized by the body's immune system as an alien material, leak through the capsule. The phagocytized material obstructs the trabecular meshwork. The IOP can be very high.

Regarding *therapy*, lens removal is indicated, preceded by medical treatment to lower the IOP and reduce the vascular engorgement.

---

6 Lens swelling may also cause late-onset glaucoma, although an early (acute) IOP rise is morel likely (see above).

7 A prolapsed vitreous may contribute to the blockage.

2.18.4.1.1.2.3.3 Phacoanaphylactic[8]

The pathophysiology is similar to that described above, but uveitis dominates the clinical picture; even a (pseudo)hypopyon may be present.[9]

Regarding *therapy*, lens removal and anti-inflammatory treatment are indicated.

2.18.4.1.1.2.4 Aqueous Misdirection ("Malignant Glaucoma")

In this poorly understood condition, which typically follows intraocular surgery but can also occur after contusion [33], the aqueous is misdirected posteriorly: rather than streaming toward the angle, it is flowing into or behind the vitreous. The increased intravitreal fluid volume pushes the lens/iris complex forward, resulting in a very shallow AC.

Regarding *therapy*, cycloplegics, antiglaucoma medications, and YAG hyaloidotomy may be attempted, but the most promising approach is surgical, which is fairly complex. Vitrectomy, anterior hyaloidectomy, zonuloidectomy, iridectomy, and lens removal [29] need to be performed, which reopen the original channel for aqueous outflow.

Pearl

Radical combined anterior- and posterior segment surgery is the most effective treatment for eyes with aqueous misdirection. The conservative approach has a much lower success rate [13].

2.18.4.1.2 Open Globe Injury

The incidence of secondary glaucoma in eyes with open globe injury is 2.7% in the USEIR [11]. The independent risk factors[10] are:

- Inflammation
- Lens injury

8 Also called phacoantigenic glaucoma or lens-related uveitis.

9 The differential diagnosis therefore includes endophthalmitis and even sympathetic ophthalmia.

10 In decreasing order.

- Initial visual acuity of <20/200
- Older age

In addition to the many conditions listed above under contusion, the following consequences of an open globe injury can lead to elevated IOP.

2.18.4.1.2.1 Anterior Synechiae

Abnormal adhesion forms between the iris and the cornea as a result of inflammation or aqueous leak through an open wound and consequently flat AC. The consequence is reduced aqueous access to the angle.

Therapy proceeds according to the etiology: surgical closure of the wound; corticosteroids to reduce the inflammation; or breaking of the synechiae (see Chap. 2.5).

2.18.4.1.2.2 Posterior Synechiae

As a result of inflammation, adhesion develops between the iris and the anterior lens capsule. The pupil is partially or totally immobile, and its shape is irregular. Communication between the posterior chamber and the AC is reduced. If the block is complete, the iris is bulging forward between its root and the pupillary margin (iris bombans), pushed by the aqueous that cannot reach the angle (see Chap. 2.5).

Regarding *therapy*, iridectomy or synechiolysis (see Chap. 2.5) is used. If the inflammation is still present, topical corticosteroids must be used.

2.18.4.1.2.3 Epithelial Downgrowth or Fibrous Ingrowth

The spreading epithelial blanket or scar tissue covers the outflow channels. The condition may develop due to the injury itself or from surgery; the IOP elevation can be fairly high and difficult to treat. Prevention is crucial, avoiding full-thickness sutures in limbal wound repair (see Chap. 2.2) and placing the paracentesis slightly central to the limbus (see Chap. 2.5).

Regarding *therapy*, surgery is the primary weapon: cyst/cell/scar tissue removal; cryopexy; and endodiathermy [25, 37]. Removal of a scar must be done very carefully to avoid tissue rupture and bleeding (see Chap. 2.5).

2.18.4.1.2.4 Toxicosis

Both a ferrous (siderosis) and a copper (chalcosis) IOFB can cause IOP elevation (see Chap. 2.13).

Regarding *therapy*, if recognized early, the IOFB can be removed and result in IOP normalization; otherwise, antiglaucoma medications, or even filtration surgery, may be needed. With time the ciliary body may be destroyed by the disease, which can also help lower the IOP [7].

2.18.4.2 Chemical Trauma

The IOP shows an initial spike after the injury (probably due to tissue shrinkage and increased uveal blood flow), followed by a period of normal or even low IOP if there is extensive ciliary body damage. Finally, chronic IOP elevation is found, due to inflammation and scarring of the angle.

Regarding *therapy*, in addition to the specific therapy for the chemical injury itself (see Chap. 3.1), proper antiglaucoma medications (see above) have to be used, along with anti-inflammatory treatment and cycloplegia. Surgery is needed if the IOP cannot be controlled medically.

2.18.4.3 Orbital Hypertension

The typical underlying condition is hemorrhage, whether caused by trauma or a retro- (para-) bulbar injection; systemic anticoagulant therapy is a risk factor [8].[11] In the worst cases, even the LP may be lost.

Regarding *therapy*, emergency lateral canthotomy may have to be performed if the IOP is so high that the central retinal artery is compressed.

2.18.4.4 "Iatrogenic": Following Closure of a Cyclodialysis Cleft

Once the detached ciliary body is reattached, the previously low IOP can rapidly reach extreme values (see Chap. 2.8).

11 In rare cases, the cause is orbital congestion in patients undergoing hydration therapy in cases of severe thermal burn. Another very rare etiology may be emphysema from one of the sinuses after an orbital fracture.

Regarding *therapy*, prophylactic treatment using topical beta blockers and oral carbonic anhydrase inhibitors is recommended to avoid such an IOP spike [19].

2.18.4.5 Sympathetic Ophthalmia

The IOP elevation may develop as part of the severe uveitis [21].

Regarding *therapy*, anti-inflammatory treatment for sympathetic ophthalmia should be sufficient, but antiglaucoma medications may also have to be applied.

DO:

- follow the IOP closely after a serious injury, especially if risk factors for the development of secondary glaucoma are present
- if medical treatment is inefficient to bring the IOP down, consider surgery early

DON'T:

- be overconfident that treatment of a certain pathology (i.e., removal of a hyphema) will solve the IOP problem; other etiologies (i.e., ghost cell formation) may contribute as well and may also require treatment
- forgo consulting a glaucoma specialist if the IOP elevation persists

Summary

Glaucoma is probably a far more common complication of closed or open globe trauma than presumed. The treatment may be simple, eliminating the underlying cause, but it may also be complex and difficult: the IOP elevation may be nonresponsive to medical treatment and require surgical intervention. In such cases, a glaucoma specialist must be consulted.

References

[1] Abu el-Asrar AM, al-Obeidan SA (1995) Pars plana vitrectomy in the management of ghost cell glaucoma. Int Ophthalmol 19: 121–124

[2] Anmarkrud N, Bergaust B, Bulie T, Sand AB (1987) Argon laser trabeculoplasty: 5 years experience from a local eye department. Acta Ophthalmol (Suppl) 182: 34–36

[3] Beckman H, Fuller TA (1979) Carbon dioxide laser scleral dissection and filtering procedure for glaucoma. Am J Ophthalmol 88: 73–77

[4] Blanton FM (1964) Anterior chamber angle recession and secondary glaucoma. A study of the aftereffects of traumatic hyphemas. Arch Ophthalmol 72: 39–43

[5] Campbell DG (1981) Ghost cell glaucoma following trauma. Ophthalmology 88: 1151–1158

[6] Canavan YM, Archer DB (1982) Anterior segment consequences of blunt ocular injury. Br J Ophthalmol 66: 549–555

[7] Chandra M, Sharma V, Ghose S, Kashyap S, Pushker N (2003) Phthisis bulbi with a large protruding foreign body: a rare complication of penetrating injuries. Orbit 22: 145–149

[8] Chorich LJ, Derick RJ, Chambers RB, Cahill KV, Quartetti EJ, Fry JA, Bush CA (1998) Hemorrhagic ocular complications associated with the use of systemic thrombolytic agents. Ophthalmology 105: 428–431

[9] DeBry PW, Perkins TW, Heatley G, Kaufman P, Brumback LC (2002) Incidence of late-onset bleb-related complications following trabeculectomy with mitomycin. Arch Ophthalmol 120: 297–300

[10] Girkin CA, McGwin G Jr, Long C, Morris R, Kuhn F (2005) Glaucoma after ocular contusion: a cohort study of the United States Eye Injury Registry. J Glaucoma 14: 470–473

[11] Girkin CA, McGwin G Jr, Morris R, Kuhn F (2005) Glaucoma following penetrating ocular trauma: a cohort study of the United States Eye Injury Registry. Am J Ophthalmol 139: 100–105

[12] Goldsmith AJ (1963) Indications for surgery in glaucoma. Secondary glaucoma. Trans Ophthalmol Soc UK 83: 233–244

[13] Greenfield DS, Tello C, Budenz DL, Liebmann JM, Ritch R (1999) Aqueous misdirection after glaucoma drainage device implantation. Ophthalmology 106: 1035–1040

[14] Haymes SA, Leblanc RP, Nicolela MT, Chiasson LA, Chauhan BC (2007) Risk of falls and motor vehicle collisions in glaucoma. Invest Ophthalmol Vis Sci 48: 1149–1155

[15] Immonen IJ, Puska P, Raitta C (1994) Transscleral contact krypton laser cyclophotocoagulation for treatment of glaucoma. Ophthalmology 101: 876–882

[16] Joussen AM, Walter P, Jonescu-Cuypers CP, Koizumi K, Poulaki V, Bartz-Schmidt KU, Krieglstein GK, Kirchhof B (2003) Retinectomy for treatment of intractable glaucoma: long term results. Br J Ophthalmol 87: 1094–1102

[17] Kim DD, Moster MR (1999) Transpupillary argon laser cyclophotocoagulation in the treatment of traumatic glaucoma. J Glaucoma 8: 340–341

[18] Kivela T, Puska P, Raitta C, Immonen I, Tarkkanen A (1995) Clinically successful contact transscleral krypton laser cyclophotocoagulation. Long-term histopathologic and immunohistochemical autopsy findings. Arch Ophthalmol 113: 1447–1453

[19] Kronfeld PC (1954) The fluid exchange in the successfully cyclodialyzed eye. Trans Am Ophthalmol Soc 52: 249–263

[20] Lerner SF (1997) Small incision trabeculectomy avoiding Tenon's capsule. A new procedure for glaucoma surgery. Ophthalmology 104: 1237–1241

[21] Makley TA, Azar A (1978) Sympathetic ophthalmia. A long-term follow-up. Arch Ophthalmol 96: 257–262

[22] Melamed S, Ashkenazi I, Gutman I, Blumenthal M (1992) Nd:YAG laser trabeculopuncture in angle-recession glaucoma. Ophthalmic Surg 23: 31–35

[23] Mooney D (1973) Angle recession and secondary glaucoma. Br J Ophthalmol 57: 608–612

[24] Palimeris G, Moschos M, Chimonidou E, Velissaropoulos P (1976) Some observations on the use of cyclocryopexy in the treatment of various forms of glaucoma. Klin Monatsbl Augenheilkd 169: 439–441 [in German]

[25] Peyman GA, Peralta E, Ganiban GJ, Kraut R (1998) Endoresection of the iris and ciliary body in epithelial downgrowth. J Cataract Refract Surg 24: 130–133

[26] Raivio VE, Immonen IJ, Laatikainen LT, Puska PM (2001) Transscleral contact krypton laser cyclophotocoagulation for treatment of posttraumatic glaucoma. J Glaucoma 10: 77–84

[27] Read J (1975) Traumatic. hyphema: surgical vs medical management. Ann Ophthalmol 7: 659–670

[28] Schlote T, Derse M, Zierhut M (2000) Transscleral diode laser cyclophotocoagulation for the treatment of refractory glaucoma secondary to inflammatory eye diseases. Br J Ophthalmol 84: 999–1003

[29] Sharma A, Sii F, Shah P, Kirkby GR (2006) Vitrectomy-phacoemulsification-vitrectomy for the management of aqueous misdirection syndromes in phakic eyes. Ophthalmology 113: 1968–1973

[30] Sihota R, Sood NN, Agarwal HC (1995) Traumatic glaucoma. Acta Ophthalmol Scand 73: 252–254

[31] Sivak-Callcott JA, O'Day DM, Gass JD, Tsai JC (2001) Evidence-based recommendations for the diagnosis and treatment of neovascular glaucoma. Ophthalmology 108: 1767–1776; quiz 1777, 1800

[32] Tesluk GC, Spaeth GL (1985) The occurrence of primary open-angle glaucoma in the fellow eye of patients with unilateral angle-cleavage glaucoma. Ophthalmology 92: 904–911

[33] Theelen T, Klevering BJ (2005) Malignant glaucoma following blunt trauma of the eye. Ophthalmologe 102 77–81 [in German]

[34] Thomas M, Parrish R, Feuer W (1986) Rebleeding after traumatic hyphema. Arch Ophthalmol 104: 206–210

[35] Tonjum AM (1968) Intraocular pressure and facility of outflow late after ocular contusion. Acta Ophthalmol (Copenh) 46: 886–908

[36] Verma N (1996) Trabeculectomy and manual clot evacuation in traumatic hyphaema with corneal blood staining. Aust N Z J Ophthalmol 24: 33–38

[37] Viestenz A, Kuchle M, Naumann GO (2003) Block excision of epithelial ingrowth after cataract surgery: report on 15 patients. Klin Monatsbl Augenheilkd 220: 465–470 [in German]

[38] Vijaya L, Mukhesh BN, Shantha B, Ramalingam S, Sathi Devi AV (2000) Comparison of low-dose intraoperative mitomycin-C vs 5-fluorouracil in primary glaucoma surgery: a pilot study. Ophthalmic Surg Lasers 31: 24–30

[39] Walton W, Hagen S von, Grigorian R, Zarbin M (2002) Management of traumatic hyphema. Surv Ophthalmol 47: 297–334

[40] Wolff SM, Zimmerman LE (1962) Chronic secondary glaucoma. Associated with retrodisplacement of iris root and deepening of the anterior chamber angle secondary to contusion. Am J Ophthalmol 54: 547–563

[41] Zaidman GW, Wandel T (1988) Transscleral YAG laser photocoagulation for uncontrollable glaucoma in corneal patients. Cornea 7: 112–114

2.19 Hypotony

Ferenc Kuhn

2.19.1 Introduction

Normal IOP is a "conditio sine qua non" for maintaining the size and visual function of the eye. If the IOP is permanently below a certain value,[1] the globe is prone to shrink in size (phthisis) and eventually lose vision even if the retina is healthy. The hypotony may be caused by an increase in outflow or a decrease in aqueous production.

2.19.2 Evaluation

In addition to a low IOP reading, certain slit lamp and ultrasonographic findings may also be present. Some of these are the consequences, others possibly the cause, of the low IOP:

- Corneal edema with folds
- Scleral folding [5]
- Shallow AC
- Greenish-grayish discoloration of the iris
- Cataract
- Chorioretinal effusion, thickening, and folds
- Tortuosity of retinal vessels
- Retinal detachment
- Edema of the disc and macula ("hypotony maculopathy")

---

1 Approximately 4–6 mmHg

2.19.3 Treatment

Hypotony and phthisis are not diseases: they are the consequence of a certain intraocular pathology. It is this pathology that requires treatment (see below). If the underlying cause responsible for hypotony cannot be cured, silicone oil implantation remains the only hope for preventing phthisis. If the IOP is restored, the visual function can improve substantially [3].

2.19.4 Specific Conditions Responsible for Hypotony

2.19.4.1 Increased Aqueous Outflow

2.19.4.1.1 Wound Leak

The wound is usually easy to find, although occasionally an occult rupture or exit wound (see Chap. 2.12) is responsible. If a corneal wound has spontaneously closed, the diagnosis may be difficult, but Seidel positivity (see Chap. 2.2) is a telling sign.

The treatment is straightforward: surgical wound closure.

2.19.4.1.2 Ciliochoroidal Detachment

The pathomechanism of how the detachment and hypotony interrelate is not absolutely clear [2], but a vicious circle may be caused by the hypotony leading to inflammation, transudation, and decreased aqueous secretion with consequent hypotony. The suprauveal fluid may be a transudate or blood.

The *treatment* is primarily anti-inflammatory (topical cycloplegics and corticosteroids); paradoxically, CAIs may be given to speed up the absorption of the suprauveal fluid. Viscoelastics can be injected into the AC [1], the ciliary body reattached with sutures, or the suprauveal fluid drained (see Chap. 2.8).

2.19.4.1.3 Retinal Detachment

The pathomechanism of increased fluid removal by the RPE is unknown. The *treatment* is reattachment of the retina (see Chap. 2.9).

2.19.4.1.4 *Retinectomy*

In eyes with a large area of denuded RPE, hypotony ensues; this has even been utilized in bringing down the IOP in blind eyes with otherwise intractable glaucoma (see Chap 2.18).

The *treatment* is destruction of the RPE in the area of retinectomy to prevent aqueous drainage, or silicone oil implantation to prevent aqueous access. A blunt-tipped diathermy probe is used for choroid (RPE) destruction; it is much more difficult and risky to use scissors or the vitrectomy probe for this purpose.

2.19.4.1.5 *Choroidal Detachment*

In this poorly understood condition, fluid collects in the suprachoroidal space via effusion. The choroid remains separated from the sclera and the fluid reaccumulates after drainage.

As a *treatment* option, the eye can be filled with silicone oil (see below) or retinal tacks can be used to affix the choroid to the sclera (see Chap. 2.9). The primary cause of the hypotony needs to be addressed.

With regard to cyclodialysis, see Chap. 2.8.

2.19.4.2 Reduced Aqueous Secretion

2.19.4.2.1 *Inflammation*[2]

Anterior uveitis, verified by the presence of flare and cells in the AC and signaling the breakdown of the blood–aqueous barrier, causes ciliary body edema. Another possible mechanism is increased uveoscleral outflow [6].

The *treatment* is anti-inflammatory (see above).

2.19.4.2.2 *Ciliary Body "Shock"*

Following a contusion, the ciliary body may temporarily halt aqueous production without the presence of any of the pathologies described in this

2 Inflammation can also elevate the IOP (see Chap. 2.18).

chapter or Chap. 2.8.[3] The AC is shallow and the cornea may show foldings of Descemet's membrane.

The *treatment* is injection of viscoelastics into the AC, repeatedly if necessary. It may take months for the ciliary body to recover.

2.19.4.2.3 Ciliary Body Destruction

The etiology is the same as above, except that there is true and visible damage to the ciliary epithelium and processes. The ciliary processes are shortened, may have lost some of their pigment content, and can dramatically shrink with time (Fig. 2.19.1). The pathomechanism is probably vascular occlusion. Commonly there is a serious iris abnormality as well.[4]

There is no treatment for the condition, although phthisis may be preventable (see below). Anterior PVR can also destroy the ciliary body if the scar is not removed in time (see Chap. 2.8).

2.19.5 Consequence of Chronic Hypotony: Phthisis[5]

The difference between an eye in "prephthisical" vs "phthisical" stage is that in the latter, tissue disruption is evident; the condition results from the cessation of aqueous production. If treatment of all known pathologies, including that of anterior PVR,[6] has been exhausted and the eye starts to shrink, there are two options left besides eye removal (see below).

3 This is the clinician's observation; there is no explanation for the phenomenon in the available literature.
4 Major iris damage is an indicator of ciliary body trauma (see Chap. 2.6).
5 The term means "wasting away".
6 Meticulous removal of membranes covering the ciliary body should be attempted even in late cases. The phthisis is not reversible but stoppable if the intervention was not too late – but this can be determined only after the attempted scar removal has failed, and should not serve as an excuse not to attempt scar removal.

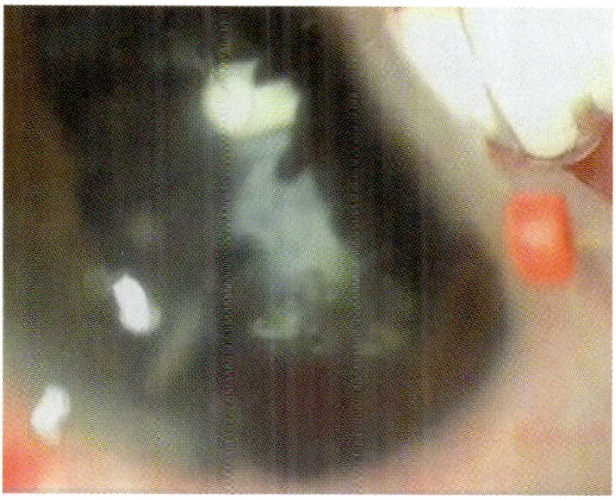

Fig. 2.19.1 Intraoperative image of repair for ciliary body destruction. This 8-year-old boy had a rupture with vitreous hemorrhage. He underwent several surgeries and eventually the eye was given up on. He developed iris scarring into the wound; there was no pupil, the retina was detached, the visual acuity was light perception, and the axial length of the previously emmetropic eye was 21 mm. After a pupil was created, the ciliary body was debulked, the pre- and subretinal scars were removed, and silicone oil was implanted (restricted to the vitreous cavity). There was no anterior PVR. The most probable explanation for the partial destruction of the ciliary processes (*arrow*) is that the posterior lens capsule was not removed originally. Twelve months after surgery, the IOP is normal, the eye has stopped shrinking, the retina is attached, and the visual acuity has improved to 20/40

2.19.5.1 Permanent Keratoprosthesis

Implanting such a device (see Chaps. 2.15, 3.1) may not only preserve the eye but actually improve function [4].

2.19.5.2 Silicone Oil Fill

The purpose of silicone oil implantation is different here from that in all other indications, in which the surgeon's aim is to achieve a 100% fill in the vitreous cavity without silicone oil prolapse into the AC.

Pearl

The goal of silicone oil implantation in the prevention or "treatment"[7] of phthisis management is to achieve a "101%" fill: the entire globe, not only the vitreous cavity, is filled, and the IOP is set at a higher-than-normal value to mechanically prevent globe shrinkage.[8]

The surgical steps are as follows:

- Perform a complete vitreous removal if this has not yet been done.
- Remove the lens in its entirety if the eye is still phakic. If the eye is pseudophakic, remove the IOL and the capsule.
- Perform a large inferior iridectomy.
- Do a fluid–air exchange.
- Be patient until the BSS is completely evacuated from the eye.
- Do a total air–silicone oil change: the AC must also be filled[9] (Fig. 2.19.2). High-viscosity oil (i.e., 5000 centistokes) may be used, but because intraocular movement of the silicone oil is prevented, the emulsification risk is lower than usual.
- Set the IOP at 30–35 mmHg.

The cornea is expected to tolerate the silicone oil touch for many months, even years, but eventually it will gradually opacify. When zonular opacity appears, there is ample time to decide whether PK with an "oil change" is performed, or the blind, potentially painful, and cosmetically unappealing eye is removed (enucleation or evisceration). This decision is best made by the patient (see Chap. 1.4).

7 This is not truly treatment but rather a prophylaxis of further deterioration.

8 Based on the principle that fluids are incompressible.

9 The goal is to prevent any aqueous that may still be produced to access the cornea. The endothelium will survive longer if silicone is able to prevent "aqueous touch."

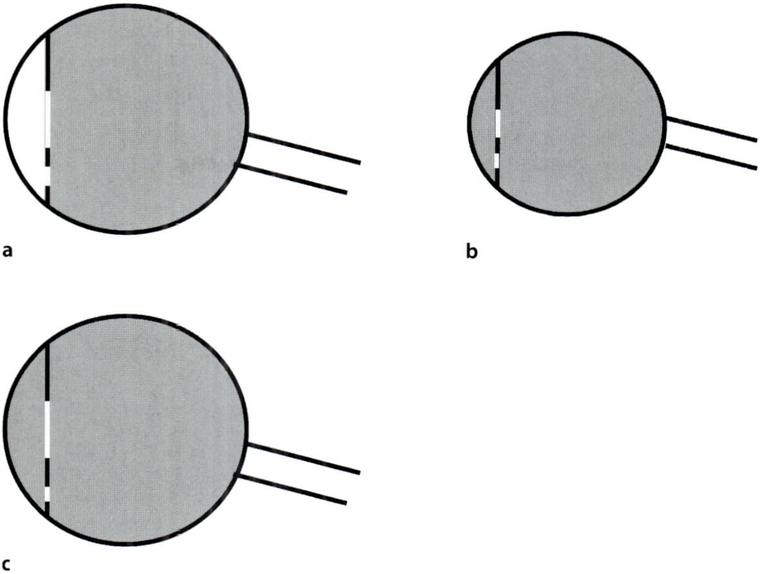

Fig. 2.19.2 Silicone oil implantation for phthisis. **a** The typical silicone oil fill is intended to be 100% in the vitreous cavity and 0% in the AC. **b** If there is no aqueous production, the globe starts to shrink. This is stopped when the internal volume of the eye equals that of the silicone oil. **c** If the eye is completely filled with silicone oil (i.e., the vitreous cavity as well as the AC), globe shrinkage is prevented

DO:

- intervene early if the IOP is low after an injury
- restore normal ciliary body anatomy as soon as possible since this almost always restores normal aqueous production; anterior PVR is the most common preventable cause of enucleation due to phthisis

DON'T:

- give up on the eye even if shrinking of the globe has already started; although phthisis is irreversible, further shrinkage can be halted

Summary

A chronically low IOP is incompatible with visual function, threatening even the normal size of the eye. Some of the pathologies that cause hypotony are treatable, others result in inexorable damage. Early recognition and treatment are usually able to prevent phthisis.

References

[1] Bellows AR, Chylack LT Jr, Hutchinson BT (1981) Choroidal detachment. Clinical manifestation, therapy and mechanism of formation. Ophthalmology 88: 1107–1115

[2] Berkowitz RA, Klyce SD, Kaufman HE (1984) Aqueous hyposecretion after penetrating keratoplasty. Ophthalmic Surg 15: 323–324

[3] Delgado MF, Daniels S, Pascal S, Dickens CJ (2001) Hypotony maculopathy: improvement of visual acuity after 7 years. Am J Ophthalmol 132: 931–933

[4] Dohlman CH, D'Amico DJ (1999) Can an eye in phthisis be rehabilitated? A case of improved vision with 1-year follow-up. Arch Ophthalmol 117: 123–124

[5] Loewenstein A, McKinnon S, DiBernardo C (1997) Echographic diagnosis of scleral fold in hypotony. Am J Ophthalmol 124: 260–261

[6] Toris CB, Pederson JE (1987) Aqueous humor dynamics in experimental iridocyclitis. Invest Ophthalmol Vis Sci 28: 477–481

2.20 Endoscopy

Claude Boscher and Ferenc Kuhn

2.20.1 Introduction

The very first use of an endoscope in ophthalmology was reported in 1934; the indication was ocular trauma [6]. Significant recent technological advances, such as reduced size, increased resolution, and probe resterilization[1] and disposability, may make endoscopy a mainstream option in the diagnosis and treatment of eyes with a variety of diseases [3, 4, 7], including PVR [8] and injury [1, 2].

2.20.2 Technical Overview[2]

Figure 2.20.1 shows the assembled system. The quality and thus usefulness of the visual information available for the surgeon depend on several parameters:

- Number and quality of fibers dedicated to image transmission
- Focal distance of the handpiece's lens(es)
- Distance of the handpiece from the target
- Angle of illumination

1 Autoclave.

2 While description of the equipment and its operational setup are not among the goals of this book, this brief exception is made here to facilitate understanding of the technology.

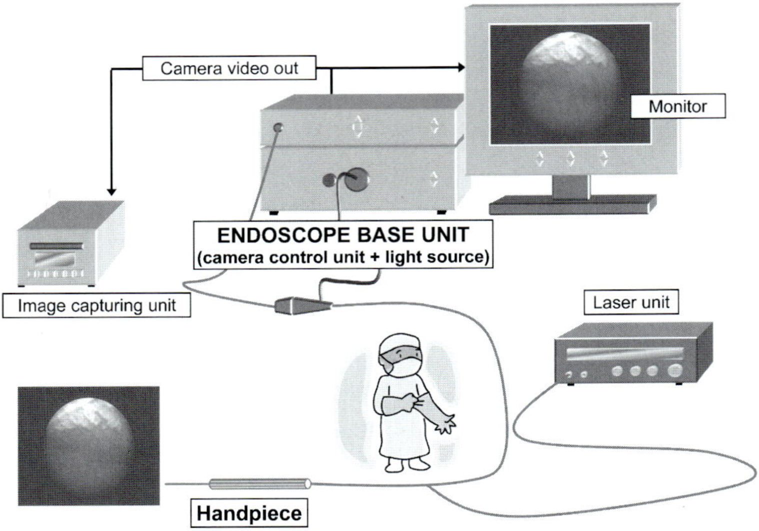

Fig. 2.20.1 An assembled endoscopy system.[1] The fiber optics transmission probe is connected to a three-chip CCD camera equipped with an ultrasensitive automatic shutter. The probe is fully autoclavable.[2] Universal connections are used so that the probe can be connected to endoscopic cameras as well as light and laser sources already available in the OR. This more than offsets the original costs of the technology

[1] OS Endoskopie, Jesi, Italy

[2] As required by WHO rules. This is especially important in traumatology, where surgery can be time-consuming and with an increased risk of endophthalmitis.

- Magnification
- Resolution of the camera
- Size of the operative field and of the targeted image
- Attributes of the light source and the distribution of the light
- Size, quality, and settings of the video monitor

2.20.3 Advantages and Capabilities of Endoscope Use in Ocular Traumatology

The advantages and capabilities of endoscope use are as follows:

- With endoscopy, the timing of surgery is determined by the condition of the injured tissues, not by the clarity of the media. If visualization of the posterior segment is severely compromised by the corneal damage and vitrectomy is urgent, the surgeon may want to forgo using the TKP (see Chap. 2.15). Endoscopic bypassing of the anterior segment opacities [1, 3] spares the patient of the potential complications of performing PK on an acutely injured eye. If PK becomes necessary subsequently, it can be scheduled so that the risk of transplantation-related intra- and postoperative complications is reduced.
- During EAV, progressive intraoperative opacification of the cornea or lens does not jeopardize surgical success.
- The endoscope helps identify the site for ideal sclerotomy placement, including that for the infusion cannula. The proper position of the cannula's port[3] can be confirmed before the infusion is opened.
- Endoscope use allows inspection of intraocular spaces that are impossible or very difficult to view by traditional methods: the posterior surface of the iris; the lens capsules, bag, and the IOL behind the iris; the zonules and capsulozonular complex; and the ciliary body.
- The endoscope makes it unnecessary to employ scleral indentation, regardless of whether it would be used to examine or treat the crucial peripheral structures[4]. Foregoing scleral indentation means that pathologies, such as ciliary body detachment or vitreoretinal traction, are inspected "in vivo", i.e., without physical distortion. The presence of anterior PVR or cyclitic membranes [2, 3] is not only easier to recognize, but their true effect on the normal tissues can be observed.

---

3 i.e., is it in front of, rather than underneath, the retina and uvea.

4 i.e., anterior retina, pars plana, ciliary body.

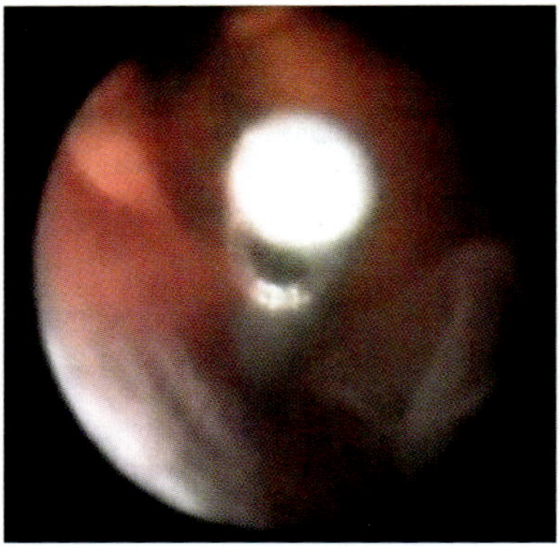

Fig. 2.20.2 Endoscopic peeling of the anterior vitreous base. This eye had an IOFB injury, and the retina was also detached. Endoscopy-assisted vitrectomy was performed 20 days later. Blood, adherent to the pars plana, is being dissected and removed

- With proper technique,[5] complete and unhindered intraoperative inspection is achieved, both circumferentially (360° visualization of all anterior structures; see Chap. 2.8) and antero-posteriorly (from the retrolental to the subretinal space). Endoscopy thus has unique significance in eyes whose injuries involve the posterior eye wall (see Chaps. 2.9, 2.14).
  - The endoscope is not simply a diagnostic tool: with its high-magnification and high-resolution image and tangential approach it allows performing surgical tasks (e.g., EAV) that would be difficult or impossible to accomplish with traditional viewing techniques. An incomplete list of such tasks includes:
  - Dissection of the vitreous base area to remove vitreous, blood (Fig. 2.20.2), proliferative cells, stem cell ingrowth [9], scar tissue, and cyclitic membranes [2, 3]
  - Releasing traction to help reattach the retina, choroid, and ciliary body (Figs. 2.20.3, 2.20.4)
  - Complete removal of the vitreous from behind the lens

5 i.e., using multiple sclerotomies in the presence of a clear lens.

– Freeing the iris (see Chap. 2.6) from scar tissue grown over its posterior surface or "unrolling" of a retracted iris [8]
– Repositioning subluxated or luxated IOLs

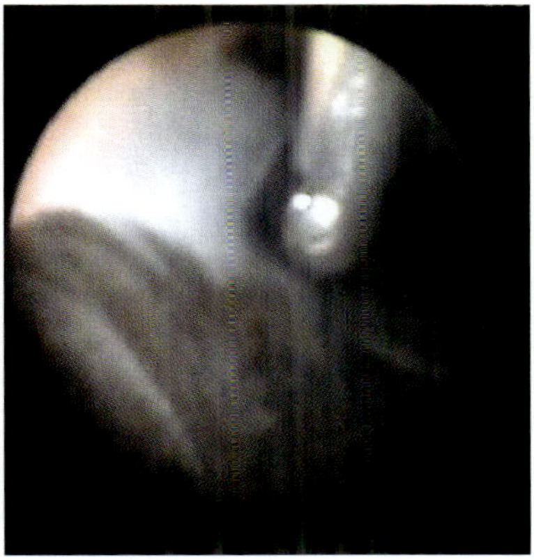

Fig. 2.20.3 Endoscopy-assisted vitrectomy revision of the ciliary body area after failure of conventional vitrectomies. A thick cyclitic membrane is adherent to a corneal wound, and there is ciliary detachment. The iris and cornea are visible at the top of the image. The flow is raised up to 14 ml/m to allow grasping of the elastic membrane. Even though complete removal was not possible, the remnants could be dissected from the ciliary epithelium

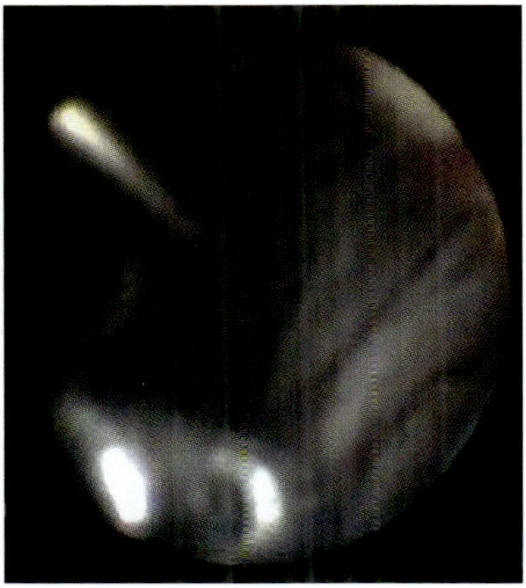

Fig. 2.20.4 Endoscopy-assisted vitrectomy revision of complex posttraumatic anterior segment pathologies. Tangential, high-magnification view of the peeling of adhesions between the ciliary body and vitreous, which is also incarcerated into the corneal wound. The retracted iris and cornea are visible on the right side of the image

2.20.4 Disadvantages and Difficulties of Endoscope Use in Ocular Traumatology

When switching from microscopic to endoscopic (video monitor) viewing, the learning curve is quite steep, due to the following:

- Difference in image composition. Instead of observing the inside of the eye *and* the intraocular instruments through the microscope's eye-pieces, the image is shown on the video monitor.[6] This image corresponds to what is found in front of the endoscope's tip inside the eye,[7] and the endoscope itself is not visualized.
- Loss of stereopsis.
- Lack of visual feedback of the surgeon's hand motions and the endoscope's position.

Pearl

Alternatively observing the video monitor or the microscope-provided image helps with orientation and probe manipulation by allowing identification of anatomical landmarks such as the lens or the optic disc. Switching the view is especially important for the less experienced surgeon.

- Different method of establishing position. Like in B-scan ultrasonography, the endoscope's orientation determines the orientation of the image, e.g., simple rotation of the probe between the surgeon's fingers changes what is up or down.
- Different method of moving along the operative field. This is done no more via directing the microscope along the x–y axis with a foot pedal but by moving the endoscope inside the eye.

6 Once the endoscope is introduced through the pars plana, the surgeon observes the inside of the eye and all intraocular maneuvers on the video monitor, not through the microscope.

7 It is as if the surgeon's very eyes were placed inside the patient's eye.

- Different method of changing the magnification. Bringing the endoscope closer to the target makes the image larger, and vice versa.
- Inability to perform bimanual surgery.[8]
- Difficulty in dealing with major fresh bleeding if it covers the endoscope's tip.

Cave

Endoscope use and especially EAV can be much more difficult in ocular traumatology than for other indications and are best left for the surgeon already experienced in endoscopic *and* trauma surgery.

2.20.5 Issues Related to Surgical Technique

The initial step is to introduce the endoscope through a standard sclerotomy[9] to determine the ideal sites for the infusion cannula, the working instruments, such as the vitrectomy probe, and, possibly, the endoscope itself.[10]

Pearl

The initial sclerotomy for the endoscope should be at no more than 3 mm from the limbus. This reduces, although does not eliminate, the risk of iatrogenic retinal injury during endoscope introduction.

8 This is significant when tissues with high resistance, such as mature cyclitic membranes, are encountered; tearing of the underlying ocular tissues (e.g., ciliary epithelium, iris root) is a real risk. With advances in technology, bimanual surgery will likely become possible in the future, making these maneuvers easier and less risky.

9 Preoperative B-scan ultrasonography, the UBM, or transcleral illumination may help identify the most optimal site for the initial entry (see Chap. 2.16).

10 i.e., if it is found that the initial entry site is not ideal.

- If the eye is hypotonous, intravitreal injection of BSS or air[11] can restore the IOP and make endoscope insertion easier.[12]

Further difficulties[13] and important issues include:

- Loss of visibility of the normal anatomical landmarks
- Detachment of the ciliary body, choroid, and/or retina
- Anterior displacement of the vitreous base/retina
- Massive fresh hemorrhage that interferes with or completely blocks visualization
- A long (6 or 7 mm) infusion cannula should be used; it must be sharp[14] since choroidal, ciliary body, and retinal detachment, and thick, elastic cyclitic membranes adherent to the pars plana are not uncommon (Fig. 2.20.3). Self-retaining cannulas require special attention so they do not get expelled.[15]
- Loss of view intraoperatively. If blood covers the probe's tip, the endoscope should be withdrawn and cleaned. This may have to be done repeatedly, if necessary.
- Number of sclerotomies. If the eye is phakic and the lens is to be preserved, a fourth sclerotomy may be needed to avoid lens injury. This is especially important if extensive manipulations at the vitreous base are required to prevent or treat an anterior PVR.[16]
- Core vitreous. This is the initial step of vitrectomy. The direction of vitreous removal is antero-posterior (see Chap. 2.9), and it usually starts in the visual axis. In a severely traumatized eye, even without a purulent infection, it may difficult, if not impossible, to distinguish between a

11 This is a good advice for any eye with low IOP. The maneuver nevertheless requires experience so that the needle does not inflict further tissue damage and the fluid or air is not injected under the retina.

12 If visibility allows, an AC maintainer can also be used.

13 These are not necessarily specific to endoscopy.

14 The track created with the MVR blade can rapidly close due to tissue elasticity.

15 The risk is higher during EAV than in conventional vitrectomy because of the rotation of the eye during peeling at the vitreous base.

16 Obviously, complete scar removal takes precedence of lens preservation (see Chap. 2.9).

detached and necrotic retina and layers of vitreous tainted with streaks of blood and coated with fibrin (see Chaps. 2.12, 2.17). Preoperative ultrasonography may have been unfeasible, or yielded erroneous (see Fig. 1.9.5) or undecipherable information. With its high magnification, the endoscope has a good chance of allowing recognition of the retina[17] before it is penetrated.

- Posterior cortical vitreous. Its detachment and removal is crucially important and represents the second step of vitrectomy. Separation may be aided by PFCL use. The endoscope-provided control increases safety and efficacy. The surgeon should also be familiar with the type, parameters, and settings of his vitrectomy machine. To avoid undue traction on the retina, a machine with flow control[18] is preferred; when working in close proximity to the retina, the flow should be low (1–2 ml/m) and the cutting speed set at below 15 cpm or even "cut by cut."
- Peripheral vitreous. The last phase of vitrectomy is to remove as much of the vitreous, hemorrhage, fibrin, membranes, or scar tissue in the periphery as possible. Avulsion of the anterior vitreous base or ciliary detachment is not uncommon: the endoscopic hyaloido-capsulo-zonulo-ciliary dissection must therefore be performed cautiously to avoid injuring the zonular system or the ciliary epithelium. One of the surgeon's hands holds the endoscope that doubles as a light pipe while the other hand operates the usual vitrectomy instruments. A complete, 360° job can be accomplished by utilizing all sclerotomies and repeated switching of the hands as needed. The endoscope also allows complete cleansing of the sclerotomies, assuring that no tissue remains or gets incarcerated. The vitrectomy machine's settings may have to be similar to those described above. Helpful additional tricks include the following:
  - Blood, accumulated between various tissues, can be used as a marker to help delineating boundaries and cleavage plans, thus facilitating dissection.

17 Nevertheless, this may remain a challenge even for the experienced surgeon.

18 i.e., using a peristaltic, not Venturi, pump.

- Tissues and membranes located superiorly[19] can be dissected under direct visualization by placing the endoscope in an inferior sclerotomy, or the area is approached tangentially by alternating the endoscope between the two superior sclerotomies.
- The membranes may be so thick and elastic as to allow true dissection at the level of the Wieger ligament or ciliary epithelium only if a flow-control vitrectomy machine is used. The cut rate and flow should be adapted to each individual case.
- Air or PFCL is often necessary to exert counter pressure on tissues to avoid iatrogenic injury to the ciliary epithelium or retina[20] while performing complete dissection (see Chap. 2.9). The endoscope provides unique, high-magnification visual feedback.
- For the thick proliferative membranes the flow may have to be tripled to allow relieving at least some of the circumferential traction. The endoscope's high magnification and access to any intraocular space offers the best chance of freeing the ciliary body from cyclitic membranes and subsequent hypotony/phthisis (see Chap. 2.19). Radial cuts into the membranes may be the only option if the endoscope-relayed image shows that dissection is impossible. Radial cuts can also alleviate the need for a prophylactic encircling scleral buckle.

In addition to removal of the vitreous and peripheral membranes, EAV also allows performing virtually the entire arsenal of intravitreal maneuvers, including:

- Lensectomy/phacofragmentation
- Removal of EMPs and the ILM[21]
- Removal of subretinal membranes and blood

19 i.e., between 11 and 1 o'clock.

20 Especially if the retina is detached.

21 Staining of the ILM is necessary.

- Cryopexy[22], laser, diathermy, retinotomy, and retinectomy
- Exchanges between BSS, air/gas, silicone oil, PFCL as well as removal of these substances, even if trapped subretinally

DO:

- consider endoscopy/EAV in severely traumatized eyes if the cornea (AC, lens, pupil) interferes with visualization of the posterior segment
- create as many sclerotomies as necessary to do a complete job and avoid injuring a lens that would otherwise be preserved
- be thorough with the removal of vitreous, blood, fibrin, inflammatory debris, etc.
- make full use of the opportunity the endoscope offers to completely clean the vitreous base and ciliary body

DON'T:

- use the endoscope if you are inexperienced in both EAV and the vitrectomy management of severely injured eyes
- limit endoscope use to diagnostic purposes
- try to perform surgery on cases that would benefit from bimanual surgery
- operate blindly

Summary

Endoscopy provides a means to "bypass" a nontransparent anterior segment and thus allow for timely vitrectomy. The endoscope is not just a diagnostic tool: it can be utilized to perform virtually any and all maneuvers the vitreoretinal surgeon using the microscope would carry out. Endoscopy-assisted vitrectomy (EAV) requires the ocular traumatology expert to also be experienced in every aspect of endoscope use.

22 Cryopexy is to be avoided because of its risks of inducing PVR (see Chap. 2.9).

References

[1] Boscher C (1998) Endoscopic vitreoretinal surgery of the injured eye. In: Alfaro D, Liggett P (eds) Vitreoretinal surgery of the injured eye. Lippincott-Raven, Philadelphia, pp 301–314

[2] Boscher C (2002) Endoscopy. In: Kuhn F, Pieramici D (eds) Ocular trauma: principles and practice. Thieme, New York, pp 414–418

[3] Hammer ME, Grizzard WS (2003) Endoscopy for evaluation and treatment of the ciliary body in hypotony. Retina 23: 30–36

[4] Koch FH, Luloh KP, Augustin AJ, el Agha MS, Guembel H, Ohrloff C, Grizzard WS, Hammer ME, Sinclair S (1997) Subretinal microsurgery with gradient index endoscopes. Ophthalmologica 211: 283–287

[5] Park S, Marcus D, Duker J, Pesavento R, Topping P, Frederick A, D'Amico D (1995) Posterior segment complications after vitrectomy for macular hole. Ophthalmology 102: 775–781

[6] Thorpe H (1934) Ocular endoscope: instrument for removal of intravitreous non magnetic foreign bodies. Trans Am Acad Ophthalmol Otolaryngol 39: 422–424

[7] Uram M (1992) Ophthalmic laser microendoscope endophotocoagulation. Ophthalmology 99: 1829–1832

[8] Boscher C (2001) Endoscopy for anterior PVR. American Academy of Ophthalmology Subspecialty Day, New Orleans

[9] Cuenca N, Martinez-Navarrete GC et al. (2004) Process of differentiation of retinal neurons from stem cells in the peripheral retinal margin of primates. Association for Research and Vision in Ophthalmology, Ft. Lauderdale

SECTION III

3.1 Chemical Injuries

Norbert Schrage and Ferenc Kuhn

3.1.1 Introduction

Most chemical injuries cause only limited[1] damage, and patients tend to rinse their eye themselves, usually with water. The duration of contact between eye and agent[2], and the agent's characteristics, are the primary factors in determining the outcome.

3.1.2 Evaluation

An acute chemical injury is one of the few conditions when virtually all patients voluntarily and immediately disclose the incident. A chemical burn[3] is also an exception because the ophthalmologist should not appreciate *history-taking* as his initial goal; instead, he must "shoot first and ask later": details of injury are asked during or after the initial irrigation. Table 3.1.1 shows the questions the ophthalmologist should raise.

1 It is sensible to use this term rather than "mild," reflecting that with delayed/improper treatment, a mild injury can rapidly become severe (see endophthalmitis classification in Chap. 2.17).

2 i.e., the time between injury and agent removal.

3 The terms "chemical injury" and "chemical burn" are alternatively used in this chapter, referring to the same condition.

Table 3.1.1 Taking a history in a patient with chemical burn

What happened?
When did it happen?
What is the name of the agent that caused the injury?
What characteristics (e.g., pH, concentration) does this agent have and how much got onto the eye?
Was this a work-related injury? If yes, was a witness present? Was a report filed?
Was the injury self-inflicted or the result of assault[1] [6]?
Was the eye irrigated after the injury? If yes, with what and for how long?
What therapy has been employed for the injury so far?
How much pain is there now?
How has vision been effected?

It must be emphasized again that these questions are asked only *during* or *after* the initial irrigation, not beforehand (see text for more details)

[1] Unfortunately, this is not uncommon in certain societies.

Pearl

If the patient has a chemical injury, the taking of a detailed history should never precede the irrigation.

Pain may be a somewhat misleading symptom. The cornea is involved in nearly all cases, and the pain and severity of the damage are often inversely proportional[4].

Cave

Severe chemical injuries tend to cause little pain because of the destruction involving the nerve endings. A lack of pain in an eye with severe morphological damage is therefore indicative of a very severe injury with poor prognosis.

4 Similar to that seen with mechanical injuries to the cornea (see Chap. 2.2).

Following the initial irrigation, a *penlight* is used to search for remnants of the agent[5] on the lids, in the palpebral fissure, and in the deep fornices; the latter requires double eversion of the upper lid (see Chap. 2.1). *Slit lamp* examination follows to determine the damage to anterior segment structures and grade the injury (Table 3.1.2). Since viability of the limbal vascular arcades has prognostic importance, this must carefully be evaluated. The visual acuity and the IOP[6] should also be taken. Secondary glaucoma can rapidly develop and cause severe optic nerve damage. Checking the pH of the conjunctival cul-de-sac at the end of the initial rinsing period helps determining when the situation has been stabilized.

Pearl

After a chemical injury, evaluation and irrigation may have to be alternated: if further rinsing is deemed necessary, the examination is interrupted and continued only after the irrigation has been repeated.

3.1.3 Treatment[7]

3.1.3.1 Primary Intervention and Postirrigation Management

Certain aspects of the injury are beyond physician control: the agent starts causing tissue destruction upon contact. The ophthalmologist-controlled factors in determining the prognosis are the *time* from patient arrival to irrigation [9] and the *quality* of rinsing [3, 13][8]. If the irrigation is painful, topical anesthetics must be instilled without delay: brief rinsing with xylocain 2% eliminates the pain and doubles as an initial irrigation.

5 e.g., pieces of lime.

6 Applanation tonometry on the burnt cornea is *not* contraindicated.

7 See also Table 2.10.1.

8 i.e., the quality of the fluid used and how thorough the rinsing is.

Table 3.1.2 Grading ocular burns

	Grade			
	I	II	III	IV
Timing				
Immediately	Erosion, hyperemia	Erosion	Erosion	Deep ischemia, involving >240°
		Ischemia in <120°	Ischemia in 120–240°	Conjunctival necrosis
		Chemosis	Red chemosis	
			Turbid cornea	Porcelain-white cornea
				Iris atrophy
				Fibrin exudate in AC
Re-grading on day 2	Regeneration	Restored circulation	Persistent erosion	Anterior segment melting
		Regeneration	Corneal ulceration	Proliferation
			Vascularization	Large ulcerations
			Scar formation	Cataract
				Glaucoma
				Diffuse scar formation

Pearl

Chemical eye burns require immediate rinsing, continued for at least 15 min[9]. Any consumable solution suffices if it is not alcoholic or acidic; preferably, it should be of room temperature. Ophthalmologists are strongly encouraged to educate all ER personnel regarding the techniques of irrigation.

Typically, water or saline is used for rinsing. If available, a polyvalent, hypertonic, amphoteric compound, such as Diphoterine[10] [4], is preferred, which is effective against acids, alkali, and agents with oxidative or redox activity. If both eyes have been burned, the irrigation must be done alternatively on both sides. Should the cornea be opaque and the iris discolored, the AC must also be irrigated with BSS (see Chap. 2.5). Irrigation improves the prognosis even if hours have elapsed since the injury [3].

3.1.3.1.1 Irrigation

The process of irrigation should proceed as follows:

- Explain to the patient what will take place. This is especially important in children who are scared and would not cooperate (see Chap. 2.16).
- Use anesthetics if necessary (see above).
- Carefully separate the lids. Placement of a lid retractor is preferred, although manual separation (see Chap 1.9) is also acceptable.
- Gently rinse the cornea and the fornices using an infusion line (Fig. 3.1.1); the infusion bottle should be 30–80 cm above eye level.
- Remove all particles[11] with a cotton-tipped applicator or forceps.
- Proceed with the irrigation even if the injury is open globe. Closure with sutures should *follow*, not precede, rinsing.
- Rinse the palpebral conjunctiva and the fornices as well; the latter requires double eversion (Fig. 3.1.2).

9 ANSI-Standard Z358.1-2004.

10 Prevor GmbH, Köln, Germany.

11 These are usually calciferous.

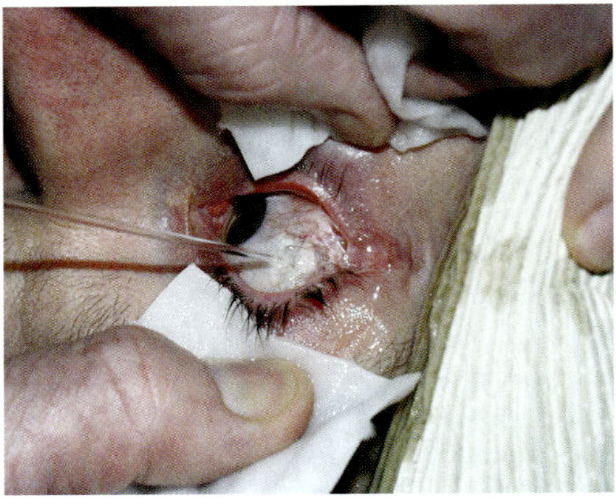

Fig. 3.1.1 Rinsing the eye after a chemical injury. The flow of the rinsing fluid is low and soft, the eye is turned away from the stream, the lids are held open with fingers pressuring the bones not the eyeball, and a paper drain is used to try to keep the patient's clothing dry

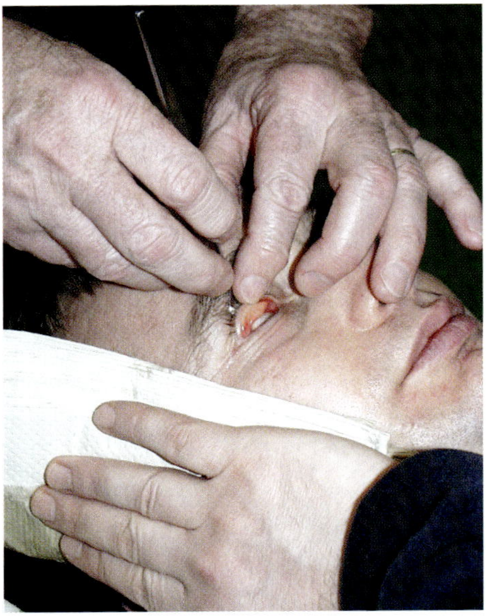

Fig. 3.1.2 Double eversion of the upper lid with a Desmarres retractor. The upper fornix is completely visible and accessible, making particle removal easy to perform. The patient is instructed to look straight downward, and his forehead is positioned low to permit free flow of the irrigation fluid

3.1.3.1.2 *Additional Steps to be Taken*

- Perform slit lamp examination, take the visual acuity and the IOP (oral acetazolamide treatment must be initiated if the IOP is elevated), measure the pH of the ocular surface, and *grade the injury*.
- If the injury is Grade I or II, topical therapy should be used: corticosteroids [17]; ascorbic acid [5, 16]; and antibiotics. Admission is not mandatory,[12] but daily evaluations are recommended until the corneal epithelium is healed.
- If the injury is Grade III or IV,[13] the irrigation must be continued, using phosphate-free solutions such as Isopto Max[14] or Corti-biciron[15] [17], and the patient should be admitted.
- All efforts are aimed at rescuing the limbal stem cells [19] by reducing the inflammation and scar formation (and by subsequent surgery, see below). Hourly[16] drops of corticosteroids, ascorbic acid, and antibiotics, continued for up to 2 weeks, are employed.
- Superficial debridement should be done twice daily by rinsing the eye with ringer lactate solution.
- A round-tipped glass rod should be rolled across the upper and lower fornices to prevent adhesion development.
- If insufficient limbal regeneration is seen within the first 4 days, an amniotic graft should be placed to secure the corneal surface and improve healing.
- At least 2 days after the injury, the demarcation of necrotic areas is well appreciated. The necrotic tissue should be surgically removed; if the necrosis involves large areas of the limbus and conjunctiva, an initial tenonplasty is required [12]. Tenon's capsule is bluntly dissected; its soft sheets are advanced up to the limbus (Fig. 3.1.3) and fixed to the

12 This also depends on factors such health insurance system, the patient's socioeconomic and hygienic situation, and financial circumstances.
13 The prognosis is poor, mostly because of the damage to the limbal stem cells.
14 Alcon Pharma GmbH, Freiburg, Germany
15 S&K Pharma, Perl, Germany
16 Ointment is used for nighttime.

sclera by full-thickness sutures (similar to that in scleral patching; see Chap. 2.3).

- In Grade IV burns, the primary goal of treatment is to prevent secondary damage such as glaucoma or ulceration with perforation.

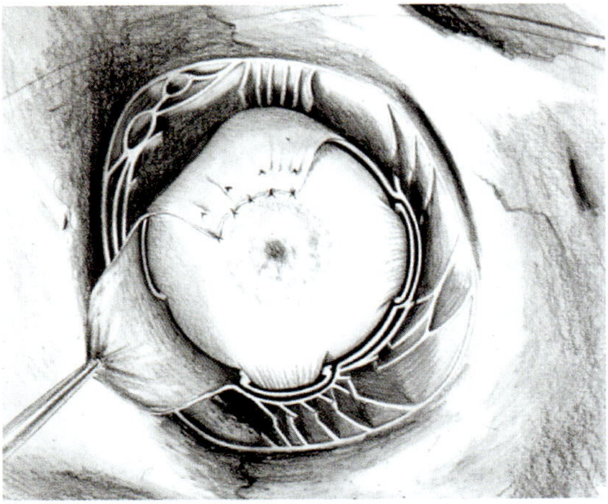

a

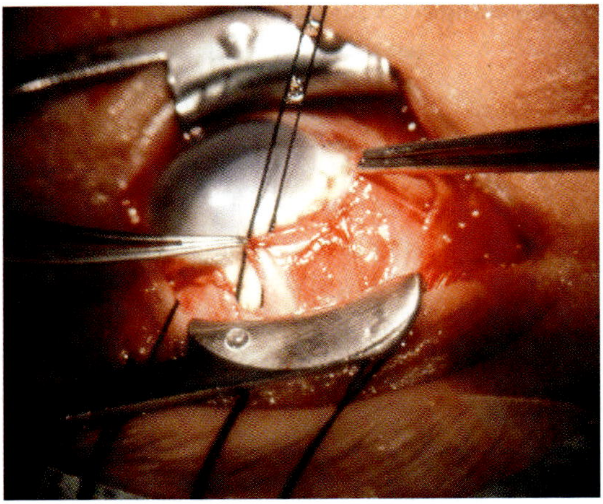

b

Fig. 3.1.3 Prochaska–Marburg tenonplasty. The epibulbar tissues are liberated and advanced up to, and sutured to, the limbus. **a** Schematic drawing. **b** Intraoperative photograph

Once the acute phase is passed and the surface of the eye is stable, the patient can be discharged on topical corticosteroids, antiglaucoma medications, and antibiotics; these are used until the redness diminishes.

3.1.3.2 Secondary Intervention

With the appearance of pale scars, *ocular surface restoration* becomes possible via a step-by-step approach.

3.1.3.2.1 Lid Reconstruction

Scars must be removed, normal lid position restored (anti-entropium or ectropium surgery), and the normal eyelash configuration restored (anti-distichiasis or trichiasis surgery). If required, the lid skin must be reconstructed [10, 17].

Pitfall

Ocular surface reconstruction is likely to fail if it has not been preceded by restoration of the normal lid anatomy.

3.1.3.2.2 Symblepharon Management

Although symblepharon development is more common after heat than after chemical injury, it does represent a significant problem, which needs to be addressed:

- In eyes *without conjunctival shortening*, incision and conjunctivoplasty are sufficient.
- In eyes *with shortened fornices*, the scars need to be removed and bucchal mucosa or amniotic membrane transplanted [11]. To prevent rolling up of the donor tissue, two silicone bands must be secured, sandwiching the lid: one over the graft internally and one over the skin externally.

3.1.3.2.3 Ocular Surface Restoration

The process of ocular surface restoration is as follows:

- *Implantation of amniotic membranes, limbal autografts, or cultured stem cells* [14].[17] In the postoperative period, topical, preservative-free corticosteroids are used and a soft bandage contact lens needs to be placed.
- *Lamellar keratoplasty* has the advantage of sparing the patient of the risks of open globe surgery, but the development of an intracorneal (interfacial) scar is a potential complication. Deep lamellar keratoplasty may be combined with autologous limbal grafting [20].
- *Penetrating keratoplasty* requires epithelial regeneration from the limbus to prevent superficial ulceration.
  - The "umbrella" technique can be used in early cases, serving tectonic as well as surface reconstruction purposes [8].
  - In the "horseshoe" technique the donor tissue, containing 120° of the limbus, is eccentrically placed [18].
  - Both of these are high-risk grafts and thus topical as well as systemic[18] immunosuppressive therapy is required. Nevertheless, graft rejection remains common; if several grafts have been rejected, the permanent keratoprosthesis remains the last alternative.
- *Permanent keratoprosthesis* use is not without risk,[19] but they are the best option for severely damaged eyes. The device can provide structural stability and often permit the preservation of vision. Several types are available (e.g., Osteo-Odonto-Keratoprosthesis [2], Boston keratoprosthesis [1, 15], and ACTO Tex-KPRO [7] (Figs 3.1.4, 3.1.5), and all require long-term follow-up. A specialist experienced in the field needs to be consulted.
- *Additional interventions*, such as cataract extraction or antiglaucoma surgery, are performed as required.

17 From the fellow eye, a patient's relative, or another donor.

18 e.g., mycophenolic acid (Myfortic; Novartis AG, Basel, Switzerland).

19 e.g., extrusion, inability to measure the IOP, endophthalmitis.

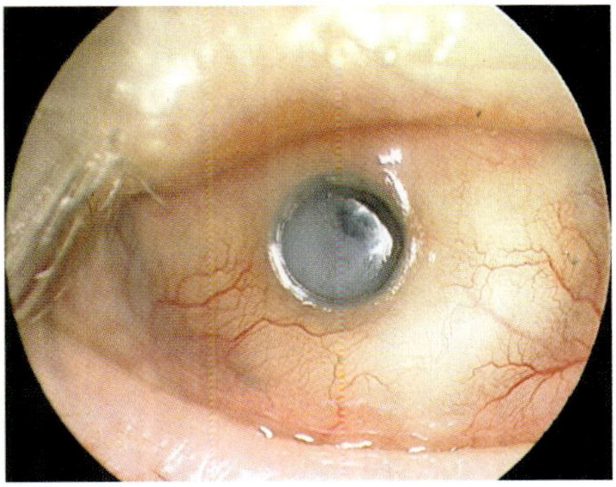

Fig. 3.1.4 Fjodorov keratoprosthesis. The device has a titan ring and a PMMA optic. A rigid retroprosthetic membrane has occurred, but a central hole still allows some vision

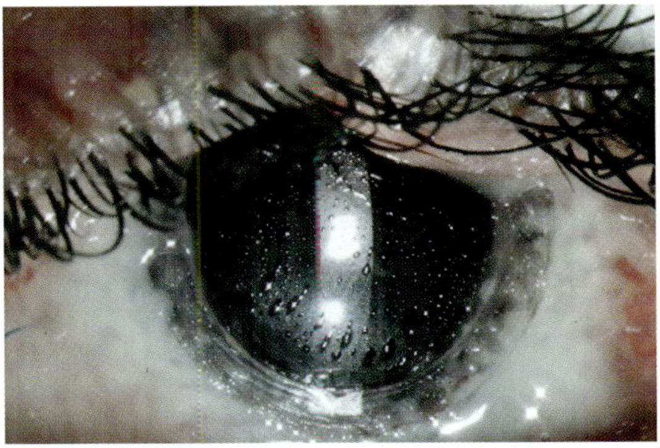

Fig. 3.1.5 ACTO Tex-KPRO keratoprosthesis. Implanted 8 months previously, this device allows 0.4 visual acuity; the retina is reattached under silicone oil, and the IOP is 15 mmHg

DO:

- consider irrigation the most important element of the treatment
- use any neutral fluid for irrigation and irrigate both the visible, easily accessible areas as well as the upper fornix, and remove all agent particles mechanically
- admit patients with Grade III or Grade V injuries
- administer topical corticosteroids and antibiotics long-term to prevent infection, and to reduce inflammation and scarring
- surgically reconstruct the severely damaged anterior segment

DON'T:

- delay irrigation to take a detailed history
- forgo the irrigation even if the injury is not fresh: it may still improve the final outcome
- neglect the IOP: if elevated, it can quickly make the prognosis much worse
- try to restore the ocular surface without first addressing lid and eyelash position abnormalities

Summary

A chemical injury is one of the very few conditions in which the prognosis may be determined literally by minutes: if the irrigation is delayed or done inappropriately, the damage can be irreversible.

References

[1] Dohlman CH, Doane MG (1994) Some factors influencing outcome after keratoprosthesis surgery. Cornea 13: 214–218

[2] Falcinelli G, Falsini B, Taloni M, Colliardo P, Falcinelli G (2005) Modified osteo-odonto-keratoprosthesis for treatment of corneal blindness: long-term anatomical and functional outcomes in 181 cases. Arch Ophthalmol 123: 1319–1329

[3] Gerard M, Merle H, Chiambaretta F, Rigal D, Schrage N (2002) An amphoteric rinse used in the emergency treatment of a serious ocular burn. Burns 28: 670–673

[4] Hall AH, Blomet J, Mathieu L (2002) Diphoterine for emergent eye/skin chemical splash decontamination a review. Vet Hum Toxicol 44: 228–231

[5] Heckelen A, Hermel M Kondring B, Schrage NF (2004) Ascorbic acid reversibly inhibits proliferation of retinal pigment epithelial cells. Acta Ophthalmol Scand 82: 564–568

[6] Ho W, Ying S, Chan H, Chow C (2001) Assault by burning: a reappraisal. Burns 27: 471–474

[7] Kompa S, Redbrake C, Langefeld S, Brenman K, Schrage N (2001) The Type II Aachen-Keratoprosthesis in humans: case report of the first prolonged application. Int J Artif Organs 24: 110–114

[8] Krause A, Tost M, Schlaffer G (1995) [Putschkowaskaja corneal protection]. Klin Monatsbl Augenheilkd 206: 161–164

[9] Kuckelkorn R, Kottek A, Schrage N, Reim M (1995) Poor prognosis of severe chemical and thermal eye burns: the need for adequate emergency care and primary prevention. Int Arch Occup Environ Health 67: 281–284

[10] Kuckelkorn R, Schrage N, Becker J, Reim M (1997) Tarsoconjunctival advancement: a modified surgical technique to correct cicatricial entropion and metaplasia of the marginal tarsus. Ophthalmic Surg Lasers 28: 156–161

[11] Kuckelkorn R, Schrage N, Redbrake C, Kottek A, Reim M (1996) Autologous transplantation of nasal mucosa after severe chemical and thermal eye burns. Acta Ophthalmol Scand 74: 442–448

[12] Kuckelkorn R, Schrage N, Reim M (1995) Treatment of severe eye burns by tenonplasty. Lancet 345: 657–658

[13] Merle H, Donnio A, Ayeboua L, Michel F, Thomas F, Ketterle J, Leonard C, Josset P, Gerard M (2005) Alkali ocular burns in Martinique (French West Indies) Evaluation of the use of an amphoteric solution as the rinsing product. Burns 31: 205–211

[14] Rama P, Bonini S, Lambiase A, Golisano O, Paterna P, Luca M de, Pellegrini G (2001) Autologous fibrin-cultured limbal stem cells permanently restore the corneal surface of patients with total limbal stem cell deficiency. Transplantation 72: 1478–1485

[15] Ray S, Khan BF, Dohlman CH, D'Amico DJ (2002) Management of vitreoretinal complications in eyes with permanent keratoprosthesis. Arch Ophthalmol 120: 559–566

[16] Reim M, Beil KH, Kammerer G, Krehwinkel S (1982) Influence of systemic ascorbic acid treatment on metabolite levels after regeneration of the corneal epithelium following mild alkali burns. Graefe's Arch Clin Exp Ophthalmol 218: 99–102

[17] Reim M, Kottek A, Schrage N (1997) The corneal surface and wound healing. Progr Ret Eye Res 16: 183–225

[18] Reinhard T, Sundmacher R (1994) Lamellar horseshoe sclerokeratoplasty and thermoplasty in keratoconus with peripheral ectasia of the cornea. Klin Monatsbl Augenheilkd 205: 305–308 [in German]

[19] Tsai RJ, Tseng SC (1994) Human allograft limbal transplantation for corneal surface reconstruction. Cornea 13: 389–400

[20] Yao YF, Zhang B, Zhou P, Jiang JK (2002) Autologous limbal grafting combined with deep lamellar keratoplasty in unilateral eye with severe chemical or thermal burn at late stage. Ophthalmology 109: 2011–2017

3.2 Electromagnetic Trauma

Yaniv Barkana, Michael Belkin, Ferenc Kuhn

3.2.1 Introduction

Electromagnetic waves, both in the visible and invisible spectrum, are able to damage the eye. With the increasing availablity of intense light sources and interest in laser weapons, the significance of such trauma for individuals and society is expected to rise. In this chapter we describe the interaction of electromagnetic waves with the eye and the clinical course of consequent injuries. In the absence of effective treatment for most conditions, prevention is the best option against vision loss.

3.2.2 Evaluation

In some cases, the patient himself seeks medical attention because of pain (e.g., welder's photokeratitis; see Chap. 2.2). In other cases the source is more difficult to identify (e.g., light damage sustained during eye surgery). Reliable history may also be difficult to obtain in certain cases (e.g., self-inflicted damage, children's solar trauma, or if the patient was unaware of the exposure). The ophthalmoscope is the most important diagnostic tool.

3.2.3 Specific Conditions

3.2.3.1 Light-induced Damage (Photic Eye Injury)

Light, especially if powerful (direct viewing of the sun or an atomic bomb explosion, even if it is many miles away [4]) and concentrated, such as that coming from artificial sources,[1] can cause permanent ocular damage [2]. The cornea and lens refract and focus the visible and near IR light onto the retina, which is thus uniquely vulnerable since its irradiance is 10,000 times higher than that of the cornea. The extent of the photic damage depends on the following:

- Wavelength of the radiation. Rapidly absorbed by organic tissues are photons of wavelengths shorter (UV) or longer (IR) than the visible spectrum. These do not reach the retina but may cause corneal injury.
- Duration and intensity of the exposure.
  - *Thermal* damage occurs when heat is produced faster than it can be dissipated [15]. An increase of at least 10°C causes denaturation and coagulation of proteins with ensuing cell death, necrosis, and scarring[2].
  - *Mechanical* damage occurs when the energy transfer is in the pico- to nanosecond range: the tissue disintegrates into plasma [15] and a compressive pressure pulse (explosion) irradiates and disrupts the surrounding tissues.[3]
  - *Photochemical* damage occurs when the delivery of energy is slow and without significant heat build-up [8]. Single photons induce chemical reactions in the absorbing molecules, breaking bonds in nucleic acids and proteins.[4]
- Tissue involvement and specific location of injury. This is the most important factor in determining the extent and importance of the sensory damage.
  - A *foveal* lesion causes immediate and significant visual loss, even if subsequent improvement is possible.
  - A *parafoveal* lesion's initial effect[5] may persist via the spreading of neural cell degeneration into the fovea.

1 e.g., ophthalmic instruments and laser systems.
2 This is the basis for argon laser photocoagulation of the retina.
3 This is the basis for YAG laser photodisruption of the iris.
4 This is the basis for excimer laser use in the cornea.
5 Edema and inflammation, which can extend over several times the diameter of the original burn.

  - Lesions elsewhere in the retina cause a scotoma only,[6] unless blood vessels are also disrupted and intraocular bleeding occurs [1].
- Presence or absence of defenses, such as refractive error (i.e., ametropia), blink, and aversion reflexes to bright light.

3.2.3.2 Solar Retinopathy

Whether self-inflicted [6], caused by ignorance (not wearing suitable eye protection during a solar eclipse[7] [21]), or being influenced by religious rituals [5] or hallucinogenic drugs [22], gazing at the sun can quickly lead to photochemical damage to the photoreceptors and RPE.

3.2.3.2.1 Clinical Features

The clinical features are as follows:

- Most patients present within a few days postinjury, although some people delay their visit to the ophthalmologist for months or even years.
- The most common initial symptoms are decreased visual acuity[8], central scotoma[9], and a negative afterimage of the sun, which may last several hours. The damage may be bilateral or unilateral (usually in the dominant eye).
- The typical ophthalmoscopic lesion is a small, yellow-grayish spot in or near the fovea, surrounded by macular edema. The edema resolves in days or weeks, after which the macula may look normal or show minor pigmentary disturbance. Foveolar depression or pseudohole may be observed, but a true macular hole is rare [9].
- The FLAG is usually normal, although a macular window defect is occasionally observed.

---

6 It can be much larger if focal damage to the nerve fiber layer has also occurred.

7 Retinal damage has been reported following direct observation of the sun through sunglasses, smoked glass, or exposed film, and even after exposures lasting only a few seconds.

8 Visual acuity worse than 20/80 is exceptional.

9 Can be identified even in the presence of 20/20 acuity.

- There is no known therapy for acute solar retinopathy. Corticosteroids are sometimes given, but their efficacy is unknown.
- Early visual improvement is the rule, occurring mostly within a few weeks or months. Final acuity is typically 20/25 or better, but a small central or paracentral scotoma may persist. The outcome is less favorable in atypical severe cases with low initial acuity. Late complications are rare.

Pearl

The safest way to observe the sun or its eclipse is *indirect*: looking at the image of the sun projected onto a piece of paper through a pinhole aperture in a cardboard.

3.2.3.3 Iatrogenic Injury from Ophthalmic Light Sources

Light from the operating microscope [17] or vitrectomy endoilluminator [11] can cause a retinal burn.

- The incidence of photic maculopathy during cataract surgery can reach 7%.
- Prolonged operation time is a significant risk factor.
- The symptoms and prognosis depend on the location and severity of the lesion.
- After anterior segment surgery, complaints are rare since the visual acuity is not significantly affected. Even when a paracentral scotoma is documented, it may improve with time [14].
- After vitrectomy, the complaints and outcome may be substantially worse since the light is held much closer to the retina and its position can be stationary for extended periods[10] [11]. This is an increasingly serious threat today with the light sources becoming stronger (see Chap. 2.9).

10 e.g., peeling of an EMP or the ILM.

- Ophthalmoscopically, the typical finding is a perifoveal, round to oval area of RPE change.[11] The shape of the lesion corresponds to the shape of the illuminating source.[12] The lesion is usually inferior to the fovea and outside the foveal avascular zone. Progressive pigmentation of the lesion may be observed over the next several months, distinguishing the acute maculopathy from an old scar.
- The FLAG shows a sharply demarcated, mottled hyperfluorescent lesion.

Table 3.2.1 provides a summary of recommendations to prevent iatrogenic photic retinal trauma from ophthalmic light sources.

3.2.3.4 Welding Arc-related Retinopathy

In marked contrast to the commonly encountered photokeratitis, injury to the retina from radiation emitted by welding arcs is rare [18]. The clinical features are very similar to those described above in acute solar retinopathy.

3.2.3.5 Laser-induced Eye Injuries

The laser's light beam is coherent, monochromatic, monodirectional, and minimally divergent. Accidental injuries threaten (Fig. 3.2.1) if proper safety precautions are not implemented. The injury occurs *directly* (the victim looking at the laser source) or *indirectly* (reflection from a mirror or another nearby object[13]). Unexpected discharge of the laser device has also been reported [7].

---

11 The early and therefore rarely observed sign is a grayish lesion at the level of the RPE.

12 e.g., a horizontally oval lesion if the microscope illuminator has horizontally oriented filaments

13 e.g., photographic paper or a plastic membrane.

Table 3.2.1 Prevention of iatrogenic photic retinal trauma from ophthalmic light sources

Minimize the length of surgery
Use as low a light intensity[1] as possible
Use noncoaxial microscope light when possible. Oblique illumination will place the intense image of the illuminating beam at the retinal periphery rather than in the foveal area
Use selective filters to eliminate UV and IR wavelengths[2]
Use corneal shields against retinal exposure whenever possible
If using an endoilluminator during vitrectomy, minimize direct exposure to the fovea by:
– Reducing the power (using too much power is especially tempting in the "Photon[3] era" and with small-gauge surgery)
– Increasing the distance between the probe and the retina
– Intermittently illuminating the fovea and parafoveal areas, instead of keeping the – light over the same site for extended periods of time
– Directing the light away from the fovea whenever possible

[1]Whether it is the indirect ophthalmoscope, operating microscope, or the endoilluminator during vitrectomy

[2]Filters are commonly used but their benefit has not adequately been tested

[3]i.e., the endoilluminator for vitreous surgery (Synergetics, East Windsor Hill, Conn.)

Pearl

Individuals at high risk of laser exposure should undergo ophthalmoscopic screening prior to employment as well as after its termination, mainly for legal reasons. Lacking effective treatment, periodic eye examinations are not indicated.

3.2.3.5.1 Clinical Features

The clinical features are as follows:

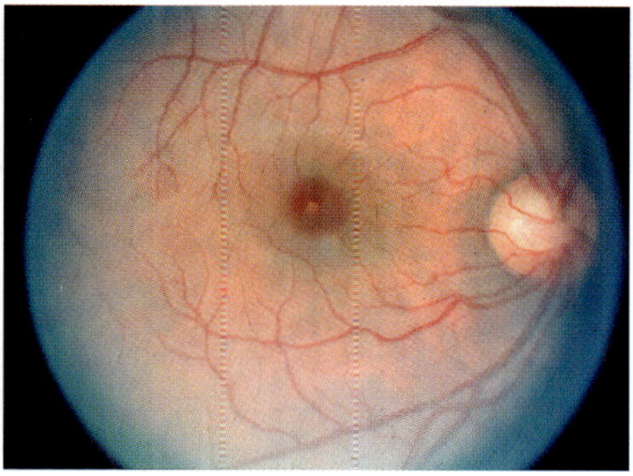

Fig. 3.2.1 Macular injury caused by laser. Note the spread of the lesion from less than 0.1 mm (original beam diameter) to over 1.5 mm. The spread explains why the vision eventually deteriorates in eyes with a parafoveal laser-induced retinal injury

- Almost all of the reported injuries were caused by short-pulse lasers,[14] explaining why the clinical courses are so similar.
- The victim experiences a sudden and severe, monocular visual disturbance, often preceded by a visible flash of bright-colored light. An audible "pop" is common but pain is unusual [3].
- The visual acuity is markedly decreased[15] and a visual field defect is present. The anterior segment is typically unaffected and the IOP is normal. On ophthalmoscopy, one or more localized areas of retinal edema, burns, or holes are seen, typically in or near the macula, with or without accompanying subretinal, subhyaloid, or vitreous hemorrhage.
- Over the next few days to weeks there is marked improvement, mainly due to clearing of the hemorrhage accompanied by waning of the inflammation.

14 Mostly YAG, operating in the visible and near-IR spectrum, and emitting a few tens of millijoules per pulse of duration in the nanosecond range.

15 Commonly to 20/200 or worse.

- Long-term the visual acuity remains stable, although it may also worsen due to late complications such as chorioretinal scarring, or the development of a macular hole or EMP.
- While there is no treatment of the laser-induced trauma itself,[16] certain complications (e.g., EMP) may improve with proper treatment.

Controversial

It remains to be determined whether early intervention (see Chap. 2.9) or just observation should be recommended for a laser-induced macular hole [19].

3.2.3.5.2 Laser Pointers

Laser pointers emit a continuous, narrow beam of usually red light of up to 5 mW of power. If shone directly into an immobile eye for at least 10–20 s, retinal injury occurs since the retinal irradiance is similar to that caused by sun gazing [16]. Under normal circumstances, however, long exposure and thus retinal damage are unlikely[17]. While the risk of eye injury from these inexpensive and widely available devices is negligible, their use for flash blinding may lead to accidents.[18]

Since visible radiation is not absorbed by tissues at the front of the eye, pain or irritation should not be blamed on laser pointers.[19]

16 Corticosteroids and "neuroprotective" compounds have been attempted, but their benefit has never been proven.

17 Due to the blink reflex and aversion response.

18 Convictions in criminal court have followed the directing of laser pointers into airplane cockpits.

19 If these occur, they are most likely due to eye rubbing.

3.2.3.5.3 Military Lasers

Representing an increasingly important hazard, lasers can be employed as *adjuncts* to weapons[20] or as *weapons*[21]. Certain military-type lasers are available even over the Internet, and may become a serious medical/societal problem in the future.

3.2.3.5.4 Prevention

Prophylaxis against laser-induced retinal trauma is relatively simple in the civilian environment by wearing proper protective goggle. There is no effective defense against military lasers unless the wavelength of the weapon the enemy uses is known[22].

3.2.3.6 Heat-induced Damage

In experimental models damage to the blood-retina barrier and the photoreceptors by electromagnetic radiation has been reported [10, 13].

3.2.3.7 Lightning-induced Trauma

A whole array of symptoms and pathologies can be caused by a lightning strike, including temporary blindness, keratitis, uveitis, cataract, macular edema and hole, RPE and photoreceptor damage, and optic neuropathy [12, 20]. The treatment depends on the type of damage; the prognosis after cataract extraction is generally good.

---

20 e.g., for range finding and target identification.

21 e.g., jamming of enemy equipment, damaging sensors, blinding combatants, physically destroying targets.

22 The emitted beam can be made to reach a circle of a few meters at a distance of a few kilometers from the source.

DO:

- explain to the public how observation of a solar eclipse should and should not be observed
- prevent iatrogenic photic damage to the retina from ophthalmic illumination sources

DON'T:

- try to predict the visual outcome after a laser-induced macular injury since the vision can both improve or worsen

Summary

Electromagnetic waves can cause a variety of ocular consequences; some of these are very painful but insignificant (e.g., welder's keratopathy), others can cause permanent blindness. The ophthalmologist's intervention options are unfortunately very limited.

References

[1] Blankenstein M, Zuchlich J, Allen R, Davis H, Thomas S, Harrison R (1986) Retinal hemorrhage thresholds for Q-switched neodymium-YAG laser exposures. Invest Ophthalmol Vis Sci 27: 1176–1179

[2] Boettner E, Wolter J (1962) Transmission of the ocular media. Invest Ophthalmol Vis Sci 1: 776–783

[3] Boldrey E, Little H, Flocks M, Vassiliadis A (1981) Retinal injury due to industrial laser burns. Ophthalmology 88: 101–107

[4] Buettner K, Rose H (1953) Eye hazards from atomic bomb light. Sight Sav Rev 23: 1

[5] Cangelosi G, Newsome D (1988) Solar retinopathy in persons on religious pilgrimage. Am J Ophthalmol 105: 95–97

[6] Ewald R, Ritchey C (1970) Sun gazing as the cause of foveomacular retinitis. Am J Ophthalmol 70: 491–497

[7] Foroozan R, Buono LM, Savino PJ (2003) Traumatic cataract after inadvertent laser discharge. Arch Ophthalmol 121: 286–287

[8] Ham WT Jr, Ruffolo JJ Jr, Mueller HA, Guerry D III (1980) The nature of retinal radiation damage: dependence on wavelength, power level and exposure time. Vision Res 20: 1105–1111

[9] Jacobs NA, Headon M, Rosen ES (1985) Solar retinopathy in the Manchester area. Trans Ophthalmol Soc UK 104 (Pt 6): 625–628

[10] Kiryu J, Ogura Y, Moritera T, Yoshimura N, Honda Y (1993) Breakdown of the blood-retinal barrier after radiofrequency-induced ocular hyperthermia. Ophthalmologica 206: 107–110

[11] Kuhn F, Morris R, Massey M (1991) Photic retinal injury from endoillumination during vitrectomy. Am J Ophthalmol 111: 42–46

[12] Lagreze W, Bomer T, Aiello L (1995) Lightning-induced ocular injury. Arch Ophthalmol 113: 1076–1077

[13] Liggett PE, Pince KJ, Astrahan M, Rao N, Petrovich Z (1990) Localized current field hyperthermia: effect on normal ocular tissue. Int J Hyperthermia 6: 517–527

[14] Lindquist T, Grutzmacher R, Gofman J (1986) Light-induced maculopathy: potential for recovery. Arch Ophthalmol 104: 1641–1647

[15] Marshall J (1970) Thermal and mechanical mechanisms in laser damage to the retina. Invest Ophthalmol Vis Sci 9: 97–115

[16] Marshall J (1998) The safety of laser pointers: myths and realities. Br J Ophthalmol 82: 1335–1338

[17] McDonald H, Irvine A (1983) Light-induced maculopathy from the operating microscope in extracapsular cataract extraction and intraocular lens implantation. Ophthalmology 90: 945–951

[18] Naidoff M, Sliney D (1974) Retinal injury from a welding arc. Am J Ophthalmol 77: 663–668

[19] Newman DK, Flanagan DW (2000) Spontaneous closure of a macular hole secondary to an accidental laser injury. Br J Ophthalmol 84: 1075

[20] Norman ME, Albertson D, Younge BR (2001) Ophthalmic manifestations of lightning strike. Surv Ophthalmol 46: 19–24

[21] Ridgway A (1967) Solar retinopathy. Br Med J 3: 212–214

[22] Schatz H, Mendelblatt F (1973) Solar retinopathy from sun-gazing under the influence of LSD. Br J Ophthalmol 57: 270–273

3.3 The Effects of Systemic Trauma on the Eye

Wolfgang Schrader and Ferenc Kuhn

3.3.1 Introduction

Certain systemic injuries even if the eye is not directly involved, may indirectly cause ocular pathologies, usually by one of the following mechanisms:

- Changes in rheologic conditions
- Hypoxia
- A sudden increase of the intravascular pressure.

  Because of a great variety of retinal findings and a still somewhat vaguely understood retinal response, the pathomechanisms are not completely understood. The retinal findings may be caused by:
- Embolic damage (e.g., air, blood products, fat)
- Increased intraluminal pressure with endothelial vascular damage
- Mechanical forces acting at the vitreoretinal interface

Pearl

All physicians, and especially those working in the ER, should know that bodily trauma can cause sight-threatening ocular complications even in the absence of direct eye involvement.

Patient complaints about visual loss whether voiced hours or months after the trauma, should result in an instant referral to an ophthalmologist. If the patient is unconscious or mentally incompetent, ophthalmological examination should be initiated to rule out a direct or indirect traumatic retinopathy. The findings should be meticulously documented for medical and legal purposes (see Chap. 1.8).

3.3.2 Evaluation

The most important diagnostic tool is the ophthalmoscope; FLAG plays more of a role in these injuries than in a typical, direct eye injury. Specific diagnostic information is provided below with each condition (see Chap. 1.9 for further details).

3.3.3 Specific Injuries

3.3.3.1 Heavy Blood Loss

Massive or recurrent blood loss, especially from the gastrointestinal system, can lead to anemia and secondary arterial hypotension. AION is the consequence that is responsible for the visual loss [12] via, presumably, a sudden decrease of the arterial blood pressure and release of endogenous factors [10].

3.3.3.1.1 Symptoms

Following a serious bleeding, the patient may notice a temporary visual loss, with a recovery after several minutes. A few days later (occasionally weeks) the patient notices bilateral, acute, irreversible visual loss, ranging from a small, usually inferior, visual field defect to complete blindness.

3.3.3.1.2 Evaluation

On *ophthalmoscopy*, the typical appearance of an AION is seen, with disc edema in the acute phase and an optic atrophy in the late phase. The *FLAG* is not very helpful; the peripapillary choroidal and retinal perfusion may be decreased [10].

3.3.3.1.3 Treatment

There is no effective therapy for AION treatment; further vasoconstriction should be avoided or medically reversed (with angiotensin-converting enzyme inhibitors).

3.3.3.2 High-altitude Retinopathy

Hypoxia at high altitudes (typically above 4000 m[1]) causes increased retinal blood flow and blood volume possibly via autoregulatory mechanisms.[2] Physical strain with Valsalva maneuvers (e.g., during mountain climbing) compounds the condition via increased retinal venous pressure. A hypoxic retinal capillary bed exposed to increased retinal venous pressure predisposes to intraretinal hemorrhage.

3.3.3.2.1 Symptoms

Although up to 60% of mountaineers develop high-altitude retinopathy in altitudes above 4000 m [20], usually no symptoms are noted unless vitreous hemorrhage occurs.

3.3.3.2.2 Evaluation

On *ophthalmoscopy*, a marked increase of retinal vessel diameters with tortuosity of arterioles and venules are seen, along with hyperemia or edema of the disc. The intra- or preretinal hemorrhages often spare the macular area.

3.3.3.2.3 Treatment

The retinal changes disappear within weeks. To prevent high altitude retinopathy, ascending slowly and the use of supplemental oxygen are recommended.

3.3.3.3 Hyperbaric Trauma

Not only a hypobaric, but also a hyperbaric, environment can cause ocular damage, usually during diving, but also following hyperbaric oxygen

1 Approximately 13,000 feet.

2 Those sensitive to the decreased atmospheric pressure may also have difficulty in flying airplanes at high altitudes or in unpressurized airplanes: vasodilatation and intraocular hemorrhages may occur. The low pressure must also be taken into consideration when intraocular gas tamponade is used: gas expansion occurs with a spike in the IOP.

therapy. The term "hyperbaric trauma" summarizes three different injuries: barotrauma; decompression disease; and air embolism.

The eyes are directly exposed to pressure changes with the diver wearing an air-filled head gear. When the diver is deep in the water, a negative pressure in the mask may cause lid edema and conjunctival hemorrhages. Conversely, a diver may suffer from Caisson disease after too fast a decompression. Because the intracorporal air pressure may decrease by more than one bar, air bubbles can develop in the vessels and cause vascular occlusions [2]. If lung alveoli rupture, air bubbles may directly enter the vessels and cause occlusions in the central artery or in the intracranial arteries.

3.3.3.3.1 Evaluation

Lid edema and subconjunctival hemorrhages may be visible at the slit lamp. On ophthalmoscopy, signs of retinal vascular occlusions can be found.

3.3.3.3.2 Treatment

The vaso-occlusive changes may be irreversible and unresponsive to medical treatment.

3.3.3.4 Purtscher's Retinopathy

Described in 1868, this distinctive retinal pathology can be caused by head trauma, chest compression[3], fracture of a (long) bone, orbital and liver trauma, angiography, and surgery[4].

3.3.3.4.1 Evaluation

Although unilateral cases have also been reported [27], the symptoms are usually bilateral, even if asymmetrical. They present within a few hours, but no later than 4 days, after the trauma. The patients complain about decreased vision, typically between CF and 20/200.

On ophthalmoscopy (Fig. 3.3.1), the following symptoms are found:

---

3 The most common etiology is an MVC.

4 Carotid, thoracic, renal.

- Superficial retinal hemorrhages
- Serous macular detachment
- Dilated and tortuous vasculature
- Numerous white patches or confluent cotton wool spots around the optic disc
- Disc edema

On *FLAG* the characteristic signs are:

- Focal areas of arteriolar obstruction
- Patchy capillary nonperfusion
- Disc edema
- Dye leakage from retinal arterioles, capillaries, and venules [27]
- Blockage of background choroidal fluorescence but usually normal choroidal filling in the acute stage
- Late perivenous staining and/or partial vein obstruction
- Disc edema

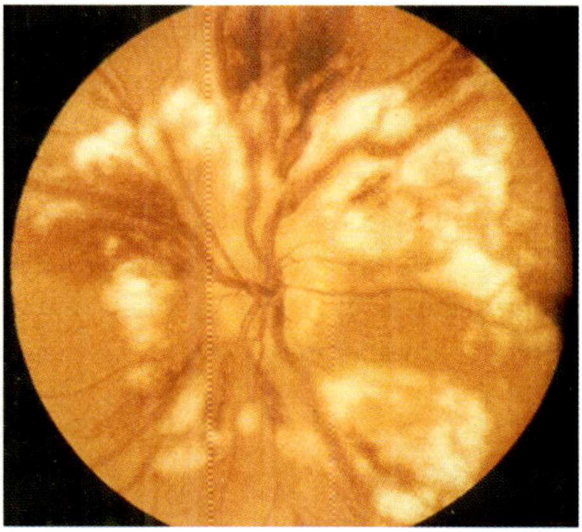

Fig. 3.3.1 Purtscher's retinopathy. Hemorrhages and multiple cotton-wool spots are visible in the posterior pole in this patient who was injured in an MVC

3.3.3.4.2 Treatment

Observation is sufficient. The retinal lesions resolve over a period of weeks to a few months. After resolution, the fundus may appear normal, but pigment migration and optic atrophy can occur [3]. Visual acuity returns to normal or near normal in most eyes. Initially, visual field defects may occur, including central, paracentral, segmental, or annular scotomas. The visual field defects usually resolve completely, although, particularly if optic atrophy has occurred, they may be permanent [3]. Careful documentation is needed to be able to subsequently prove that the damages are trauma related.

3.3.3.5 Shaken Baby Syndrome

3.3.3.5.1 Introduction

The traumatic sequelae of nonaccidental injuries occurring in infants and young children as a consequence of violent shaking are called shaken baby syndrome.[5] The reported mortality rate of 15% underscores the importance of recognizing this form of child abuse [19]. In central Europe, 3.5% of parents confessed to having used violence against their children so that it might have resulted in severe injury and 10% of children admitted to hospital due to injury showed evidence of physical violence; less than 5% of abused children become known to the authorities. The typical victim of shaken baby syndrome is a male infant younger than 6 months of age[6] who is alone with the perpetrator at the time of injury [16]. The injury is unrelated to race, gender, socioeconomic status, or education [16].

An infant is more likely to suffer from intracranial and intraocular bleeding as a result of shaking [7] because the head is proportionately larger and heavier relative to the body than that of an older child or adult, and the still weak neck muscles provide less stability and protection.

---

5 Synonyms include whiplash shaken infant syndrome, battered child syndrome, and child abuse syndrome.

6 Two-thirds of the abused children are babies.

3.3.3.5.2 Evaluation

The diagnosis of child abuse requires a high index of suspicion. The history of shaking is characteristically lacking, and there may be minimal external signs of trauma.

Cave

The leading sign of child abuse is ocular in 4–6% of cases, but the vast majority of abused children have some eye involvement.

While after accidental head injuries nearly all children under 3 years of age have no abnormality on fundus examinations, most babies with nonaccidental head injuries show retinal hemorrhages of varying degree, occurring in 11–23% of all physically abused children and in 50–80% of shaken babies [9, 18, 24].

On ophthalmoscopy, intraocular hemorrhage can be present in various locations: subretinally; intraretinally; preretinally (subhyaloidally); and intravitreally [17]. The blood is concentrated in the posterior pole region and is usually bilateral. The amount of intraocular blood correlates with the degree of the acute neurological damage [29]. Cotton-wool spots, white-centered hemorrhages (Roth's spot), macular edema, disc edema, and retinoschisis are less common [6, 30].

On CT or MRI, the intracranial pathology includes subarachnoid or intracerebral hemorrhage, cerebral edema, and cerebral atrophy. Elevated intracranial pressure is often present. A variety of neurological symptoms can occur: irritability; lethargy; seizures; and coma. Death should not be an unexpected consequence [31].

3.3.3.5.3 Differential Diagnosis

In infants retinal hemorrhages are most common post partum or in shaken babies: 19–32% of eyes show retinal hemorrhage in one or both eyes 24 h after a normal birth. By 72 h the rate drops to ~13%, and these hemorrhages usually completely resolve within 6 weeks. If intravitreal or retinal hemorrhages are found in a child older than 6 weeks, this is most likely due to abuse.

3.3.3.5.4 Management Strategy

Suspicion of a child abuse requires a multidisciplinary approach and a careful documentation (e.g., photography and ultrasonography) of all findings. If violence is suspected, a detailed systemic examination has to be performed. The ophthalmologist has a key role because of the pathognomic appearance of the fundus (other causes of retinal hemorrhages have to be carefully ruled out; Table 3.3.1).

Table 3.3.1 Differential diagnosis of traumatic retinopathy. (Modified after [3])

	Contusion retinopathy	Purtscher's retinopathy	Purtscher's retinopathy (fat embolism)	Purtscher's retinopathy (traumatic asphyxia)	Valsalva retinopathy
Type of trauma	Directly to the eye	Chest compression, head injury	Fracture of long bones, multiple injuries	Chest compression	Valsalva maneuver
Accompanying systemic picture	None	None	Pulmonary and cerebral signs, petechial hemorrhages	Blue-black discoloration of upper body	None
Onset of systemic picture	None	None	Symptom-free interval for a few days	Immediate	None
Initial vision	Normal to CF	Variable	Normal	Normal to NLP	Normal to CF
Duration of reduced vision	Several days	Several weeks	Several days	Several weeks	Several weeks

Table 3.3.1 *(continued)* Differential diagnosis of traumatic retinopathy. (Modified after [3])

	Contusion retinopathy	Purtscher's retinopathy	Purtscher's retinopathy (fat embolism)	Purtscher's retinopathy (traumatic asphyxia)	Valsalva retinopathy
Final vision	Usually normal, sometimes impaired	Usually normal, sometimes impaired	Normal	Normal to NLP	Usually normal, sometimes impaired
Eye's external appearance	Normal to contused	Normal	Normal to petechial conjunctival hemorrhages	Subconjunctival hemorrhages	Normal to conjunctival hemorrhages
Fundus picture acutely	Retinal whitening	Exudates and hemorrhages	Exudates and hemorrhages, retinal edema	Normal or hemorrhages, rarely exudates	Retinal hemorrhage, sub-ILM blood
Time from trauma to fundus changes	Within a few hours	Within 4 days	After 1 or 2 days	Immediate or 2 days	Acutely

Pearl

The ophthalmologist must be familiar with the retinal manifestations of child abuse and act as an expert witness as part of a multidisciplinary approach to the diagnosis and management of abused children. Even without visible retinal damage, visual loss can occur in a third of children with subdural or subarachnoidal hemorrhage [11].

The treatment is usually supportive. The hemorrhages spontaneously absorb within a few months. Late manifestations include perimacular retinal folds, chorioretinal atrophy or scarring, optic atrophy, and retinal detachment [8, 17]. A retinal detachment or a nonclearing vitreous hemorrhage requires surgical treatment (see Chaps. 2.9, 2.16).

3.3.3.5.5 Prognosis and Outcome

The clinical course of shaken baby retinopathy ranges from complete resolution to severe visual loss due to optic atrophy or macular scarring [21]. Postmortem examination of the optic nerves in shaken babies often reveal perineural hemorrhage, which may contribute to the poor outcome in survivors through nerve fiber compression and optic atrophy [15, 22]. A 50% incidence of gazing disorders is reported in shaken baby syndrome, reflecting nervous system insults [19].

3.3.3.6 Terson Syndrome

Terson syndrome (Fig. 3.3.2) is defined as a vitreous hemorrhage occurring in association with any form of acute intracranial[7] hemorrhage; the incidence reaches 8% [14]. Other types of intraocular bleeding is found in up to 20% of eyes [5, 30]. Subarachnoid bleeding from a cerebral aneurysm, in particular an aneurysm of the anterior communicating artery, is the most common underlying cause in adults [5], but traumatic subdural bleeding in children (see Chap. 2.16) [14].

3.3.3.6.1 Evaluation

On ophthalmoscopy, multiple preretinal, intraretinal, and subretinal hemorrhages can be seen if the vitreous hemorrhage allows inspection of the retina. A dome-shaped accumulation of blood is found at the macula in 39% of eyes, two-thirds of which is underneath the ILM [14].[8] Ultrasonography allows preoperative identification of the hemorrhagic macular cyst, and surgical intervention may have to be performed more urgently in such cases.

7 Subarachnoidal or subdural, occasionally intracerebral.

8 Hemorrhagic macular cyst.

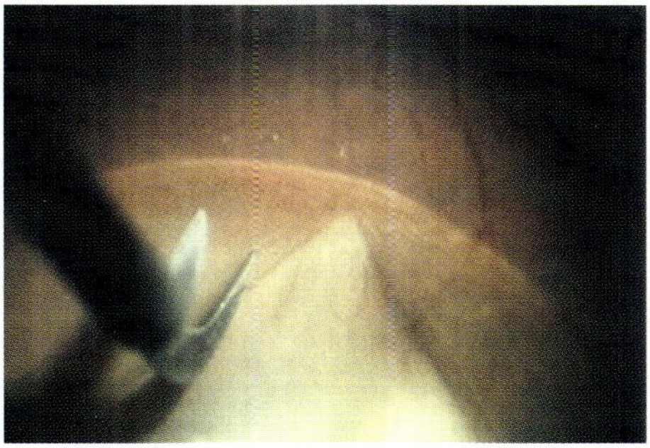

Fig. 3.3.2 Terson syndrome. Intraoperative image of an eye with a submembranous hemorrhagic cyst in the macula. The cyst's border is clearly visible, delineated by a white line representing the ILM's reinsertion into the retina. The cyst still contains blood, which is degenerated and has turned white. The scissors is used to open the ILM for complete blood evacuation (R. Morris, Birmingham, Alabama)

Cave

The amount of intraocular hemorrhage directly correlates with the rapidity and magnitude of intracranial pressure elevation. The presence of intraocular hemorrhage is associated with increased morbidity and mortality [4, 28].

3.3.3.6.2 Management

The final visual outcome may be good without pars plana vitrectomy [25], but surgery is able to achieve rapid visual rehabilitation and prevent PVR and retinal detachment [14, 28]. Vitrectomy is especially useful if a hemorrhagic macular cyst is present or if the patient is in the amblyopic age.[9]

The decision whether to observe or operate should be discussed with the patient, family, neurologist, and the physical therapist (see Chap. 1.4).

9 This is true even if the prognosis is much worse in children than in adults.

3.3.3.7 Valsalva Retinopathy

A rapid rise in abdominal pressure, especially against a closed glottis, is called a Valsalva maneuver. It may occur during heavy lifting, coughing, vomiting, blowing balloons, or other straining activities. As the veins above the heart have no valves, a Valsalva maneuver induces a rapid rise in the intravenous pressure and may cause a rupture of the superficial retinal or conjunctival capillaries and a hemorrhagic retinopathy. Underlying conditions, such as diabetic retinopathy, retinal telangiectasis, arterial macroaneurysms, pregnancy, and sickle cell disease, may exacerbate the development of a hemorrhage, as does anticoagulant therapy.

3.3.3.7.1 Evaluation

A history of straining can usually be identified. The amount of visual impairment depends on the extent of the foveal hemorrhage.

On slit lamp, the anterior segment is mostly normal, although subconjunctival hemorrhage may be present.

On ophthalmoscopy, retinal hemorrhages are seen, including subhyaloidal bleeding and the typical hemorrhagic macular cyst underneath the ILM [6]. A meniscus may be observed as the blood settles inferiorly. Vitreous hemorrhage may also develop if the blood breaks through.

3.3.3.7.2 Treatment

The preretinal/sub-ILM hemorrhage usually clears spontaneously. If the hemorrhage does not resolve within a few weeks, it can be drained with a pulsed YAG-laser [23]. Vitrectomy is often necessary (see Chap. 2.9).

3.3.3.8 Whiplash Syndrome

Whiplash injury occurs via an acceleration–deceleration energy transfer to the neck.[10] It is most often seen in a person involved in rear-end or side-impact MVC. The bone and soft tissue trauma (whiplash injury) in turn may lead to a variety of clinical manifestations (whiplash-associated disorders).

10 Violent flexion that is followed immediately by an extension of the neck.

The visual disturbance may be caused by the sequealae of a direct injury to the cervical or carotid artery, or by an accompanying Purtscher type of trauma (see above).

3.3.3.8.1 Symptoms

The complains include the following:

- Mild to severe neck pain (88–100%) and headache (54–66%) [26].
- Mild reduction in visual acuity[11] (8–26%; [1, 26]), which presents acutely. The symptoms are bilateral and resolve over a period of a few days.
- Horner's syndrome (miosis, ptosis, and pseudo-endophthalmitis) [3].

3.3.3.8.2 Evaluation

On external inspection, temporary palsy of cranial nerves with diplopia may be found if the brain has suffered a concussion [3]. On ophthalmoscopy, a grayish swelling of the foveal area is seen right after the injury. A crater-like depression of less than 100 μm in diameter with slight RPE disturbance develops and can remain unchanged even if the patient's visual symptoms have improved [13]. On the FLAG, a small area of hyperfluorescence may be observed [13].

3.3.3.8.3 Management

There is no known treatment. The visual acuity usually returns to 20/20, although it can also remain diminished. The clinical appearance and course may be similar to those of contusion retinopathy or solar retinopathy [6]. The findings should be precisely documented and photographed because the patient may later seek compensation for the injury (see Chap. 1.8).

11 Usually ~20/30

DO:

- carefully examine the child if foul play is suspected
- weigh all options, consider the benefits and risks, when deciding whether or not to intervene for a vitreous or macular hemorrhage caused by bodily trauma

DON'T:

- refuse vitrectomy just because the prognosis is "generally poor": surgery can nevertheless be beneficial to the particular individual

Summary

A variety of ocular sequelae can be caused by injuries to the body. The ocular consequences may be inconsequential but can also be severe, and the bodily trauma can be fatal in an abused infant. For many of the ocular complications there is no known treatment.

References

[1] Burke JP, Orton HP, West J, Strachan IM, Hockey MS, Ferguson DG (1992) Whiplash and its effect on the visual system. Graefe's Arch Clin Exp Ophthalmol 230: 335–339

[2] Duke-Elder S, Leigh AG (1965) System of ophthalmology, vol VIII: Diseases of the outer eye. Mosby, St. Louis, pp 995–1003

[3] Duke-Elder S, MacFaul P (1972) System of ophthalmology. Injuries, part I: Mechanical injuries, vol XIV. Henry Klimpton, London

[4] Frizzel R, Kuhn F, Morris R, Quinn C, Fisher W (1997) Screening for ocular hemorrhages in patients with ruptured cerebral aneurysms: a prospective study on 99 patients. Neurosurgery 41: 529–534

[5] Garfinkle AM, Danys IR, Nicolle DA, Colohan AR, Brem S (1992) Terson's syndrome: a reversible cause of blindness following subarachnoid hemorrhage. J Neurosurg 76: 766–771

[6] Gass J (1987) Stereoscopic atlas of macular disease: diagnosis and treatment. Mosby, St. Louis

[7] Greenwald MJ, Weiss A, Oesterle CS, Friendly DS (1986) Traumatic retinoschisis in battered babies. Ophthalmology 93: 618–625

[8] Han DP, Wilkinson WS (1990) Late ophthalmic manifestations of the shaken baby syndrome. J Pediatr Ophthalmol Strabismus 27: 299–303

[9] Harley RD (1980) Ocular manifestations of child abuse. J Pediatr Ophthalmol Strabismus 17: 5–13

[10] Hayreh SS (1987) Anterior ischemic optic neuropathy. VIII. Clinical features and pathogenesis of post-hemorrhagic amaurosis. Ophthalmology 94: 1488–1502

[11] Hollenhorst RW, Stein HA (1958) Ocular signs and prognosis in subdural and subarachnoid bleeding in young children. AMA Arch Ophthalmol 60: 187–192

[12] Johnson MW, Kincaid MC, Trobe JD (1987) Bilateral retrobulbar optic nerve infarctions after blood loss and hypotension. A clinicopathologic case study. Ophthalmology 94: 1577–1584

[13] Kelley JS, Hoover RE, George T (1978) Whiplash maculopathy. Arch Ophthalmol 96: 834–835

[14] Kuhn F, Morris R, Mester V, Witherspoon C (1998) Terson's syndrome. Results of vitrectomy and the significance of vitreous hemorrhage in patients with subarachnoid hemorrhage. Ophthalmology 105: 472–477

[15] Lambert SR, Johnson TE, Hoyt CS (1986) Optic nerve sheath and retinal hemorrhages associated with the shaken baby syndrome. Arch Ophthalmol 104: 1509–1512

[16] Lancon JA, Haines DE, Parent AD (1998) Anatomy of the shaken baby syndrome. Anat Rec 253: 13–18

[17] Levin AV (1991) Ocular complications of head trauma in children. Pediatr Emerg Care 7: 129–130

[18] Levin DB, Bell DK (1977) Traumatic retinal hemorrhages with angioid streaks. Arch Ophthalmol 95: 1072–1073

[19] Ludwig S, Warman M (1984) Shaken baby syndrome: a review of 20 cases. Ann Emerg Med 13: 104–107

[20] McFadden DM, Houston CS, Sutton JR, Powles AC, Gray GW, Roberts RS (1981) High-altitude retinopathy. J Am Med Assoc 245: 581–586

[21] Mushin AS (1971) Ocular damage in the battered-baby syndrome. Br Med J 3: 402–404

[22] Rao N, Smith RE, Choi JH, Xu XH, Kornblum RN (1988) Autopsy findings in the eyes of fourteen fatally abused children. Forensic Sci Int 39: 293–299

[23] Raymond LA (1995) Neodymium:YAG laser treatment for hemorrhages under the internal limiting membrane and posterior hyaloid face in the macula. Ophthalmology 102: 406–411

[24] Riffenburgh RS, Sathyavagiswaran L (1991) Ocular findings at autopsy of child abuse victims. Ophthalmology 98: 1519–1524

[25] Schultz PN, Sobol WM, Weingeist TA (1991) Long-term visual outcome in Terson syndrome. Ophthalmology 98: 1814–1819

[26] Spitzer WO, Skovron ML, Salmi LR, Cassidy JD, Duranceau J, Suissa S, Zeiss E (1995) Scientific monograph of the Quebec Task Force on Whiplash-Associated Disorders: redefining "whiplash" and its management. Spine 20: 1S–73S

[27] Teichmann KD, Gronemeyer U (1981) Unilateral morbus Purtscher with poor visual outcome. Ann Ophthalmol 13: 1295–1299

[28] Velikay M, Datlinger P, Stolba U, Wedrich A, Binder S, Hausmann N (1994) Retinal detachment with severe proliferative vitreoretinopathy in Terson syndrome. Ophthalmology 101: 35–37

[29] Wilkinson WS, Han DP, Rappley MD, Owings CL (1989) Retinal hemorrhage predicts neurological injury in the shaken baby syndrome. Arch Ophthalmol 107: 1472–1474

[30] Williams DF, Mieler WF, Williams GA (1990) Posterior segment manifestations of ocular trauma. Retina 10: S35–S44

[31] Wygnanski-Jaffe T, Levin AV, Shafiq A, Smith C, Enzenauer RW, Elder JE, Morin JD, Stephens D, Atenafu E (2006) Postmortem orbital findings in shaken baby syndrome. Am J Ophthalmol 142: 233–240

Subject Index

D

E